Transmission Electron Microscopy Sample Preparation

Rajender Singh

Transmission Electron Microscopy Sample Preparation

From Specimen to Micrograph

Springer

Rajender Singh
Central Instrumentation Laboratory
(CIL)/Sophisticated Analytical
Instrumentation Facility (SAIF)
Panjab University
Chandigarh, India

ISBN 978-3-031-82969-7 ISBN 978-3-031-82967-3 (eBook)
https://doi.org/10.1007/978-3-031-82967-3

This Springer imprint is published by the registered company Springer Nature Switzerland AG
The registered company address is: Gewerbestrasse 11, 6330 Cham, Switzerland

Foreword

It is a great pleasure that I am writing the foreword to this outstanding contribution in the field of Transmission Electron microscopy (TEM) by *Rajender Singh*. The book, *Transmission Electron Microscopy Sample Preparation*, is presented as an ultimate guide with connecting the crucial gaps between theory and practical through knowledge and expertise of author.

TEM technique has proven to be one of powerful tools for imaging at molecular and atomic level innovative exploration which extended respective application to material science, structural biology and nanotechnology areas. Successful TEM imaging is not just limited to sophisticated instrumentation, but also equally guided and eased through skillful sample preparation. This is where *Rajender Singh's* book *Transmission Electron Microscopy Sample Preparation* offered a comprehensive roadmap from basic to precise sample preparation for perceptive micrographs. *Rajender Singh* incorporated his full knowledge and technical experience to text of this book project. He has written chapters of this book extensively explaining and summarizing all facts and figures related to basic TEM instrumentation, operation and precise sample preparation. While writing each and every detail in the book, he was very attentive and aware to make it valuable for novice researchers as well to veteran practitioner.

This book presents a well balance adjustment between the theoretical background and practical applications w.r.t. electron microscopy. Right from first chapter to last chapter, each and every existing and proposed EM hypothesis related instrumentation, powder, liquid, biological, etc., specimen, imaging dynamics with troubleshooting skills has been authenticated with practical examples. This will reflect the *Rajender Singh's* deep understanding w.r.t. ideal operation of TEM and precise sample handling. For any researcher, working in the field of electron microscopy, this book will be surely playing a torch-bearer role. I am sure that this text book will have long-lasting impact on scientific community and will be referred in the community and generations of microscopists.

In conclusion, *Transmission Electron Microscopy Sample Preparation*, book must be read by everyone who wants to learn, explore and master, something exciting and innovative in the field of electron microscopy. I congratulate, *Rajender Singh* on this remarkable achievement and highly recommend this book for students and scientific professionals.

Prof. Ganga Ram Chaudhary
Professor, Department of Chemistry/
Director, Department of CIL/SAIF
Panjab University
Chandigarh, India

Preface

The objective to write the book, *Transmission Electron Microscopy Sample Preparation*, is to sensitize and communicate electron microscopy (EM)-related information with users/researchers/scientists from college, university to industry, from basic to advance level. This book comprised total 11 chapters w.r.t. TEM instrumentation, sample preparation for living to non-living samples, high-end EM instrumentation, ideal imaging, dynamic troubleshooting, with unique case studies' discussion for novel insights.

Chapter 1, "**Introduction to Transmission Electron Microscopy (TEM)**", covers fundamental information w.r.t. EM historical background, basic working of TEM, different modes of operation with imaging and application capabilities.

Chapter 2, "**Fundamentals of TEM Sample Preparation**", highlighted the classification of different samples types, basics of TEM sample preparation with different practical challenges.

Chapter 3, "**Techniques for Thin Specimen from Bulk Samples**", explores about importance of thin specimen surface with respect to pre and post requisite requirements, different specimen thinning techniques with probable challenges, and troubleshooting has been comprised.

Chapter 4, "**TEM Sample Preparation for Powder and Liquid Formulations**", focuses on broad categories of powder and liquid samples, w.r.t. respective characterization under TEM and HRTEM. Further, different operational, processing and imaging parameters w.r.t. respective challenges have been discussed.

Chapter 5, "**Sample Preparation for Soft Matters (Non Biological) and Biological Samples**", addresses broad samples categories including soft and biological specimen, best possible ways of respective sample preparation, requirement related to thin sectioning with probable challenges and respective troubleshooting.

Chapter 6, "**Introduction to Cryo-TEM and Related Sample Preparation**", presents the basic and working of Cryo-TEM, detail classification of samples belongs of life science including soft specimen and importance of respective techniques. Detailed sample preparation related to Cryo-TEM technique including wide varieties of applications also has been presented in current chapter.

Chapter 7, "**In-situ TEM: Principle, Working, Application and Challenges**", discusses basics of In-situ TEM with principle, working, features of dynamic specimen holder, probable challenges with respective troubleshooting and innovative application.

Chapter 8, "**Sample Preparation for Quantitative Analysis Under TEM**", introduces the importance of quantitative analysis with different modes of TEM, respective application and challenges.

Chapter 9, "**Correlative Light and Electron Microscopy (CLEM) Sample Preparation**", focusses on basic principle, working and importance of CLEM, with respective integration capabilities, application and probable challenges with troubleshooting aspect has been summarized.

Chapter 10, "**Ideal TEM Imaging, Analysis and Troubleshooting Tricks**", covers summary of pre and post requisite requirement related to TEM technique with major and minor beam alignments followed by respective basic to advance troubleshootings and precise sample preparation has been discussed. Further, with correlation of EM technique with other microscopy techniques also has been comprised.

Chapter 11, "**Unique Case Studies in TEM Instrumentation, Analysis and Interpretation**", provides practical insights related to EM instrumentation requirements, unique specimens analysis.

Through above-mentioned detail discussion w.r.t. different aspects of TEM, HRTEM, quantitative mode of operation, Cryo-TEM, In situ-TEM, CLEM, ideal imaging with respect to specific case studies has been presented. Respective insightful data analysis and interpretation will equip and train any novice and establish EM practitioner towards next level of expertise in field of electron microscopy.

Chandigarh, India Rajender Singh

Acknowledgements

Writing this book *Transmission Electron Microscopy Sample Preparation*, has been a rewarding journey through my cumulation of passion for understanding the complex details of microscopic world. I would like to extend my heartiest gratitude to everyone who supported and encouraged directly and indirectly me throughout this journey.

Firstly, I am grateful to my mentors *Prof. Ganga Ram Chaudhary, Prof. Gaurav Verma, Prof. J. S. Sherawat, Prof. Nagesh Thakur, Prof. Vir Singh Rangra, Prof. Ramesh Sharma, Prof. Dheeraj Sharma, Prof. H. P. S. Kang, Prof. Anil Kumar, Prof. Poonam, Prof. Devender Mehta, Prof. S. K. Mehta, Prof. Sanjay Kaushik, Prof. Prashant Gautam, Prof. Arun Thakur, Prof. Manu Sharma, Prof. Pankaj Sharma, Prof. Vineet Sharma, Prof. P. B. Barman, Prof. Ragini Raj Singh, Dinesh Sharma*, for their precious continuous support and guidance. I am also grateful to my colleagues Dr. Deepika Jamwal, Dr. Pawan Kumar, Dr. Rajinder Kumar, Dr. Hitanshu, Dr. Bandana, Dr. Moondeep Chauhan, Dr. Neha Kondal, Dr. Rohini Sharma, Dr. Sangeeta, Dr. Bunty Sharma, Dr. Preeti, Prerana, Dr. Ajay Sharma, Dr. Amit Thakur for their valuable discussion and support. I am also thankful to Anuj Kumar, Anoop, Neeraj, Subash Magoon, Manish, Maninder, Rimpal, Jagtar Singh, Anit Kumar, Anitha, Mohinder Singh, Balbir Singh, Navjot, Sarbjeet, Prashant Gupta, Rajeev Bhatia, Sunil Mehta, Surjeet, Roshni, Puspa for their moral support.

I would like to say special thanks to *Vice chancellor, Panjab University, Chandigarh, Prof. Renu Vig*, for providing access to valuable electron microscopy facilities. I would like thanks to *Director, CIL/SAIF, and Registrar, Prof. Y. P. Verma, Panjab University, Chandigarh*, for providing moral support in transforming this dream project into realistic domain.

I have no words for the contribution of my loving wife *Poonam* and charming son *Aniket Chandel*, for unwavering support, patience and love, which have been the greatest source of inspiration and strength during this project. I would like to thanks my beloved late grandfather and grandmother respected father Sh. Udham Singh, mother Smt. Brahmi Devi, uncle ji, aunty ji, sisters for their continuous blessings. Your constant support during whole project will be always a true inspiration during long hour writing and researching time.

Finally, I wish to acknowledge the scientific community all over the globe for their continuous contribution and advancements in the field of electron microscopy. I hope this book will contribute little more in the field of electron microscopy.

Contents

About the Author

Rajender Singh holds a Master degree of Science in Physics from Barkatullah University, Bhopal, Madhya Pradesh, in year 2006 and earned Ph.D. degree in Physics and Material Science from Jaypee University of Information of Technology, Waknaghat, Solan, Himachal Pradesh, in year 2018. With the over 13 years of extensive experience in the field of electron microscopy, he has developed extensive expertise in managing and operating advanced instruments including, Scanning electron microscope (SEM), Field emission scanning electron microscope (FESEM), Transmission Electron Microscope (TEM), High-Resolution Electron Microscopy (HRTEM), Ultramicrotome and critical point drying (CPD) systems. Earlier in his carrier, author has worked in Himachal Pradesh University Shimla as a Technician overseeing the operation and maintenance of SEM FEI Quanta 250 with EDS, and X-ray diffraction Xpert Pro (Powder and Thin film) (XRD) instrument. Since March 2014, author has been working as Scientific Officer in Department of central instrumentation laboratory (CIL)/sophisticated analytical instrumentation facility (SAIF), Panjab University Chandigarh, India. In this role, author is responsible for handling and upkeep of TEM H7500 (Hitachi) 120 KV, HRTEM JEM2100 Plus LaB_6 200 KV with diffraction, EDS, STEM modes, FESEM SU8010 with EDS, Ultramicrotome UC7 (Leica), CPD 300 (Leica). In addition, author is actively involved imparting practical training and mentorship to students across the school, colleges and universities. Moreover, to above routine instrumentation responsibilities, author has also published 15 research articles in international journals.

Through combination of hands-on experience, deep technical knowledge, and passion for mentoring next-generation scientists with good research publications record, Rajender Singh has made significant contributions in the field of electron microscopy. Their commitment to advancing research and shared technical expertise will ensure long-lasting impact on the scientific community for novice and experience researchers.

Abbreviations

ABF	Annular Bright Field
ACD	Anticontamination Device
ADF	Annular Dark Field
API	Active Pharmaceutical Ingredient
ARM	Atomic Resolution Microscope
ASEM	Atmospheric Scanning Electron Microscope
BF	Bright Field
BSA	Bovine Serum Albumin
BSE	Back Scattered Electron
CBED	Convergent Beam Electron Diffraction
CCD	Charge Couple Device
CEMOVIS	Cryo-Electron Microscopy of Vitreous Sections
CLEM	Correlative Light Electron Microscopy
CLR	Core Loss Region
CMOS	Complementary Metal Oxide Semiconductor
CPD	Critical Point Drying
CYRO-ET	Cryo-Electron Tomography
CYRO-TEM	Cryo-Transmission Electron Microscopy
DDE	Direct Electron Detector
DED	Direct Electron Direction
DF	Dark Field
DF-TEM	Dark Field-TEM
DP	Diffusion Pump
DPC	Differential Phase Contrast
DQE	Detection Quantum Efficiency
EDS	Energy Dispersive Spectroscopy
EELS	Electron Energy Loss Spectroscopy
EM	Electron Microscopy
EMBL	European Molecular Biology Laboratory
EMDB	Electron Microscopy Data Bank
EMI	Electromagnetic Interference

ETEM	Environment TEM
FEG	Field Emission Gun
FIB	Focused Ion Beam
FS	Freeze Substitution
GIF	Gatan Energy Filter
HAADF	High Angle Annular Dark Field
HAADF-STEM	High Annular Dark Field Scanning TEM
HF	Hydrofluoric Acid
HMDS	Hexamethyldisilane
HPF	High Pressure Freezing
HRTEM	High-Resolution Transmission Electron Microscopy
IC	Integrated Circuit
LC	Liquid Crystal
LIB	Lithium Ion Battery
LLR	Low Loss Region
LM	Light Microscopy
MEMS	Micro Electro Mechanical System
NBED	Nano-beam Electron Diffraction
NEMS	Nano Electromechanical System
NMs	Nanomaterials
NPs	Nanoparticles
PALM	Photo-activated Localization Microscopy
PLD	Pulse Laser Deposition
PS	Polystyrene
rGO	Reduced Graphene Oxide
RP	Rotary Pump
SACT	Small Angle Cleavage Technique
SAED	Selected Area Electron Diffraction
SEM	Scanning Electron Microscopy
SEND	Scanning Electron Nano-Diffraction
SIC	Silicon Carbide
SIP	Sputter Ion Pump
SLC	Sealed Liquid Cell
SNR	Signal to Noise Ratio
SOP	Standard Operating Protocol
SPR	Single Particle Reconstruction
SPRF	Self-Pressurized Rapid Freezing
STED	Stimulated Emission Depletion
STEM	Scanning Transmission Electron Microscopy
STORM	Stochastic Optical Reconstruction Microscopy
TEM	Transmission Electron Microscopy
TMP	Turbo Molecular Pump
UPS	Uninterrupted Power Supply
ZLP	Zero Loss Peak

Chapter 1
Introduction to Transmission Electron Microscopy (TEM)

The Electron Microscope reveals to us the complex and intricate architecture of matter, opening new dimension for scientific discovery
*by **Ernest Ruska** (Lobel Laureate) Co-inventor of TEM*

Abstract Summarizing simple to complex facts and figures related to transmission electron microscopy (TEM) technique will be the torchbearer approach towards germination of innovative and insightful information of specimen analysis at atomic and molecular scale. Right from historical background with evolution stages of electron microscopy, respective fundamentals, working with different modes of operation including bright field (BF), dark field (DF), high angle annular dark field imaging (HAADF), cryo-TEM, environmental-TEM (ETEM) etc., has been discussed. In addition, quantification modes including energy dispersive spectroscopy (EDS), electron energy loss spectroscopy (EELS), and electron diffraction (ED), also have been summarized under current chapter. Efficient utilization of TEM with maximum potentialities will be functionalized through utilization of 3 M, i.e. man, machine and money in an appropriate manner. Application of TEM technique has been extended from material science to biological sciences, including analysis of cellular structure, macromolecules, to medical research with device failure mechanisms to upgrade in respective technologies. This chapter will definitely lay the stout foundation towards the building of innovative database through EM imaging.

Keywords Transmission electron microscopy · Dark field · Bright field · HAADF · EDS · EELS

1.1 Introduction

The hidden details of materials belongings to living and non-living specimens within the realm of transmission electron microscopy (TEM) will be guided in the current introductory chapter. We are going to discuss the journey of TEM by tracing

R. Singh, *Transmission Electron Microscopy Sample Preparation*,
https://doi.org/10.1007/978-3-031-82967-3_1

through its stages of development towards dynamic tools in research and development progress. With comprehensive aspects of TEM instrumentation and respective diverse applications from living to non-living specimens, current chapter highlighted the importance of microscopic arena. Respective approaches have covered the crystalline or amorphous structure of specimens belonging to material science to the delicate behavior of biological science. The main objective behind writing the current valuable book was to highlight the TEM mysterious instrumentation, importance of sample preparation with demystifying steps from raw specimens to quality micrographs through electron microscopy (EM). This foundation chapter will set the learning stage for a new EM user or an experienced researcher/scientist on their transformative journey of TEM from basic to advanced instrumentation with precise sample preparation followed by critical explanation of respective data [1].

This chapter mainly focuses on the historical background of electron microscopy (EM), respective roles of key contributors in respective development, followed by its principles and working with the area of application w.r.t. research and development needs.

Figure 1.1, has highlighted the TEM broad area of applicability in different fields, through which TEM users can understand and correlate level of TEM dominated information can be extracted from a specimen during respective analysis and get correlated with other techniques like Xray-diffractometers or spectroscopy.

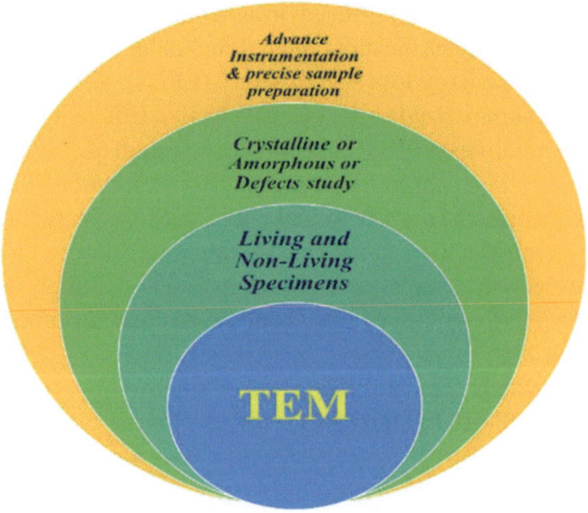

Fig. 1.1 General representation having TEM with area of study

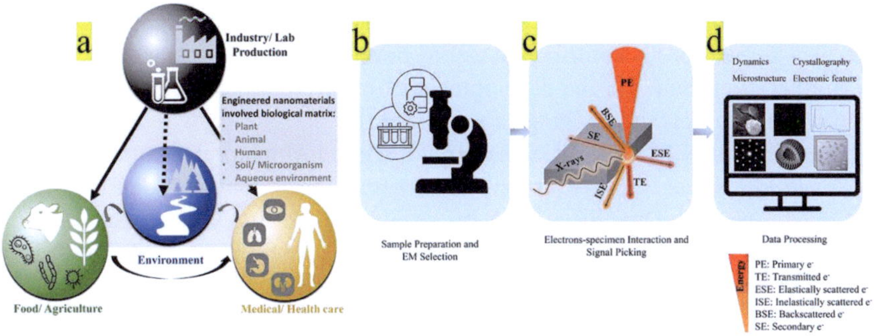

Fig. 1.2 **a** Images shows production of nanomaterials and their application, **b** sample preparation for appropriate EM selection, **c** signal generation during electron-material interaction, **d** respective data processing and interpretation (Reprinted with permission from Ye et al. [7] under open access)

1.2 Historical Background of TEM

1.2.1 Early Discoveries and Theoretical Foundations

Quantum mechanics started the basic journey of electron microscopy (EM) [2]. Scientists named Louis de Broglie and Erwin Schrodinger, inspired by Einstein's photon description, proposed the wave-particle duality of electron [3], which further laid the foundation for promising electron microscopy's basic structure in its initial age of developments [4].

1.2.2 First Electron Microscope

Well known light microscopes resolution limit, directs the use of electron in place of light revolutionized the dimension of microscopy [4, 5]. The invention of Electron Microscope has opened new possibilities in revealing the properties of material at nanoscale. The 1930 breakthrough cleared the invention of the first electron microscope in 1931 by German scientists named Ernest Ruska and Max Knoll as shown in Fig. 1.2 [6, 7].

1.2.3 Contributions of Key Developers in TEM

Name of key inventor behind the development of the first EM was '***Ernest Ruska***', who is also known as the '*Father of Electron Microscopy*' through his extraordinary contribution in the development of first electron microscope (EM). His novel contribution earned him the Nobel prize in Physics in 1986 and acknowledged the impact of EM on global scientific research [6]. **Ruska's** doctoral mentor named '***Max Knoll***' was also known for his contribution to EM development as a Ruska's collaborator. He further contributed to the development of electron optics, paving the way for improved resolution and imaging capabilities [6].

In addition to Ruska and Knoll contribution into EM major developments, many other names who has been also contributed in same area. Reinhold Rudenberg (1883–1961) who was the Director at Siemens company filed first official patent on EM in 1931. Similarly, Ernest Bruche (Berlin), Bodo von Borries (1905–1956) from Germany, an electrical engineer, also make significant contributions in respective developments [4, 6],

1.3 Evolution of TEM Techniques

1.3.1 Post-War Developments

Subsequent to World War II, rapid developments have been experienced in electron microscopy instrumentation [8]. Specifically, focused research on cold field emission sources, magnetic lenses, and improvised vacuum systems has uplifted the resolution and imaging capabilities of TEM.

1.3.2 TEM to High-Resolution TEM (HRTEM)

Visualization of atomic domains of material under TEM in the 1970's enables the researchers to think and explain beyond the existing limit of imaging. Improvements in electron sources, electromagnetic lenses, aberration correction, detectors, sample preparation techniques, etc. w.r.t. EM instrumentation bring insight into the detection of high-resolution aspect of specimen. The fast-growing technological advancements in TEM to HRTEM opened new frontiers in material science, catalyzing discoveries at atomic and molecular level [9, 10].

1.3.3 Integration with Spectroscopy Techniques

Over the years, beyond the well-known imaging regime of TEM, it has evolved with the incorporation of supporting techniques like energy dispersive spectroscopy (EDS) and electron energy loss spectroscopy (EELS). Stated expansion allowed the researchers/scientists to analyze the chemical composition, electronic properties with chemical analysis of material at micron as well as at nanoscale [7, 11].

1.3.4 Innovative Upgradation w.r.t. TEM Instrumentation

Understanding of material under EM study is incomplete until, we will not visualize possible dynamic processes in real time observations in stabilized state. Developments of in-situ TEM, cryo-TEM, liquid cell assembly, micromechanical electrical system (MEMS), etc. techniques, has analysed and interpret insightly, precisely, and authentically different physical, chemical and biological phenomenon very closely and precisely. This will lead to understand and explore the working of any device/ system during its live working state under normal or harsh environmental conditions [7, 11].

Figure 1.2a shows the fabrication of different nanomaterial and their major area of application viz. food/agriculture, medical/health and industry. In addition, Fig. 1.2b–d has depicted the signal generation during electron-material interaction, and respective data processing and interpretation w.r.t. electron microscopy technique [7].

At the stage of twentieth century, specifically TEM reflects a series of transformative milestones and collaborative efforts of revolutionary scientist in shaping the electron microscopy. It will play a vital tool for scientific examination and material characterization towards the sustainable growth of society.

1.4 Fundamental Principles of TEM

1.4.1 Wave-Particle Dual Nature

Quantum mechanics explained about the electron wave-particle dual nature principle. As TEM deals with electron, which possess wave as well particle nature. This concept of duality of electron have marked as a milestone in achieving higher resolution in comparison to optical microscope. This concept was firstly demonstrated by Davisson and Germer in 1927. Louis De Broglie proposed that wavelength is given by Eq. 1.1 [4, 9, 12, 13]:

$$\lambda = \frac{h}{p} = \frac{h}{mv} \tag{1.1}$$

where $h = 6.626 \times 10^{-34}$ Js is the Planck constant; p, m, v represents momentum, mass and speed of electron.

In case of TEM, momentum to electron will be enhanced with the increase of accelerating voltage V, which is equal to kinetic energy of electron (eV) as shown in Eq. 1.2:

$$eV = \frac{m_o v^2}{2} \tag{1.2}$$

With reference to Eqs. 1.1 and 1.2, have define the relation between accelerating voltage (V) and electron wavelength (λ) as shown below:

$$\lambda = \frac{h}{2m_o eV} \quad \text{and} \quad \lambda\, \alpha\, \frac{1}{V^{1/2}} \tag{1.3}$$

Inverse relation between wavelength (λ) and accelerating voltage (V) bring clear concept to achieve smallest wavelength at highest accelerating voltage [12].

1.5 TEM Important Aspect

1.5.1 Electron Gun

Quality electrons generated through electron gun in TEM will be accelerated through (80–300) kV voltage to pass through ~ 1 μm thick specimen. With respect to nature of specimen like polymer, biological etc., with safety aspect, < 100 kV accelerating voltage TEM will be preferred. Specialized specimen preparation and analysis as per need and compatibility with e-beam, use of energy filter bring minimum energy spread lead to quality analysis under TEM [4, 11, 14].

1.5.2 Electromagnetic Optics

The vertical dimension of TEM is longer than SEM, due to many electromagnetic lenses arranged from electron gun to detector side. The arrangement of condenser lenses before specimen will converge e-beam into focussed diameter whereas the objective lens will be helpful in generating first image and diffraction patterning. Subsequently, transmitted electron will be transferred onto detector (CCD etc.) to observe the respective imaging or diffraction pattern. Moreover, installation of more electromagnetic lenses may be present, will vary from model to model of TEM w.r.t. different manufacturer like STEM have scanning coil etc. Rising updation in TEM instrumentation w.r.t. electron source, electromagnetic optics etc., aberration corrected TEM have substantially improved the spatial resolution to < 0.05 nm [4, 11, 14].

1.5.3 Specimen Stage

Normally, most of TEM design will allow specimen with maximum 3 mm diameter size and ~ 200 μm thickness during electron beam interaction for observation.

Restriction of limited space w.r.t. specimen insertion and limited movement is due to design of electrostatic lens. Although, updated aberration corrected TEM will have extended higher specimen size limits with maintaining spatial resolution limit < 0.1 nm, through revolutionary development in objective lens design having pole piece gap upto 5 mm. The updated design in TEM instrumentation extended the ~ 5 mm diameter of specimen with transparency condition brings more diversified analysis. Specimen will be loaded on specialized holder having movement of specimen in x, y, z direction with single and double tilt holder from $\pm$ 20° to 40°. In case of 3D tomography imaging, tilt range may be needed upto $\pm$ 70° [15]. More importantly, the positioning of specimen and tilt options w.r.t. electron beam is very important in order to capture the different area imaging of specimen [4, 9, 11].

1.5.4 Detector

With respect to quality transmission of electrons through specimen, presence of respective electromagnetic lenses focuses electrons onto appropriate phosphor screen or detector generate respective area image. In comparison to older TEM photographic imaging, present time most of TEM models fitted with digital electron detection system i.e. charge couple device (CCD), direct electron detection (DED) etc., which convert sensed electron into electronic pulse/pixel. The specification of detectors fitted in TEM will capture possible information/data from respective specimen as per nature, type and specification of main TEM instrumentation [4, 9, 11].

1.5.5 TEM Operation

The story of perfect TEM technique imaging is not about to capture few images but it is about to the precise process which will be followed right from respective EM specification design, installation procedure and precise operation and maintenance. Technically, EM instrument area must be vibration and dust free, negligible electromagnetic interference (EMI) with controlled laboratory environment including temperature, humidity etc. During operation of EM machine daily, there must be certain standard steps need to followed related to electron beam current values, beam alignment, astigmatism correction etc. Moreover, the person behind the machine must be capable and well trained w.r.t. specific EM machine operation related to alignment, imaging as well the routine troubleshooting and maintenance aspects [4, 9, 11].

Collectively, Fig. 1.3 has depicted the important factors related to TEM instrumentation and operation.

Figure 1.4a, b shows the schematic representation of scanning transmission electron microscope (STEM) and TEM working [16] whereas (c) shows respective basic principle demonstration [17].

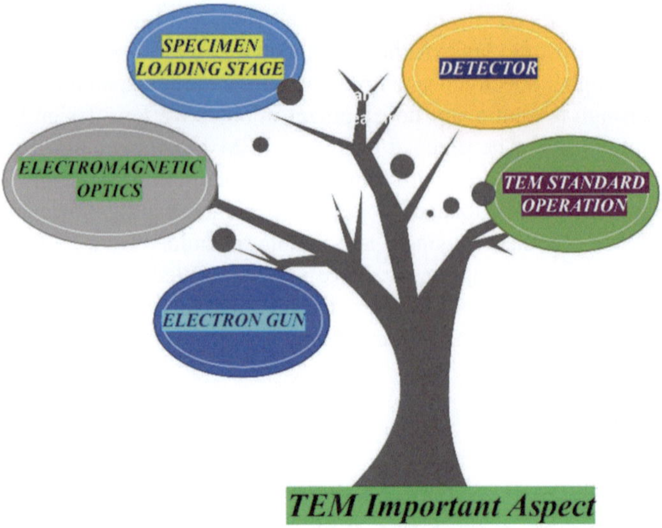

Fig. 1.3 Demonstrated the major factors related to TEM instrument

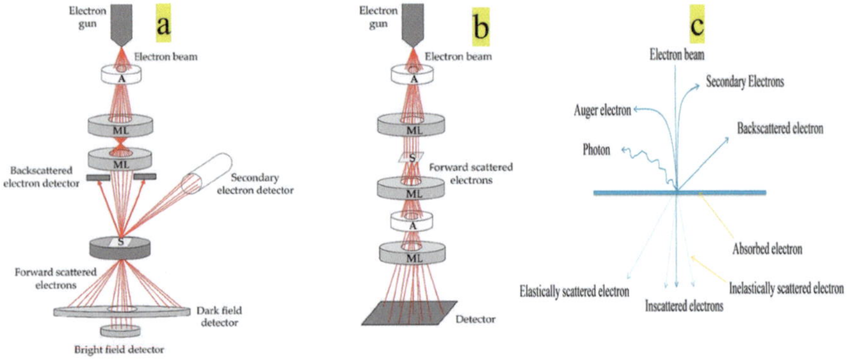

Fig. 1.4 **a** Shows schematic representation of scanning transmission electron microscope (STEM) with **b** transmission electron microscope (TEM) (S: Sample, ML: Magnetic lens, A: Aperture) (Reprinted with permission from Malenica et al. [16] under open access), depicting basic principle of TEM (Reprinted with permission from Ahmad et al. [17] under open access)

1.6 Modes for TEM Operations

Since with the invention of electron microscope in 1931, scientists have been started analysing nano regime of materials. Over the years, the continues development has been made in electron microscopy. This includes development in bright field

(BF), dark field (DF), high resolution TEM (HRTEM), electron diffraction, energy-dispersive X-ray spectroscopy (EDS), Electron energy loss spectroscopy (EELS) modes of operations [4, 7, 9, 11].

1.6.1 Bright Field Imaging

This is most common mode in TEM operation. It consists of an electron source, electromagnetic lenses for focussing the electron beam, with series of apertures and detectors [9]. This is widely used for high resolution imaging with structural analysis of materials at the nanoscale. Under this mode, transmitted electrons form a dark image with brighter background. As contrast of specimen will be guided through the mass and crystallinity of material [18], respective high-density material appears darker.

1.6.2 Dark Field (DF) Imaging

Under this mode of operation, imaging with scattered electrons due to mass with lowered background noise will be reported. DF mode will utilizes high annular dark field scanning TEM (STEM-HAADF) and dark field-TEM (DF-TEM) [9, 19]. With special beam alignment and use of specific condenser aperture, quality dark field image will be captured having dark background and brighter region of scattered electrons. Under DF-TEM at particular tilt angle, transmitted electrons will be blocked by respective aperture [18]. For example, high density nanoparticles (NPs) incorporated in any low-density material or biological material, DF imaging will image NPs having brighter appearance inside the biological matrix. Further, with the DF imaging, different type of defects and imperfections for crystalline material can be predicted. In addition, the variable density distribution of specimen can also be elaborated more precisely in DF mode of analysis.

1.6.3 Cryo-TEM

Cryo-TEM deals with analysis of water-based specimen. Imaging under current mode will be proceed rapid freezing of specimen in presence of liquid nitrogen or any other cryogenic liquid [20, 21]. This technique will be helpful in preserving the natural state of specimen with minimum damage to specimen during beam irradiation. This specialized technique is widely used to study the structural biology, biological macro-molecule, viruses and cellular structures at cryogenic conditions [20]. In addition, nanomaterial imaging having minimum artifacts will also be ensured in comparison to traditional sample preparation methods [13].

1.6.4 Environmental TEM (ETEM)

Environmental TEM deals with analysis of material under controlled environmental conditions like controlled gas atmosphere or elevated temperatures etc. [9]. This unique type of TEM will be very helpful in study the dynamic processes of material in real time. In-situ TEM will be helpful in observing the reactions and different dynamic processes of material in material science as well in nanotechnology. This technique will be also useful in investigation of catalytic reactions in real time under controlled gaseous environment [22, 23].

1.7 Quantitative Techniques w.r.t. TEM

Prior to specimen optimization via considering respective nature and properties during TEM imaging mode, specimen insightful explanation and interpretation through quantitative mode can be performed. Energy Dispersive X-ray Spectroscopy (EDS) and Electron Energy Loss spectroscopy (EELS) are two most common quantitative techniques which has been coupled with TEM [4, 9].

1.7.1 Energy Dispersive X-Ray Spectroscopy (EDS)

EDS is a technique which detect characteristic X-ray emitted by a specimen with high-energy electron beam irradiation as shown in Fig. 1.3c. X-ray's emitted are specific to every element of specimen. This will allow specimen detailed elemental quantification study with distribution of respective elements in mapping mode. For example, commercially available sunscreens or any related products claiming for presence of green synthesized Ag/TiO_2/ZnO [24, 25] etc. NPs will be authenticated through TEM coupled EDS instrument. Further, the development of liquid cell assembly have revolutionized the monitoring of nucleation and growth kinetics of nanomaterial through in-situ monitoring [26]. Although, the interference from grid material in addition to other secondary phase from formulation, need proper optimization and right explanation.

1.7.2 Electron Energy Loss Spectroscopy (EELS)

EELS is measure of the energy lost by electrons as when they pass through a specimen under inelastic scattering [27]. Under this mode of operation, observed loss in energy is specific to specific atomic energy levels which will further provide information about sample's composition and electronic structure. In addition to EELS similar quantification aspect as of EDS, EELS will detect the signal generated from core loss edge have capability to interpret same material to different existed forms [21]. EELS will be also helpful in predicting about respective elements chemical bonding, electronic valance and conduction band properties.

1.7.3 Electron Diffraction (ED)

ED technique is coupled with TEM basic instrumentation which provide diffraction data w.r.t. selected area of specimen. Through satisfying the basic condition of diffraction i.e. wavelength of source electron must be smaller than atomic spacing of specimen, respective specimen crystal structure arrangement, phase presence etc., can be predicted. Obtained SAED data i.e. polycrystalline, amorphous etc., will be corroborated through X-ray diffraction study for further authentication [4, 9, 24].

Figure 1.5 has digarmmically represented different modes of TEM operation.

With the understanding of different TEM modes of operation, one can make EM operation more interesting and insightful. Wide range of modes of operation viz.

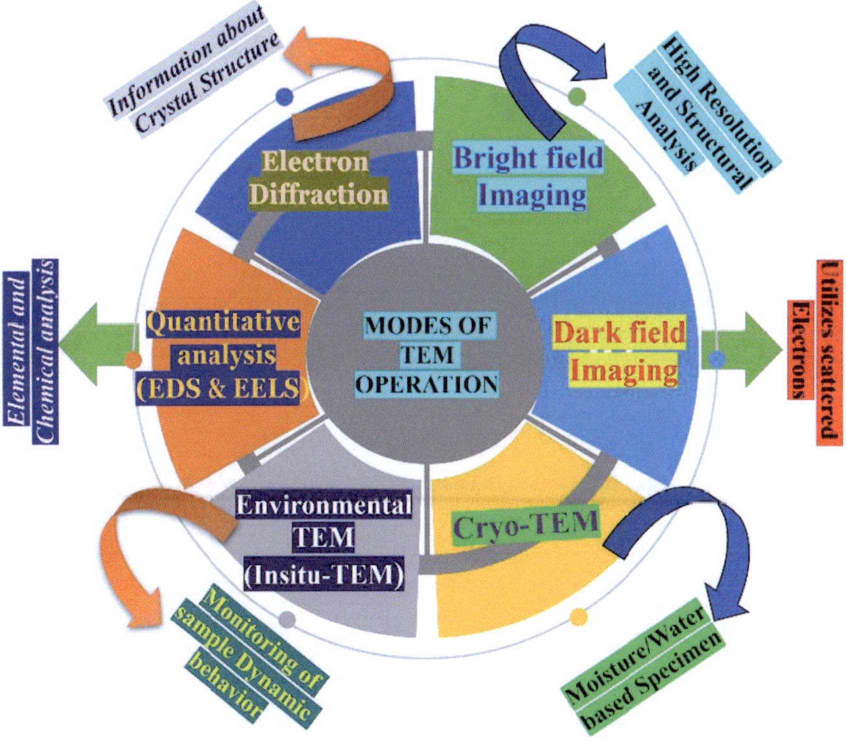

Fig. 1.5 Presented digarmmically different modes of TEM operation and their broad outcomes

imaging, diffraction and spectroscopy etc., will expand the comprehensive characterization of diverse materials and their respective structure investigations for developing novel techniques and devices.

NOTE: Choice of TEM mode will directly impact the detail of information obtained. Select right TEM mode cautiously essential for accurate analysis.

1.8 Right Sample Under Right TEM

This is the most important step which must be followed by researchers in performing TEM analysis of sample i.e. selection of appropriate features-based TEM as per sample nature and its desired applications. Below, we have summarized some points which will be helpful in performing appropriate TEM analysis:

1.8.1 Water Based Samples

Most of samples belong to life science, pharmaceutical science etc., having water as the major part of its structure, need to be processed through standardized protocols. Specimen must be processed through freeze fracture, plunge freezing, cryo-ultramicrotome etc., and must be analysed under technique like cryo-TEM or cryo-SEM etc. This approach will preserve and maintain the integrity of specimen during respective processing and imaging. Although, before inserting the specimen into cryo-TEM, researchers will have to proceed through certain chemical processes [9, 13, 28], to ensure the stability of specimen.

1.8.2 Nanomaterial (NMs)/Nanoparticles (NPs)/Thin Film

The materials (NMs/NPs) having size range i.e. bulk to nano range without water phase, one can proceed respective samples preparation through respective dispersion of appropriate solvent. It is further followed by air drying of specimen solution on TEM grid will be viewed under TEM, HRTEM, STEM-HAADF, in-situ TEM instruments as per requirement of study. Specially, specimen not having thickness in the range of ~ <100 nm, need to process appropriately before inserting into TEM machine [4, 9].

1.8.3 Resolution Requirement

Specimen growth kinetics during synthesis process will decide for range of resolution requirement (conventional TEM to HRTEM or STEM-HAADF etc.) for respective imaging process. Accordingly, the range of incident electrons wavelength through electron source will vary with higher incident accelerating voltage (from 80 to 300 kV or more) as per availability of instrument. If objective of sample analysis and imaging is around atomic scale resolution, we have to go with high resolution TEM (HRTEM) or STEM-HAADF instrumentation capabilities [4, 9, 11]. Further, if objective of study is to explore and investigate about dynamics nature of sample in live environment, environment TEM (in-situ TEM) will be preferred.

1.8.4 Structural Exploration

Quality performance of any material can be authentically claimed with in-depth analysis of respective material with best characterization techniques. TEM techniques play a very crucial role in investigation belong to living to non-living materials structural features like growth mechanism, crystal structure, defects, grain boundaries, cellular structures etc. at bulk as well at nanoscale resolution [9, 11].

1.8.5 Elemental and Chemical Analysis

Current mode of TEM operation has ability to perform sample elemental analysis with detailed quantification and distribution analysis. This ability is valuable for materials belong to materials science, geology and biology etc., for determining the probable composition as well the presence of different impurities phase. Whereas, the electronic state exploration and bonding information of material, electron energy loss spectroscopy (EELS) mode of operation can be utilized [9].

1.8.6 Use of Specialized Specimen Holders

The dynamic observations during experiment of any synthesis time or working of any functional device/material, is very crucial is difficult to perform. The use of assembly or attachment like liquid cell, gas assembly, heating stage etc., upgraded with basic TEM instrument can explore many undiscovered stories of material behaviour. In-situ TEM holder has ability to explore and understand the insights of respective material in dynamic mode like solution or gaseous environment etc. Effect of different external parameters like variable pressure of different gases, variable temperature etc. will be very out of box in understanding and finding some novel insights of material dynamics at nanoscale. This will be very much helpful for future in designing any device or sensors etc. [9].

1.8.7 Advanced Detectors

Imaging close to actual behaviour of specimen directly observed with the help of advanced TEM detectors like charged couple devices (CCDs), complementary metal oxide semiconductor (CMOS), direct electron detector (DDE) etc., having efficient signal collection and improved quality imaging. In addition, TEM with advanced low signal sensitive EDS, EELS detector etc., can be utilized in precise elemental quantification analysis with precise chemical analysis [4, 9, 11]

1.8.8 Automated User-Friendly Interfaces

TEM with user friendly interfaces and automated features will be very useful in the case where users belong to various research areas having varying level of research objectives and unexpected hypothesis.

Figure 1.6 has highlighted the importance of nature of TEM sample, respective instrumentation requirement with desired result outcomes

Before planning to purchase TEM instrument, careful evaluation in term of research needs, budget and area of expertise etc. must be taken care. Researchers must have to consider nature of samples before its processing, resolution range, environment conditions and probable research goals while planning to purchase or analyse sample under electron microscope. Prior to fulfilment of above stated considerations, EM instrument will surely satisfy the current as well future research needs with optimization of sample preparation aspect and respective acquired data analysis.

NOTE: Right combination of TEM instrumentation with rightly processed sample is the key to unlock the precise structural, morphological, elemental and chemical insights.

1.9 Application of TEM

There are following area where TEM technique applicability can be extended:

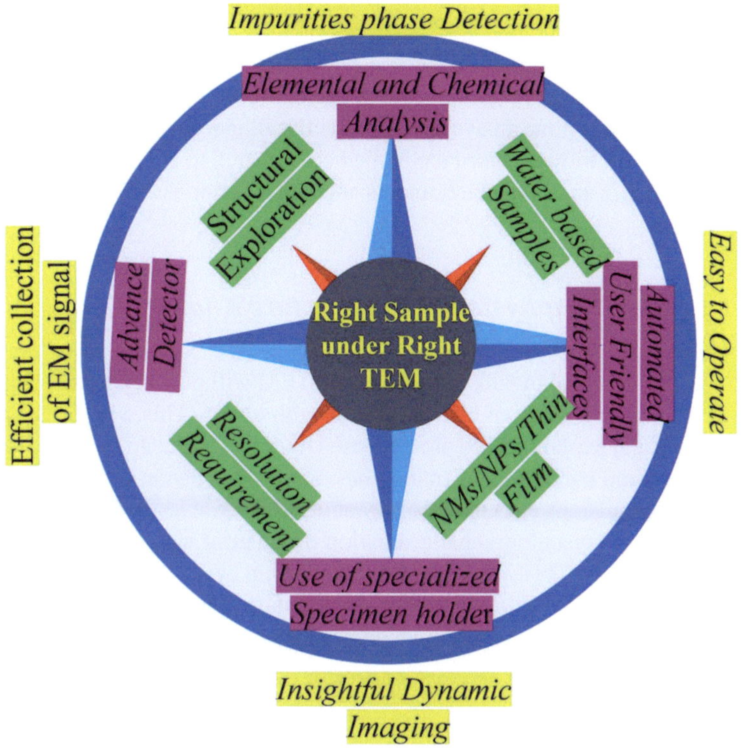

Fig. 1.6 Highlighted the importance of factors related to nature of TEM sample, instrumentation requirement and probable result outcomes

1.9.1 Biological Science

In field of biology, TEM allows researchers to visualize and study the cellular structures and provide detail information in form of images of different organelles, membranes and respective cellular components at nanoscale. Researchers will use TEM as a thoughtful inference tool for scientific community in understanding the cellular functions as well the diseases spreading as well diagnostic mechanisms [29].

1.9.2 Macromolecular Structure

Similar to structural biology, TEM technique enables the visualization of different macromolecules structures including proteins, nucleic acid etc. This will play very crucial role in understanding and applying the biomolecular interactions for advancement of targeted therapies [9].

1.9.3 Pathology and Medical Research

TEM technique will play important role in inspection of tissues and cells of living species during their routine analysis with respective diagnosis in different infections. This technique will further contribute in medical research to understand and explore the impact of drugs and related treatments at cellular and molecular levels [13].

1.9.4 Crystallography and Microstructure Analysis

The growth any material in bulk to nano-range, TEM will play key tool in visualization of respective behaviour at high resolution with clarity. This will further help in understanding and explaining the pre-proposed hypothesis related to shape, size and texture of prepared nanoparticles (nanotubes, nanowires, nanorods, nano-triangles, microspheres, emulsions etc.) morphology at ultrastructure level. Further, TEM can also be utilized in crystallographic evaluation of material via atomic arrangements of respective crystals. This will be further extended in evaluation of microstructure, defects, interfaces etc. of different materials. All stated factors will be essential and useful during optimizing the respective properties of material under TEM study for specific application [4].

1.9.5 Nanodevices Characterization

TEM will play a very crucial in the investigation of structural and components level failure of different nanodevices at nanoscale. This will include study of nanoelectronics, nano-sensors and other nano-size devices etc., under normal TEM, HRTEM, in-situ TEM instrument with micro-electromechanical system (MEMS) specimen holder [30, 31], as per requirement of study.

1.9.6 Integrated Circuit (IC) and Respective Failure Analysis

Failure analysis in semiconductor industry is a major challenge in respective industry. TEM get proven to be an ultimate milestone in the detection and analysis of defect generation or material degradation mechanism. This will be further helpful in identifying respective material problems with their rectification for future to enhance the overall efficiency of system [32].

The digrammical representation of above stated important application of TEM has been demonstrated in Fig. 1.7.

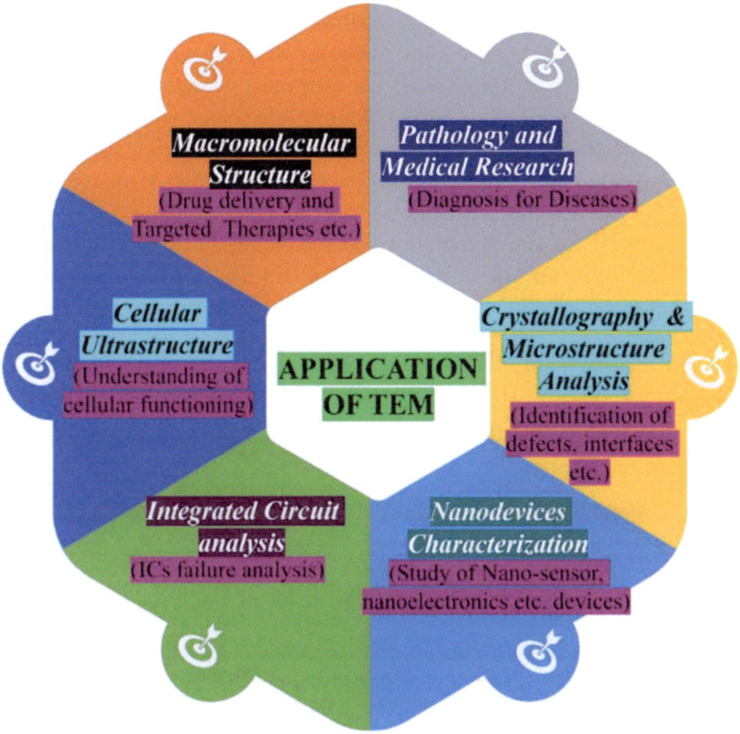

Fig. 1.7 Different probable TEM application

NOTE: The versatile nature of TEM brings indispensable advancement in Material Science, life sciences, nanotechnology and beyond fields.

1.10 Conclusion

Introduction from basics of TEM, principle, working, various modes of operation to application in diversified areas of application, brought EM novice and experience users fascinated and excited towards the amazing world of TEM *to find-out something new and novel*. We have presented the chronological explorations of TEM developments in past times, key milestones and contributions of key pioneer including *Ernest Ruska and Max Knoll*. In continuation, we have discussed about the key features of TEM, witnessing its transformative influence on the various scientific disciplines. Further, with the explanation of different modes of TEM basic to advance operation i.e. bright field, dark field, cryo-TEM, environmental TEM, EDS, EELS and electron diffraction etc., offer more outline about the respective operation and analysis. Before choosing TEM for sample analysis, user must need to prepare the optimize specimen from bulk source which may belong to life science to non-living category with accuracy and precision having minimum artefacts.

Through current introduction to TEM basics and related aspects, readers of electron microscopy science can precisely understand and correlate coming chapter i.e. importance of TEM sample preparation, very effortlessly. Join us with the transition from current chapter 'TEM basics' to domain of 'TEM sample preparation' which is going to reveals the unseen curiosities and observations at different scales of observation.

Declaration:

Author declares that there is no personal or financial conflict of interest regarding publication of this chapter.

References

1. Haguenau, F., Hawkes, P.W., Hutchison, J.L., Satiat-Jeunemaître, B., Simon, G.T., Williams, D.B.: Key events in the history of electron microscopy. Microsc. Microanal. **9**(2), 96–138 (2003). https://doi.org/10.1017/S1431927603030113
2. Dwyer, C., Paganin, D.M.: Quantum and classical fisher information in four-dimensional scanning transmission electron microscopy. Phys. Rev. B **110**(2), 024110 (2024). https://doi.org/10.1103/PhysRevB.110.024110
3. Rashkovskiy, S.A.: Quantum mechanics without quanta: the nature of the wave–particle duality of light. Quantum Stud.: Math. Found. **3**(2), 147–160 (2016). https://doi.org/10.1007/s40509-015-0063-5
4. Williams, D.B., Carter, C.B.: Transmission Electron Microscopy. Springer US, Boston (1996). https://doi.org/10.1007/978-1-4757-2519-3
5. Ruska, E.: The development of the electron microscope and of electron microscopy (Nobel lecture). Angew. Chem. Int. Ed. Engl. **26**(7), 595–605 (1987). https://doi.org/10.1002/anie.198705953
6. Shampo, M.A., Kyle, R.A.: Ernst Ruska—inventor of the electron microscope. Mayo Clin. Proc. **72**(2), 148 (1997). https://doi.org/10.4065/72.2.148
7. Ye, Y., Cota-Ruiz, K., Cantu, J.M., Valdés, C., Gardea-Torresdey, J.L.: Engineered nanomaterials' fate assessment in biological matrices: recent milestones in electron microscopy. ACS Sustain. Chem. Eng. **9**(12), 4341–4356 (2021). https://doi.org/10.1021/acssuschemeng.1c00782
8. Mukhopadhyay, R.: The rise of Instruments during World War II. Anal. Chem. **80**(15), 5684–5691 (2008). https://doi.org/10.1021/ac801205u
9. Ayache, J., Beaunier, L., Boumendil, J., Ehret, G., Laub, D.: Sample Preparation Handbook for Transmission Electron Microscopy. Springer, New York (2010). https://doi.org/10.1007/978-0-387-98182-6
10. Wang, Z.L., Lee, J.L.: Electron microscopy techniques for imaging and analysis of nanoparticles. In: Developments in Surface Contamination and Cleaning, pp. 395–443. Elsevier (2008). https://doi.org/10.1016/B978-0-323-29960-2.00009-5.
11. Egerton, R.F.: Physical Principles of Electron Microscopy: An Introduction to TEM, SEM, and AEM. Springer, New York (2005)

12. Weinert, F.D.: Germer experiment. In: Greenberger, D., Hentschel, K., Weinert, F. (Eds.) Compendium of Quantum Physics, pp. 150–152. Springer, Berlin, Heidelberg (2009). https://doi.org/10.1007/978-3-540-70626-7_45
13. Bozzola, J.J., Russell, L.D.: Electron Microscopy Principles and Techniques for Biologists. Jones and Bartlett Publishers, Inc. (1992)
14. Brydson, R. (Ed.): Front matter. In: Aberration-Corrected Analytical Transmission Electron Microscopy. Wiley (2011). https://doi.org/10.1002/9781119978848.fmatter
15. Frank, J.: Electron Tomography Methods for Three-Dimensional Visualization of Structures in the Cell, 2nd edn. Springer (2010)
16. Malenica, M., Vukomanović, M., Kurtjak, M., Masciotti, V., Dal Zilio, S., Greco, S., Lazzarino, M., Krušić, V., Perčić, M., Jelovica Badovinac, I., Wechtersbach, K., Vidović, I., Baričević, V., Valić, S., Lučin, P., Kojc, N., Grabušić, K.: Perspectives of microscopy methods for morphology characterisation of extracellular vesicles from human biofluids. Biomedicines **9**(6), 603 (2021). https://doi.org/10.3390/biomedicines9060603
17. Ahmed, S., Messali, Z., Ouahabi, A., Trepout, S., Messaoudi, C., Marco, S.: Nonparametric denoising methods based on contourlet transform with sharp frequency localization: application to low exposure time electron microscopy images. Entropy **17**(5), 3461–3478 (2015). https://doi.org/10.3390/e17053461
18. Inkson, B.J.: Scanning Electron Microscopy (SEM) and Transmission Electron Microscopy (TEM) for materials characterization. In: Materials Characterization Using Nondestructive Evaluation (NDE) Methods, pp. 17–43. Elsevier (2016). https://doi.org/10.1016/B978-0-08-100040-3.00002-X
19. Klein, N.D., Hurley, K.R., Feng, Z.V., Haynes, C.L.: Dark field transmission electron microscopy as a tool for identifying inorganic nanoparticles in biological matrices. Anal. Chem. **87**(8), 4356–4362 (2015). https://doi.org/10.1021/acs.analchem.5b00124
20. Savva, C.: A beginner's guide to cryogenic electron microscopy. Biochemist **41**(2), 46–52 (2019). https://doi.org/10.1042/BIO04102046
21. Ilett, M., Brydson, R., Brown, A., Hondow, N.: Cryo-analytical STEM of frozen, aqueous dispersions of nanoparticles. Micron **120**, 35–42 (2019). https://doi.org/10.1016/j.micron.2019.01.013
22. Takeda, S., Yoshida, H.: Atomic-resolution environmental TEM for quantitative in-situ microscopy in materials science. Microscopy (Tokyo) **62**(1), 193–203 (2013). https://doi.org/10.1093/jmicro/dfs096
23. Wagner, J.B., Cavalca, F., Damsgaard, C.D., Duchstein, L.D.L., Hansen, T.W.: Exploring the environmental transmission electron microscope. Micron **43**(11), 1169–1175 (2012). https://doi.org/10.1016/j.micron.2012.02.008
24. Jyoti, K., Baunthiyal, M., Singh, A.: Characterization of silver nanoparticles synthesized using Urtica Dioica Linn. Leaves and their synergistic effects with antibiotics. J. Radiat. Res. Appl. Sci. **9**(3), 217–227 (2016). https://doi.org/10.1016/j.jrras.2015.10.002
25. Lu, P.-J., Huang, S.-C., Chen, Y.-P., Chiueh, L.-C., Shih, D.Y.-C.: Analysis of titanium dioxide and zinc oxide nanoparticles in cosmetics. J. Food Drug Anal. **23**(3), 587–594 (2015). https://doi.org/10.1016/j.jfda.2015.02.009
26. Patterson, J.P., Proetto, M.T., Gianneschi, N.C.: Soft nanomaterials analysed by in situ liquid TEM: towards high resolution characterisation of nanoparticles in motion. Perspect. Sci. **6**, 106–112 (2015). https://doi.org/10.1016/j.pisc.2015.10.003
27. Jungjohann, K.L., Evans, J.E., Aguiar, J.A., Arslan, I., Browning, N.D.: Atomic-scale imaging and spectroscopy for in situ liquid scanning transmission electron microscopy. Microsc. Microanal. **18**(3), 621–627 (2012). https://doi.org/10.1017/S1431927612000104
28. Mielańczyk, Ł., Matysiak, N., Klymenko, O., Wojnicz, R.: Transmission electron microscopy of biological samples. In: Maaz, K. (Ed.) The Transmission Electron Microscope—Theory and Applications. InTech (2015). https://doi.org/10.5772/60680
29. Thompson, R.F., Walker, M., Siebert, C.A., Muench, S.P., Ranson, N.A.: An introduction to sample preparation and imaging by cryo-electron microscopy for structural biology. Methods **100**, 3–15 (2016). https://doi.org/10.1016/j.ymeth.2016.02.017

30. Grenier, A., Duguay, S., Barnes, J.P., Serra, R., Rolland, N., Audoit, G., Morin, P., Gouraud, P., Cooper, D., Blavette, D., Vurpillot, F.: Three dimensional imaging and analysis of a single nano-device at the ultimate scale using correlative microscopy techniques. Appl. Phys. Lett. **106**(21), 213102 (2015). https://doi.org/10.1063/1.4921352
31. Armigliato, A., Frabboni, S., Gazzadi, G.C.: Electron diffraction with ten nanometer beam size for strain analysis of nanodevices. Appl. Phys. Lett. **93**(16), 161906 (2008). https://doi.org/10.1063/1.3003581
32. Shen, F.-C., Huang, C.-Y., Lo, H.-Y., Hsu, W.-Y., Wang, C.-H., Chen, C., Wu, W.-W.: Atomic-scale investigation of electromigration with different directions of electron flow into high-density nanotwinned copper through in situ HRTEM. Acta Mater. **219**, 117250 (2021). https://doi.org/10.1016/j.actamat.2021.117250

Chapter 2
Fundamentals of TEM Sample Preparation

The art of microscopy is not in observing the details, but in preparing the sample to reveal them
by ***Ernest Ruska*** *(Lobel Laureate) Co-inventor of TEM*

Abstract Journey of quality imaging under transmission electron microscopy (TEM) for specimens belong from materials (non-living) to biological science (living) will be governed by precise sample preparation methods and techniques. With the systematic classification of specimen belong to biological, inorganic, soft specimen etc. categories, will be easy to perform respective specimens' novel analysis. Every sample under EM analysis require dedicated preparation protocol as per respective sample nature and properties. Most importantly, the remediation-oriented handling of different challenges during sample preparation w.r.t. TEM analysis viz. knowledge of material, electron beam interaction with sample, induction of artefacts, optimum specimen thickness, staining procedure, sample drying, grid handling procedure etc., need to follow. In addition, all safety guidelines must be followed during major and minor sample preparation and EM operation procedure. With this chapter, researchers will get aware about systematic handling of different sample w.r.t. precise TEM analysis with maintaining specimen integrity and achieving high-resolution features at molecular or atomic scale.

Keywords Sample preparation · Biological · Optimum thickness · Staining · Grid handling

2.1 Introduction

Transmission Electron Microscopy (TEM) work and behave as a leading imaging technique in microstructure investigation of material belong from living to non-living categories. However, the journey of respective material at atomic or molecular level is not possible without optimized sample preparation. Current chapter has focus on paramount importance of sample preparation in achieving the basic to high-resolution, dynamic ultrastructure information via high quality images. In same

R. Singh, *Transmission Electron Microscopy Sample Preparation*,
https://doi.org/10.1007/978-3-031-82967-3_2

context, the stability of samples under vacuum and with high energy beam exposure at optimum thickness (~ 100 nm) become the major challenges to perform analysis and extract informative imaging. In above race, hydrated specimens are always a challenging task for researchers to analyzed under electron microscope (EM). Such material requires complex procedures to fix the original structure of material for actual investigation under TEM or SEM analysis.

Under TEM technique, researchers have to proceed with fine dispersed powder form or thin film form (slice) having area of observation less < 3 mm diameter and ideal thickness of < 100 nm. Several sample preparation techniques have been utilized in obtaining sample thin slices to bring specimen observable under TEM. Some methods proceed with dissolution of material into electron transparent thickness whereas other follow with breaking the material into its initial smallest state. Few techniques will follow the ultra-thick cutting of specimen into electron transparent thickness for high contrast imaging.

This chapter investigates into the fundamentals of TEM sample preparation with the exploration of specimen's physical and chemical behavior. Special emphasis has been focused on the role of safety precautions while performing respective sample preparation and analysis under TEM for novel results.

2.2 Classification of Samples

TEM is one of most well-designed scientific tools which will serve in examination of wide variety of materials, ranging from biological specimens, inorganic to soft materials etc. In order to understand and explore the material ultrastructural behavior, insight knowledge about the specimen is very important. This section will explore about the unique characteristics and precautions while dealing with biological, inorganic or soft etc. materials, while analyzing under TEM technique [1–3].

2.2.1 Biological Samples

Any material (animal, plant, human etc.) which is extracted from living state is considered as biological or life science specimen. Investigation of such samples is important and crucial due to presence of water as a main component. Broadly there are two broad categories of biological materials, are summarized below:

2.2.1.1 Cell and Tissues

Cell is basic unit of living organism whereas tissue (human, animal or plant) is the group of multicellular organelles performing different functions to execute specific tasks [1]. Bacteria, virus are the category of material having unicellular functionaries. The delicacy of biological samples due to water-based network, need proper sample preparation. Chemical and physical fixation are two approaches get utilized in order to stabilize the basic structure of any organism under electron microscope (EM). Under and over fixation of specimen, during their preparations lead to generation of different artifacts [2]. Dedicated cryo-electron microscopy instrumentation and supporting sample preparation techniques can be utilized in respective imaging. Multicellular nature of specimen will be imaged under EM through heavy metal staining will be used in contrast enhancement during revealing of actual cellular structure [4].

2.2.1.2 Macromolecules

Macromolecules are the category of material belong to large and complex form of proteins, carbohydrate, lipid, nucleic acid etc. based organic molecules [1]. Normal TEM imaging will elaborate about shape and size of material with high contrast imaging. High Resolution-TEM (HRTEM) imaging will be utilized in atomic scale exploration of respective specimen ultrastructure insights, prior to their optimized specimen preparation procedure. Well stabilized specimen under low temperature conditions (cryo-stabilization), bring minimum electron beam dominated distortion, bring insightful imaging of lipids, carbohydrate or protein-based molecules [5]. Contrast enhancement techniques like negative and positive staining or metal shadowing techniques [6], will be used in precise explanations of complex macromolecule functioning. Specifically, immunolabelling technique will also be used in localizing protein complex structure [7].

2.2.2 Inorganic Materials

Current material category includes material belong to metals, metal oxide (semiconductor etc.), minerals salts etc. The specified and controlled nucleation and growth conditions (temperature, pressure etc.) of respective precursors will convert respective material into desired yield and size range.

2.2.2.1 Metals

The excellent conductivity, malleability and strength etc., features attract researchers to investigate respective behavior under appropriate TEM technique [2]. HRTEM, STEM techniques become helpful in investigation of crystal structure of metals at atomic level with evaluation of different in-built and process induced defects or dislocation effects. In addition, with the help of energy dispersive spectroscopy (EDS) or electron energy loss spectroscopy (EELS) modes, researchers will further elaborate about the elemental distribution and chemical state of the respective components [8].

This will be very much helpful during understanding about the homogeneity of material under investigation for related device fabrication [9].

2.2.2.2 Semiconductor

Due to tunable electrical, optical etc. properties of semiconductor materials, dominated demand in the communication, computing as well in energy sectors [2]. With miniaturization of material dimensions, nanoscale analysis of respective material become very important. Intermediate band gap between metal and insulator, semiconductors have significant scope in conductivity manipulations with variation in temperature, impurities or external electric field with light emission or absorption possibilities. Respective tunable electrical, optical, thermal or dielectric etc., properties bring TEM and respective modes of analysis more important. This will be helpful for researchers in understanding and exploring about the materials defects, dislocations, grain boundaries, morphology, atomic structure information insightfully at atomic scale [10]

2.2.2.3 Mineral and Ceramic

In era of fast expanding global industrialization with technological revolution, insightful study about different geological processes become very important and essential [2]. Analysis and exploration of different varieties of minerals and ceramics materials, TEM technique will play very crucial role. Identification and evaluation of minerals/ceramic's structural and morphological modification/transformation with elemental quantification and distribution under temperature, pressure etc., can be performed at atomic scale. Understanding about the minerals/ceramic's crystal structure, texture, defects/dislocations, orientation w.r.t. atomic grains and composition through TEM/HRTEM can be performed at nanoscale [11–13].

2.2.3 Soft Material

Soft materials are the category of substances having distinctive mechanical, delicate physical and chemical properties [1]. Although biological samples will also come under soft material category, but we have discussed it under separate Sect. 2.1. Unlike rigid materials, soft materials dynamically respond to external stimuli like pressure, temperature, current etc. conditions [14] very un-predictably. We have categorized samples like polymer, elastomers, gels and organic compounds under current category.

2.2.3.1 Organic Compound

The compounds which are composed of bonding between carbon and hydrogen, oxygen, nitrogen, sulfur etc. termed as organic compounds [2, 4]. Organic compound can be natural as well synthetic. This will include material named hydrocarbon, alcohol, carbohydrates, protein, active pharmaceutical ingredient (API) or lipids/ cholesterol etc. categories. Detail atomic and molecular arrangements examination of organic compounds have been performed with proper sample preparation under appropriate TEM [14].

2.2.3.2 Polymer

Polymer material will be synthesized through smallest unit called monomer, under polymerization reaction. Wide range of polymer materials will exist on the basis of their molecular weight, mechanical strength and electrical properties etc., which direct their applicability in electronics, biomedical, medicines, automotive, packaging, coatings and adhesive fields [2, 15]. Due to their light weight, flexible nature brings them at top in research investigations. Insight of polymers material properties like growth kinetics, phase segregation, crystallinity, mechanical and electrical strength etc., will be analyzed and explored very minutely with the help of TEM. The development of polymer blends with respective miscibility behavior, will also be analyzed and confirmed with TEM and related modes of operation. Cross section features of polymer material can also be explored with optimize sample preparation via technique like ultramicrotomy [9].

2.2.3.3 Gels

Co-existence any sample form in solid as well liquid state termed as Gel. Due to its dual behavior, it is demanding in medical field, cosmetics industry etc. Continuous network of liquid with three-dimensional structure of solid element, make it unique functional behavior. In addition, the high demand of variety of food and personal care products like jam, jellies, hair gel, skin care products, rises respective material in-depth authentic analysis. Specially, application of gel based topical formulations in topical drug delivery has revolutionary outcomes and challenges faced w.r.t. treatment of diseases related to skin cancer [16]. Detail mechanism has been demonstrated in Fig. 2.1a, b.

Colloidal gel, hydrogel and aerogels are the main category under gel formulations having specific applications. The presence of water as the essential part of respective gel structure, ideal imaging will be facilitated with different cryo-techniques. With prior stabilization of gel structure, actual analysis of gel network can be reported [17, 18].

The idea to classify different types of samples w.r.t. TEM analysis as per their nature and properties, is to generate and interpret observed data with minimum error

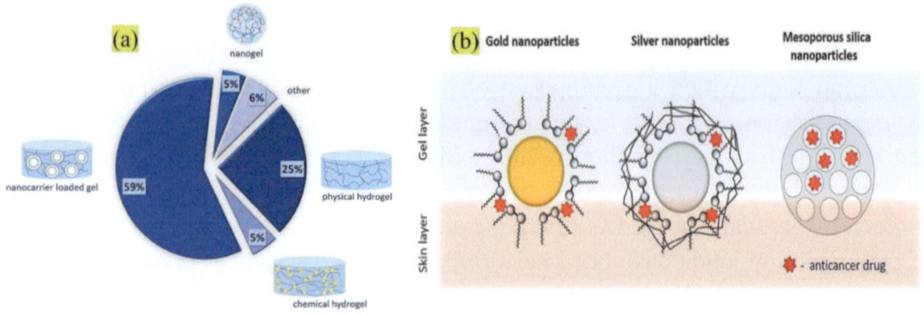

Fig. 2.1 Demonstrated use of **a** Different gels in skin cancer treatments, **b** schematic incorporation of inorganic nanoparticles in topical gel (Reprinted with permission from Slavkova et al. [16] under open access)

and mis-interpretation. Figure 2.2, have demonstrated about the broad categories of samples which can be analyzed under TEM.

NOTE: Classification of different tem samples before their preparation is important, as every sample require special handling to maintain respective integrity and precise imaging.

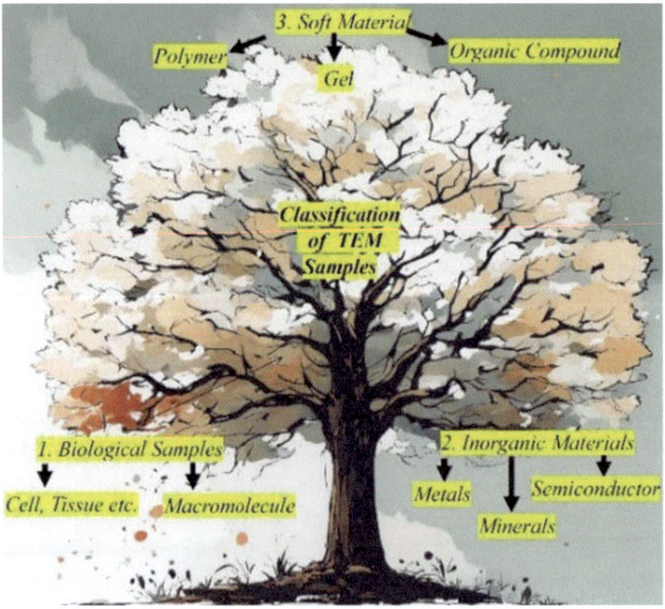

Fig. 2.2 Demonstrate about broad categories of specimens for TEM analysis

2.3 Basic Principle of TEM Sample Preparations

Synthesized sample analysis under TEM technique is not effective unless, we do not proceed prior to respective material properties analysis. Pre-planning and understanding of sample which to be analyzed under TEM, will help users to choose the appropriate protocol/procedure for TEM analysis. Without optimized and validated specimen preparation approach, one cannot expect and achieve precise and accurate TEM results. From my experience, I found many users of TEM *'which do not know and some are one do not want to know'* about their sample that *'how good it can be prepared'* or *'how badly it was prepared'*. In coming section, we have presented about some basic tricks and facts related to novel TEM sample for quality electron microscopy (EM) imaging.

2.3.1 Biological Samples (Cells, Tissues etc.)

Before discussing about biological sample preparation ways, we must have to understand broadly about its physiology and compositions [4, 5]. With the complete knowledge of specific life science specimen, EM user can decide and proceed very accurately with factors/steps like most appropriate fixation method (physical or chemical fixation), type of fixative, fixation time, fixative concentration, dehydration solvents, time span of dehydration, embedding media (epoxy), clearing reagent, infiltration time, light microscopy, ultramicrotomy, staining etc. Specifically, different fixatives (pre and post fixative) have different fixation speed irrespective of their concentration and strength as per nature of tissue/specimen. In addition to chemical fixation, use of physical fixation i.e. plunge-freezing, high pressure freezing, self-pressurized freezing etc., for any tissue sample preparation, will be depend on size of specimen, time of fixation etc. Further, the compatibility of dehydration agent and embedding media with respective tissue or cells etc., also need to validate before proceeding with any random selection. In addition, cryo-immobilization techniques are also mostly preferred for biological sample during fixation processes, just to ensure minimum dislocation of cellular components through preparation process [1].

For example, unique sample preparation and imaging process of *organ on a chip device* has been demonstrated under Fig. 2.3a–d [19].

Subsequent to fixation, dehydration and block preparation steps in specimen processing, respective specimen thin sectioning (~ 70–100 nm) is very crucial step. It is treated like *'more of an art than science'*. Fixing of appropriate specimen size in specific orientation in suitable epoxy, use of cutting knife (diamond or glass knife), cutting speed, handling of thin specimen slices etc., are the factors which need to handle and proceed with extra care and skill. Mounting of electron transparent specimen slices on TEM grids will be done with very precaution for their minimum shrinkage or folding effects. Further, specimen mounted on grid will be followed by

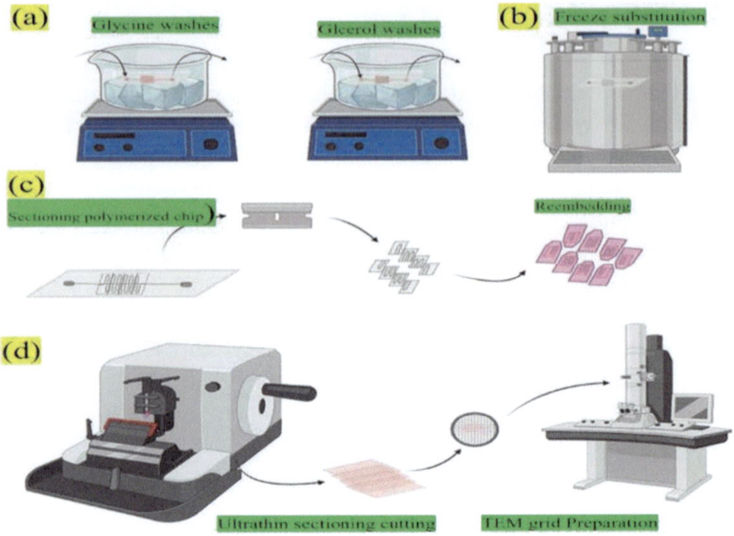

Fig. 2.3 Overview of sample preparation for organ on chip specimen, **a** specimen glycine washing followed by use of glycerol (cryoprotectant) at 4 °C, **b** freeze substitution in propane with liquid nitrogen environment, **c** Serpentine blocks re-embedding in resin for ultrathin sectioning, **d** thin section cutting process with TEM grid preparation procedure (Reprinted with permission from Mares et al. [19] under open access)

freshly prepared heavy metal stains (uranyl acetate, lead citrate, phosphor-tungstinic acid etc.), for the contrast enhancement of respective components clarity [1].

2.3.2 *Inorganic Materials*

The broad categories of inorganic materials named metals, semiconductors, minerals, ceramics etc., also need high quality precise sample preparation approach for TEM analysis. Important and utmost requirement for specimen thickness is in the range of ~ 100 nm or more better as per nature and properties of specimen. Further, a thin conductive coating of carbon etc., on material surface can be performed as an optional step to minimize the charging effects during respective imaging. Inorganic material viz. metals, semiconductors, minerals, ceramics etc., have following steps and precaution, which need to follow during TEM analysis [2]:

2.3.2.1 Metal Specimen

Any metal specimen visualization under TEM needs cutting into thin sections from thick form or metal piece with high precision saw or any other appropriate cutting tool. Initial specimen thinning process techniques like dimpling, grinding or polishing bring thickness into millimeter or micrometer range. In some case, electropolishing technique will also be very effective during conditioning of materials surface having free from artifacts, smooth and oxide free nature. Ion milling and focused ion beam (FIB) milling techniques deals with thinning of specimens in (20–100 nm) range. Specifically, FIB technique will be dedicatedly work for TEM cross-sectional sample preparation approach. Precise thinning of specimen will be proceeded by mechanical polishing including polishing through fine abrasives will be used for ultrafine smoothness with electron transparency of specimen. Mounting of metal thin slices on appropriate TEM grids (Cu, Ni, Au or Mo grid) need special care. TEM grid with specimen must be in dry form and contamination free before inserting into TEM machine for imaging purpose [4, 14].

For example in one of related study, solid state method guided metal (M) and metal oxide (M_xO_y) nanostructure synthesis has been fabricated with macromolecule complex formation i.e. chitosn-Xn and PS-co-4-PVP-MXn where X is anion accompanying cationic metal and PS-co-4-PVP will be read as poly (styrene-co-4-vinylpridine) [20] respectively. Figure 2.4a demonstrated schematic representation of solid-state method with application in process of environment remediation. Figure 2.4b–h shows detailed analysis of pyrolytic product of Chitosan-$(FeCl_3)_n$ 1:1, hematite- Fe_2O_3 materials through SEM, EDS and TEM analysis respectively. Clear presence of iron (Fe) and oxygen (o) elements in EDS has been observed with irregular and agglomerated shape dominated nanostructure in TEM imaging has been observed in Fig. 2.4b–h [20].

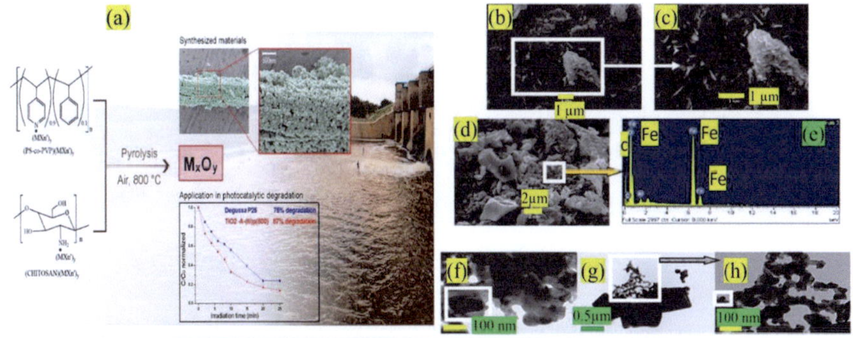

Fig. 2.4 **a** Demonstrated schematic representation of solid-state method with application in environment remediation through Fe-chitosan complex nanoparticle, **b–h** shows detailed analysis of pyrolytic product of Chitosan-$(FeCl_3)_n$ 1:1, hematite-Fe_2O_3 materials through SEM, EDS and TEM analysis respectively. (Reprinted with permission from Diaz et al. [20] under open access)

2.3.2.2 Semiconductor

Mostly similar sample preparation techniques will be followed for semiconductor analysis under EM technique as that of above discussed metallic samples. Normally, semiconductor i.e. TiO_2, ZnO, Silicon (Si), Germanium (Ge) etc., are used in variety of applications like photocatalyst etc. Respective materials will be prepared through number of techniques like electrochemical or physical or chemical reaction-based approaches. Single component-based material will be preferred due to uniform solution formation, monolayer thin film preparation in addition to specific applications. Many times, multiphase component-based semiconductor will also be preferred, in addition to having challenges like limited solubility conditions which need to optimized [5, 14]

For example, Noor Haida Mohd Kaus et al. (2021) authors have studied reduced graphene oxide (rGO)/semiconductor composite formation through different synthesis methods, for high performance photocatalysis applications in specific light region [21]. Stated process has been schematically demonstrated under Fig. 2.5.

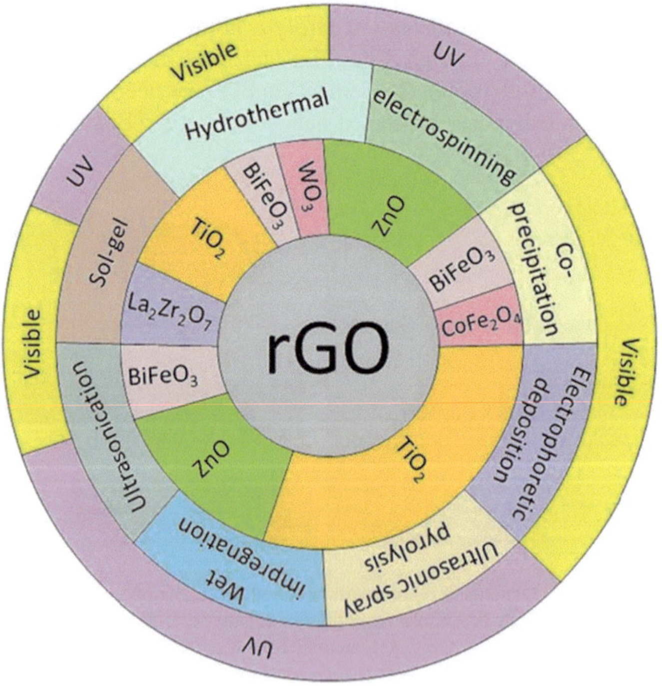

Fig. 2.5 Schematic representation of rGO/semiconductor composite with respective method of hybridization and suitable light energy region (Reprinted with permission from Mohd Kaus et al. [21] under open access)

2.3.2.3 Ceramics and Mineral

Due to presence of multiphase components in most of ceramic and minerals samples, need respective material specialized sample preparation approach. Appropriate selection of specimen with cutting into smaller piece, followed by mechanical thinning techniques like polishing, ultramicrotomy and FIB technique will be chosen for fine electron transparent specimen. Chemical, ion milling and FIB milling etc., are the techniques have an optional choice in precise thinning of specimen preparation w.r.t. TEM imaging, as per requirement (nature and type) of sample. With proper loading of thin slices on TEM grid, further carbon coating on grid, can also be executed in order to minimize the probable charging effects [11–13].

In similar work, Vry et al. [22] analyzed and reported synthesis of silicon carbide (SiC) via crosslinking of methylphenylvinylhydrogen polysiloxane preceramic polymer in presence of argon through photo-polymerization. Figure 2.6a, b confirms the polycrystalline network having faulted/twined network enclosed by fluffy phase. Further, HRTEM imaging have confirmed about SiC grains and its vicinity area visualization. Clear lattice fringes of bulk SiC has been observed with disordered arrangement at outer surface of respective material has been shown in Fig. 2.6c. Confirmation of above observation has been finished by EDS-mapping analysis (Fig. 2.6d). The outer layer of grain shows amorphous pattern as depicted by FFT image (Fig. 2.6e) whereas core area shows b-SiC cubic structure (Fig. 2.6e). In addition, inverse FFT of core SiC region as shown in Fig. 2.6g confirms stacking fault and dislocation nature of respective material.

Selection of appropriate mode of TEM operation with most suitable sample preparation protocol/procedure is very important for any EM insightful study. Solution-based nanoparticles (NPs) of metallic (Ag or Au etc.), inorganic NPs (ZnO, TiO_2

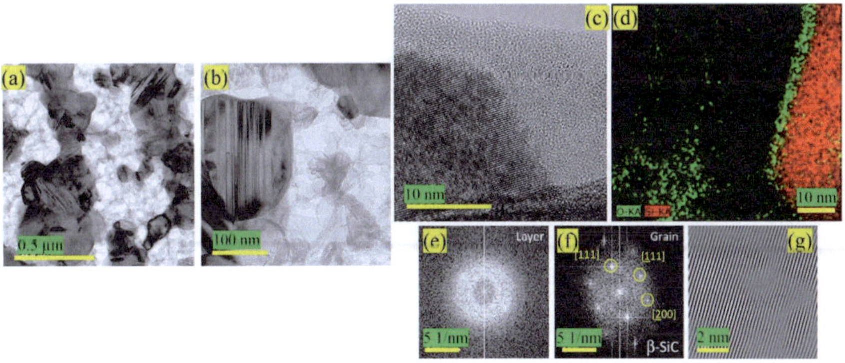

Fig. 2.6 **a** TEM image of crosslinked and pyrolyzed methylphenylvinylhydrogen polysiloxane preceramic polymer, **b** Zoomed image of respective area; **c** HRTEM image of SiC with surrounding thin layer, **d** respective area EDS mapping for Silicon and oxygen, **e**, **f** FFT pattern of surface layer and Core specimen, **g** inverse FFT pattern of SiC grains (Reprinted with permission from Vry et al. [22] under open access)

etc.), or thin film form, also demands specialized sample preparation procedure. For example, appropriate dispersion of NPs in solvent in terms of their optimum concentration, appropriate solvent, sonication time, stirring speed etc., are the factors which must be applied very cautiously while preparing the respective specimen. Selection of suitable grid (Cu, Ni, Mo or Au etc.), support material (carbon, formvar, collodion etc.) and number of meshes (100 or 200 or 300 or 400 etc.), will be decided according to size of NPs, dispersion conditions etc. In above processes, drop casting of sample solution on TEM grid will be followed with unpredictable grid drying behavior. This is the most delicate and sensitive step which need to standardized and validate according to sample type (colloidal suspension, emulsions, lipid NPs etc.)

2.3.3 Soft Materials

2.3.3.1 Organic/Polymer/Gel

Stability of soft materials like organic, polymer or gel etc. material under electron microscopy (EM) techniques stand as a prominent challenge in maintaining respective material structural integrity during EM analysis. Any material belongs to above category, need use of specialized specimen preparation protocol like drop casting, chemical fixation or physical fixation etc., as per nature of specimen.

For example, Gopiraman et al. [23] reported metal nanoparticle (Au, Ag, Ni) supported cellulose nanofiber (CNF) based composite material. Effective adhesion between CNF with Ag NPs (Fig. 2.7a–c), Au (Fig. 2.7e–g), and Ni (Fig. 2.7i–k) has been insightly demonstrated via TEM imaging. In addition, respective histogram representation has also been presented in Fig. 2.7d, h, i.

Respective specimens having water as a major constituent, need sample stabilization through chemical fixation, dehydration, embedding and infiltration steps followed by ultramicrotomy with appropriate staining. Use of optimize and validated fixative and dehydration agent, will be used after embedded material adherence with electron beam. Similarly, embedding media with optimum conditions to harden the epoxy block in presence of specimen also vary from specimen to specimen. Further, ultramicrotomy technique with nature of cutting knife, will be used as per stability aspect of sample during nano-slicing. In addition to chemical fixation protocol, many times user have to proceed with cryo-based physical fixation procedure of sample which will quickly stabilize the present water content into stable amorphous form. Further, thinning of specimen will also be proceed with technique like mechanical thinning etc. Stated protocol also needs to validate and design as per need and properties of sample under study. Obviously, smooth handling at every stage during TEM sample preparation work bring minimum artifacts-based electron transparent specimen [2, 24]. In addition, many times organic NPs (emulsion, lipid NPs etc.) need to be stained with heavy metals like uranyl acetate or phosphotungstic acid (PTA) etc., for enhancement of specimen contrast during TEM imaging.

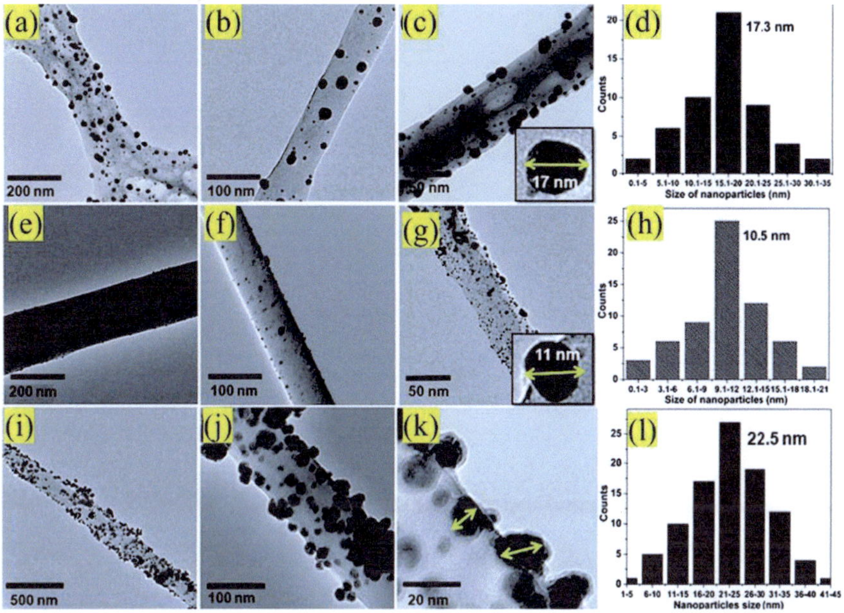

Fig. 2.7 TEM images of **a–c** Ag/CNFs, **e–g** Au-CNFs, **i–k** Ni-CNFs respectively, with respective histogram distribution (Reprinted with permission from Gopiraman et al. [23] under open access)

Artifact free analysis of gel samples, low temperature-based techniques for stabilization, can be followed. Properly stabilized gel specimen and presence of cryoprotectant like glycerol, ethylene glycol or sucrose etc., bring fixing of respective structure close to its native environment. The presence of cryoprotectants during gel stabilization process prevent the water crystal formation during specimen freezing to avoid charging or any artifacts effects [19]. Thin layer of gel specimen on specialized cryo-TEM grid, will be dried under plunge freezing in presence of liquid ethane or liquid nitrogen cooled liquid propane environment. Recent fluid cell-based TEM holder has removed many barriers for researchers to explore imaging of such specimen for future.

For reference, schematic representation of different nanovesicles based hydrophilic and hydrophilic drug incorporation on topical application of gel formulation [16] has been demonstrated in Fig. 2.8.

The knowledge about the fundamentals of TEM sample preparation, will equip any researcher with confidence and precise direction to analyze sample with accuracy. Above discussed different categories of sample w.r.t. TEM analysis i.e. biological material, inorganic material, and organic material, presented a simple, easy and latest database approach. With the help of above approach, scientist/researchers can plan or replan their research hypothesis with respect to TEM dominated novel outcomes.

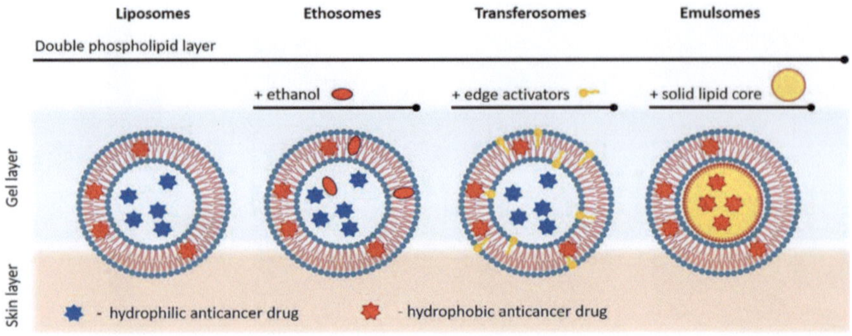

Fig. 2.8 Schematic representation of nanovesicles incorporation within topical gel (Reprinted with permission from Slavkova et al. [16] under open access)

2.4 Challenges During Sample Preparations and Possible Remedies

Ideally to perform any sample analysis or sample preparation, firstly we need to write-down the probable challenges in whole approach. Level and type of challenges will help in designing and planning related workplan approach. In similar context, preparing quality samples for TEM analysis, researchers must have to mark/highlight, all the probable challenges which may be confronted while preparing or analyzing the respective specimen. In coming paragraphs, we have tried to summarize the maximum probable factors which can directly or indirectly affect the quality sample preparation and their respective analysis under TEM for meaningful and accurate micrographs:

2.4.1 Know Your Material

As per my knowledge and experience, if we know our material's physical, chemical, thermal, mechanical etc. properties very well, we are close to achieve quality results through any techniques [2, 15]. For example, if we want to study kidney of alive rat or leaves of any plant or study of ZnO NPs or lipid based organic formulation under TEM, we must have to study about nature and properties of respective material, before preparing specimen and viewing under TEM. All stated materials are different from each other and all need separate sample preparation with respective imaging analysis. Rat kidney precise extraction from live rat or smoothly cutting of small leaf portion from parent leave/plant, followed by chemical fixation protocol, dehydration, ultramicrotomy and staining procedure. Physical fixation protocol(cryo-fixation), will also be utilized depending upon the nature and properties of specimen. At the end, imaging will be done at 70 kV or 80 kV accelerating voltage of TEM instrument.

Whereas, ZnO NPs probably need to analyse at 200 kV or 300 kV accelerating voltage with HRTEM or better instrument. Quality EM results will be supported with NPs optimized synthesis and respective effective dispersion in suitable solvent. Further, lipid-based formulations will be analysed under low temperature- TEM techniques like Cryo-TEM [2, 15] etc. In conclusion, ideally before starting EM analysis of sample, we have to '*first know our material*' then accordingly choose the respective technique like TEM, HRTEM, Cryo-TEM etc.

2.4.2 Purity and Homogeneity of Sample

Ultimate goal of quality analysis under TEM, will be guided and decided by level of purity and homogeneity of respective sample. Specimen analysed at very high magnification for atomic or molecular imaging of inorganic, metallic or biological material, the presence of any crystal defects, impurity phase or artifacts, most of time get mis-interpreted and mis-representated in respective explanation. In case of low purity and homogeneity of samples, bring deviated chemical analysis with misleading data under EM analysis [2, 15]. Researchers must have to very much careful in purity percentage aspect while choosing any fixative, chemicals, distilled water, solvents, organic reagent, cutting tools (surgical blade, glass knife, diamond knife) etc. In addition, specimen analysed under TEM, must be free from any chance of cross-contamination.

2.4.3 Sample Damage with Electron Beam

Even specimen prepared through proper procedure as per requirements of study, harsh impact of incident electron beam during TEM analysis, bring stressed/ contracted swelled images. In order to handle the current challenge of specimen actual imaging for organic formulations or biological specimen, low dose imaging, cryo-TEM or minimum exposure time etc., techniques, will be preferred. It will be utilized to ensure the minimum beam damage effect to specimen under imaging conditions [24].

2.4.4 Artifacts Generation

Right from life science to organic to inorganic specimens' preparation and analysis under TEM, challenges with different types of artifacts generation through process need to minimized through different method validation processes [25]. Specifically, improper role of fixative, respective concentration, timings of fixation, dehydration, embedding followed by infiltration procedure, staining etc., can bring multiple artifacts onto specimen. Further, thin slicing through ultramicrotomy is the most prone area to surface defects generation like wrinkles, knife marks etc. This will become more problematic due to external vibrations, acoustic noise, misaligned cutting setup, or erratic lifting of thin slices onto the TEM grids etc. Furthermore, improper compatibility of epoxy with material for slicing during infiltration bring impact like under or over fixing, leaching of specimen from epoxy. As an outcome of artifacts dominated specimen TEM imaging, bring confusion w.r.t. original features of specimen. Inappropriate use of pH and concentration of heavy metals like PTA, uranyl acetate, ammonium molybdate etc., during staining of specimen, will deteriorates the analysis of specimen. Similarly, mishandling w.r.t. TEM grid, carbon coating of grid etc., may bring unwanted issues in specimen analysis. This will need special care and handling skill w.r.t. specimen handling, to ensure minimum process and EM imaging related bad-effects [2, 15].

2.4.5 *Optimized Specimen Thickness*

Quality imaging of TEM specimen will be achieved by appropriate thickness. Specifically, TEM imaging like normal or high-resolution imaging is linked with the thickness range (~ 50–100 nm) of specimen. Thickness profile of tissue, bacteria, cells, organic, inorganic compound, metal, non-metal etc., materials under TEM, will decide the resolution of image, electron-beam interaction with specimen surface. Roughly, thickness range of specimen may vary from ~ 50 to 100 nm or better, will depend on type and nature of specimen. Specimen thickness is inversely proportional to resolution of specimen. Thicker specimen like > 100 nm thickness led to poor beam penetration and poor contrast in EM images. Unevenness in thickness profile (at nanometre), bring uneven contrast of specimen. Thinner specimen will be analysed at higher electron beam energy (high accelerating voltage like 200, 300 kV etc.) whereas thicker specimen will be preferred analysis at lower energy electron beam (lower accelerating voltage like 80 kV or 100 kV etc.) of TEM [2, 15].

2.4.6 *Staining Variability*

Non-uniformly fixed, multicellular materials have a challenge to maintain uniform contrast while explaining the physiology of specimen under EM study. In order to maintain the sufficient contrast of specimen, chemicals like uranyl acetate, lead citrate, osmium tetroxide, PTA etc. will be used in respective staining process. Selection of suitable stain, concentration, pH (acidic or basic), staining time (under or over stain), stain penetration, use of staining temperature etc. processes always need standardized.

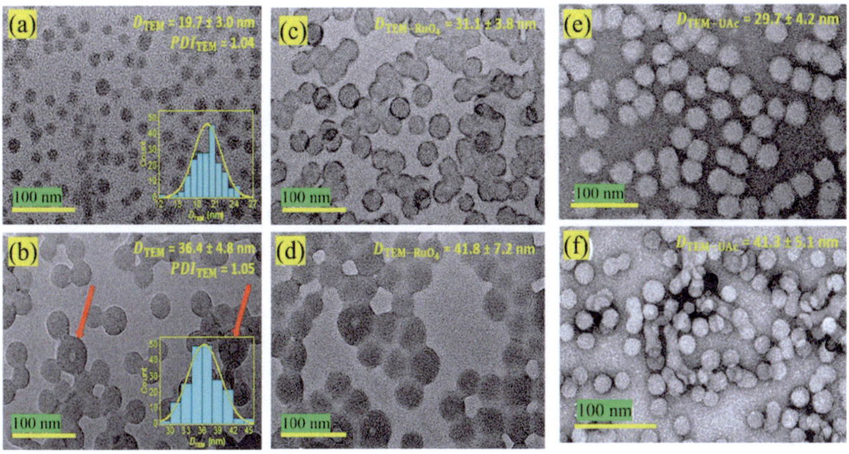

Fig. 2.9 **a** Unstained conventional TEM image of $PHEA_{85}$-b-PS_{130}, **b** $PHEA_{23}$-b-PS_{130} highlighting vesicular structure, **c** positive stain EM images of $PHEA_{85}$-b-PS_{130} and **d** $PHEA_{23}$-b-PS_{130}, **e** negative stain EM images of $PHEA_{23}$-b-PS_{130} respectively (Reprinted with permission from Tkachenko et al. [26] under open access)

Effect of staining behaviour on visualization of poly (hydroxy ethyl acrylate)-b-poly(styrene)($PHEA_x$-b-PS_y) particles has been demonstrated in Fig. 2.9a–d where x and y are the degree of polymerization of respective block [26]. Figure 2.9a, b shows the collapse of lyophilic layer of $PHEA_x$-b-PS_y upon air drying lead to misinterpreted TEM imaging. Figure 2.9c, d shows positive staining images with RuO_4 will be helpful in highlighting the boundaries of $PHEA_x$-b-PS_y polymer particles in addition to its passiveness about visualization of respective material multiphase structure. Further, Fig. 2.9e, f highlighted more better way the structure and preservation of polymer under negative staining with uranyl acetate [26].

Practically, while doing staining (positive or negative) of specimen, the occurrence of dominant background, artifacts concentration, unfixed areas, stains un-stability with e-beam, uneven thickness etc., factors will create difficulty in representing and interpreting the respective results with precision and accuracy.

2.4.7 Sample Drying

Meticulous sample drying procedures need careful considerations while preparing TEM specimen. This will minimize one of major challenge of TEM quality imaging i.e. *'Charging Effects'*. Challenge in maintaining integrity of specimen during drying procedure is the foremost objective of whole sample preparation process.

Prior to classification about type of specimen, insight about the drying methods like air drying, oven drying or freeze drying etc., is also necessary. During air drying of specimen, temperature sensitivity and degradation behaviour of specimen is very crucial. Air drying of liquid specimen will follow the thin layer deposition with slow evaporation of solvent in ventilated air on thin support-based of TEM grid, facing adverse effects of solution surface tension [27]. Normally, oven drying of specimen will be performed from ~ 40 to 60 °C range, as per thermal stability of samples. On merits, oven drying is preferred over air drying for fast evaporation of moisture or any other volatile component, without any thermal degradation.

Furthermore, solution-based sample will also be dried under rotatory evaporator [28] or vacuum concentrator [29] techniques, which works on the mechanism of lowering pressure for low temperature evaporation. In continuation, biological specimen will be dried with critical point drying (CPD) or low temperature drying (freeze drying) etc. techniques, in addition to different chemical and physical fixation techniques [30]. Use of conventional dehydration steps like gradient solvent series with acetone or ethanol etc. or dehydration agent like hexamethyl di-silane (HMDS) etc., will also be preferred as per features of specimen. Ideally, dried and processed specimen will be viewed under respective electron microscope with minimum time. Even after use of all specimen drying protocols, if specimen shows charging effects, respective TEM specimen grid will be thin layered coated of carbon under carbon coater for charge dissipation before TEM imaging.

2.4.8 Grid Handling and Transfer

This is more of practical aspect than theoretical which due to mishandling and lack of experience about its delicacy, may damage specimen as well the grid. The use of specialized wax sheet, suitable tweezers, dust free area, preservation box of grid with TEM specimen holder storage etc., are the factors which need special care while performing respective tasks [2].

Under this section, we have summarized about the probable challenges with best possible solutions for quality specimen preparation viz. sample purity, e-beam interaction with specimen, artifacts generation, staining and sample drying, grid handling etc., for novel TEM micrographs. Detail has been depicted in Fig. 2.10.

NOTE: Through study of Challenges and Remedies w.r.t. TEM sample preparation and imaging, develop effective solutions and improve the quality and accuracy of imaging.

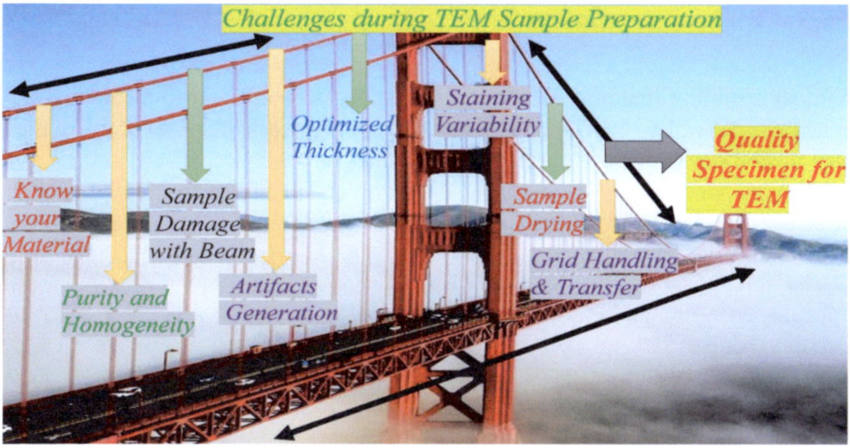

Fig. 2.10 Depicted the probable challenges during TEM sample preparation for quality EM imaging

2.5 Safety Precautions in TEM Sample Preparation

Level of researcher (individual) or a research group in any university or college, will be estimated and predicted on the basis of different safety guidelines, measure, hygiene conditions and chemicals handling and disposal procedures followed during routine working time in laboratory. Detail related to safety aspect of TEM sample preparation has been elaborated as below:

2.5.1 Use of Personal Protective Equipment (PPE)

To perform any research work or experiment, use of lab coat, hand gloves, googles. mask, closed-toe shoes etc., must be strictly used to ensure the safety of individual. Use of PPE kit must be actively used while performing task in laboratory.

2.5.2 Handling of Chemicals and Biological Samples

Accidental incidents like chemical spillage, gas leakage, skin burn or cuts etc., at laboratory workplace, needs prompt safety alarm activation arrangements at respective place. Due to incompatibility of different chemicals with sample preparation procedure, poor ventilation, lacking of biological safety cabinets, fuming hoods, safety shower and eye washer etc., lead to major risk to health and life of persons at work.

2.5.3 Waste Disposal

Without spending lucrative setups in sample preparation or instrumentation area in laboratory, well designed documented and applied waste disposal protocol must be followed in laboratory. Start with segregation of wastes according to their type i.e. chemical or biological based. Any hazardous chemical like fixative (glutaraldehyde, paraformaldehyde, osmium tetroxides etc.), heavy metals (uranyl acetate, lead citrate etc.), epoxy (Araldite, Epon, Spurr. TLV etc.), solvents (ethanol, acetone, amyl acetate, propylene oxide etc.), sharp disposals (blades, syringe etc.) etc., discarding and segregation protocol need to follow as per nature and properties of generated waste.

With the help of above-mentioned safety guidelines while performing any basic to advance research activity in any research laboratory like chemical or biological experiments etc., one can tune respective workplace for well-defined target oriented efficient research activities. It will help in protecting and strengthening environment, maintaining health hygiene with cutting-edge research outcomes.

NOTE: Implementation of safety guidelines will not only protect individual as well specimen from potential hazards but will ensure the integrity of microscopic results.

2.6 Conclusion

Soul of current chapter is in developing a strong foundation and database through electron microscopy techniques for different specimens' type in accurate structural/morphological imaging, high resolution, minimum artifacts and reproducible specimens' analysis. In beginning of current chapter, we have discussed about the different type of samples which can be analysed under TEM, includes biological (human, animal or plant, cells, bacteria, virus, macromolecules etc.), inorganic materials (metal, semiconductor, mineral etc.), soft material (organic, polymers, gel etc.). With prior knowledge to specimen properties like physical, chemical, optical, electrical or thermal etc., one can discover respective novel insights through EM analysis. Water-based structure of biological material's sample preparation for EM analysis is always an area of practice and precision. Further, sample preparation for metal, semiconductor and minerals etc., specimen also need special care and protocol. Furthermore, soft, gel and organic compound based sensitive and delicate materials, also need standardized and validated specimen preparation protocols for informative high-resolution imaging.

We have further summarized about different challenges faced by researchers during TEM sample preparation. We have precisely discussed about the importance and role of material physical and chemical properties, purity of sample, damage of specimen with electron beam, artifacts generation, controlled specimen thickness, optimized staining, different specimen drying conditions and grids handling and respective preparation procedure. Furthermore, we have also highlighted about the role of safety precautions in precise TEM analysis followed by disposal of generated waste during whole process, for maintaining hygiene in respective area. Conclusively, insight knowledge and optimized specimen preparation during TEM analysis, one can produce informative micrographs having '*thousand words explanation*'.

Declaration

Author declares that there is no personal or financial conflict of interest regarding publication of this chapter.

References

1. Bozzola, J.J., Russell, L.D.: Electron Microscopy : Principles and Techniques for Biologists. Jones and Bartlett Publishers, Inc.
2. Ayache, J., Beaunier, L., Boumendil, J., Ehret, G., Laub, D.: Sample Preparation Handbook for Transmission Electron Microscopy. Springer, New York (2010). https://doi.org/10.1007/978-0-387-98182-6
3. Hawkes, P.W., Spence, J.C.H. (Eds.) Springer Handbook of Microscopy. Springer International Publishing, Cham (2019). https://doi.org/10.1007/978-3-030-00069-1
4. Thompson, R.F., Walker, M., Siebert, C.A., Muench, S.P., Ranson, N.A.: An introduction to sample preparation and imaging by cryo-electron microscopy for structural biology. Methods **100**, 3–15 (2016). https://doi.org/10.1016/j.ymeth.2016.02.017
5. Massover, W.H.: New and unconventional approaches for advancing resolution in biological transmission electron microscopy by improving macromolecular specimen preparation and preservation. Micron **42**(2), 141–151 (2011). https://doi.org/10.1016/j.micron.2010.05.006
6. Hendricks, G.M.: Metal shadowing for electron microscopy. In: Kuo, J. (Ed.) Electron Microscopy; Methods in Molecular Biology; Humana Press, Totowa (2014), Vol. 1117, pp. 73–93. https://doi.org/10.1007/978-1-62703-776-1_5
7. Sarraf, C.E.: Immunolabeling for Electron Microscopy. Methods in Molecular Medicine: Diagnostic and Therapeutic: Antibodies 40.
8. Williams, D.B.; Carter, C.B.: Transmission Electron Microscopy. Springer US, Boston (1996). https://doi.org/10.1007/978-1-4757-2519-3
9. Rao, D.V.S., Muraleedharan, K., Humphreys, C.J.: TEM Specimen Preparation Techniques **(2010)**
10. Rai, R.S., Subramanian, S.: Role of transmission electron microscopy in the semiconductor industry for process development and failure analysis. Prog. Cryst. Growth Charact. Mater. **55**(3–4), 63–97 (2009). https://doi.org/10.1016/j.pcrysgrow.2009.09.002
11. Esquivel, E.V., Murr, L.E., Lopez, M.I., Goodell, P.C.: TEM observations of a 30 million year old mountain leather nanofiber mineral composite. Mater Charact **54**(4–5), 458–465 (2005). https://doi.org/10.1016/j.matchar.2005.01.014
12. Lee, M.R.: Transmission electron microscopy (TEM) of earth and planetary materials: a review. Mineral. Mag. **74**(1), 1–27 (2010). https://doi.org/10.1180/minmag.2010.074.1.1
13. Wang, L.M.: Applications of advanced electron microscopy techniques to the studies of radiation effects in ceramic materials. Nucl. Instrum. Methods Phys. Res. B **141** (1998)

14. Franken, L.E., Boekema, E.J., Stuart, M.C.A.: Transmission electron microscopy as a tool for the characterization of soft materials: application and interpretation. Adv. Sci. **4**(5), 1600476 (2017). https://doi.org/10.1002/advs.201600476
15. Egerton, R.F.: Physical principles of electron microscopy: an introduction to TEM, SEM, and AEM. Springer, New York (2005)
16. Slavkova, M., Tzankov, B., Popova, T., Voycheva, C.: Gel formulations for topical treatment of skin cancer: a review. Gels **9**(5), 352 (2023). https://doi.org/10.3390/gels9050352
17. Yu, G., Yan, X., Han, C., Huang, F.: Characterization of supramolecular gels. Chem. Soc. Rev. **42**(16), 6697 (2013). https://doi.org/10.1039/c3cs60080g
18. Mears, L.L.E., Draper, E.R., Castilla, A.M., Su, H., Zhuola, Dietrich, B., Nolan, M.C., Smith, G.N., Doutch, J., Rogers, S., Akhtar, R., Cui, H., Adams, D.J.: Drying affects the fiber network in low molecular weight hydrogels. Biomacromolecules **18**(11), 3531–3540 (2017). https://doi.org/10.1021/acs.biomac.7b00823
19. Glinkowska Mares, A., Feiner-Gracia, N., Muela, Y., Martínez, G., Delgado, L., Albertazzi, L., Pujals, S.: Towards cellular ultrastructural characterization in organ-on-a-chip by transmission electron microscopy. Appl. Nano **2**(4), 289–302 (2021). https://doi.org/10.3390/applnano2040021
20. Diaz, C., Valenzuela, M.L., Laguna-Bercero, M.Á.: Solid-state preparation of metal and metal oxides nanostructures and their application in environmental remediation. IJMS **23**(3), 1093 (2022). https://doi.org/10.3390/ijms23031093
21. Mohd Kaus, N.H., Rithwan, A.F., Adnan, R., Ibrahim, M.L., Thongmee, S., Mohd Yusoff, S.F.: Effective strategies, mechanisms, and photocatalytic efficiency of semiconductor nanomaterials incorporating rGO for environmental contaminant degradation. Catalysts **11**(3), 302 (2021). https://doi.org/10.3390/catal11030302
22. Vry, S., Roumanie, M., Laucournet, R., Bernard-Granger, G.: Transmission electron microscopy investigations on a polysiloxane preceramic polymer pyrolyzed at high temperature in argon. Ceramics **3**(4), 421–427 (2020). https://doi.org/10.3390/ceramics3040035
23. Gopiraman, M.: Gold, silver and nickel nanoparticle anchored cellulose nanofiber composites as highly active catalysts for the rapid and selective reduction of nitrophenols in water. RSC Adv. **8**, 3014 (2018)
24. Egerton, R.F.: Control of radiation damage in the TEM. Ultramicroscopy **127**, 100–108 (2013). https://doi.org/10.1016/j.ultramic.2012.07.006
25. Ayache, J., Beaunier, L., Boumendil, J., Ehret, G., Laub, D.: Artifacts in transmission electron microscopy. In: Sample Preparation Handbook for Transmission Electron Microscopy. Springer, New York (2010), pp. 125–170. https://doi.org/10.1007/978-0-387-98182-6_6
26. Tkachenko, V., Vidal, L., Josien, L., Schmutz, M., Poly, J., Chemtob, A.: Characterizing the core-shell architecture of block copolymer nanoparticles with electron microscopy: a multi-technique approach. Polymers **12**(8), 1656 (2020). https://doi.org/10.3390/polym12081656
27. Michen, B., Geers, C., Vanhecke, D., Endes, C., Rothen-Rutishauser, B., Balog, S., Petri-Fink, A.: Avoiding drying-artifacts in transmission electron microscopy: characterizing the size and colloidal state of nanoparticles. Sci. Rep. **5**(1), 9793 (2015). https://doi.org/10.1038/srep09793
28. Turner, J.N.: Three-dimensional ultrastructure in biology methods in cell biology. Academic Press, New York (1981)
29. Eş, I., Montebugnoli, L.J., Filippi, M.F.P., Malfatti-Gasperini, A.A., Radaic, A., De Jesus, M.B., De La Torre, L.G.: High-throughput conventional and stealth cationic liposome synthesis using a chaotic advection-based microfluidic device combined with a centrifugal vacuum concentrator. Chem. Eng. J. **382**, 122821 (2020). https://doi.org/10.1016/j.cej.2019.122821
30. Caparino, O.A., Tang, J., Nindo, C.I., Sablani, S.S., Powers, J.R., Fellman, J.K.: Effect of drying methods on the physical properties and microstructures of mango (Philippine 'Carabao' Var.) powder. J. Food Eng. **111**(1), 135–148 (2012). https://doi.org/10.1016/j.jfoodeng.2012.01.010

Chapter 3
Techniques for Thin Specimen from Bulk Samples

Thin Specimen is the essential requirement in TEM imaging to minimize the electron scattering and achieve high resolution imaging
by ***M. A. Hayat***

Abstract Ideal TEM imaging of specimen will be attained through precise electron transparent sample preparation. Importance of optimum specimen thickness during TEM imaging will revolve around optimum thickness, maximum contrast, stability and integrity of specimen. Whole approach during quality sample preparation will be guided through physical, chemical and functional properties of material/specimen under EM study. Simple to complex sample pre-thinning and fine thinning processing, will be proceed through specimen disc cutting (~ 3 mm size), electropolishing, ion milling, cross-sectioning, ultramicrotomy, chemical etching, replica, FIB etc., techniques. Optimization of challenges faced during TEM sample preparation will be attained through experience and practice w.r.t. uniform sample thickness, optimum beam exposure, specimen appropriate orientation and specimen size with ultrastructural imaging at lowest possible resolution.

Keywords Ideal Imaging · Optimum thickness · Electropolishing · FIB · Resolution limit

3.1 Introduction

Concept of quality TEM imaging will be realized with optimized thin sectioning through different techniques as per type and nature of specimen. Thickness of specimen in TEM analysis will be directly linked with the transmission of electrons, high resolution information, penetration of electron beam, image contrast having fine details etc. Thick specimen leads to maximum absorption, low penetration and high scattering of incident electrons bring poor resolution, low contrast information. Multicellular and multiple composition-based biological specimens like tissue, cells

R. Singh, *Transmission Electron Microscopy Sample Preparation*,
https://doi.org/10.1007/978-3-031-82967-3_3

etc., required uniform electron transparent specimen thickness. Specifically, biological specimens' thickness must be in ~ 50–100 nm range, to highlights and elaborate the cellular and subcellular structure of respective specimen. For material science specimens, thickness range of specimen will depend on the properties and area of interest of material.

In current chapter, we have elaborated, explained insightly about the novel quality sample preparation ways, troubleshooting w.r.t. existing challenges.

3.2 Importance of Thin Section/Layer

The ultimate approach in exploring material properties through TEM analysis at bulk or nanoscale is facilitated with allowance of transmission of incident electrons through specimen surface. Unless, we are not in the specified thickness range of specimen as per their nature of specimen like organic, metallic or biological, over scattering and burning of specimen will takes place during electron beam exposure. We want to mention that there is no rigid/fix rule on specimen's thickness requirements during TEM imaging and is depend upon the nature, properties and level of desired information from specimen. Ever-known challenge in TEM analysis is specimen homogenous thickness profiling. Wide variety of specimen slicing techniques for electron transparency range are available like ultramicrotomy, cryo-ultramicrotomy, ion milling, FIB, cryo-FIB, chemical thinning, electropolishing, laser ablation etc. All stated techniques will be used for different specimen preparation prior to their stabilization via chemical or physical fixation, dehydration, embedding and infiltration or freeze-drying steps etc. [1]. Figure 3.1, has depicted the importance factors related to thinning of specimen under TEM analysis.

NOTE: Thin Specimens in TEM analysis facilitates precise electron penetration, which is the most essential for capturing fine structural details.

3.3 Requirement w.r.t. Specimen Thin Section/Layer

3.3.1 Do I Know My Specimen

Ideally, TEM analysis of any specimen has to be electron transparent nature, representative of original sample behavior, non-magnetic, uniform surface and stability with electron beam. Detailed information w.r.t. TEM samples and related precautions has been summarized in *Chap. 2* of current book.

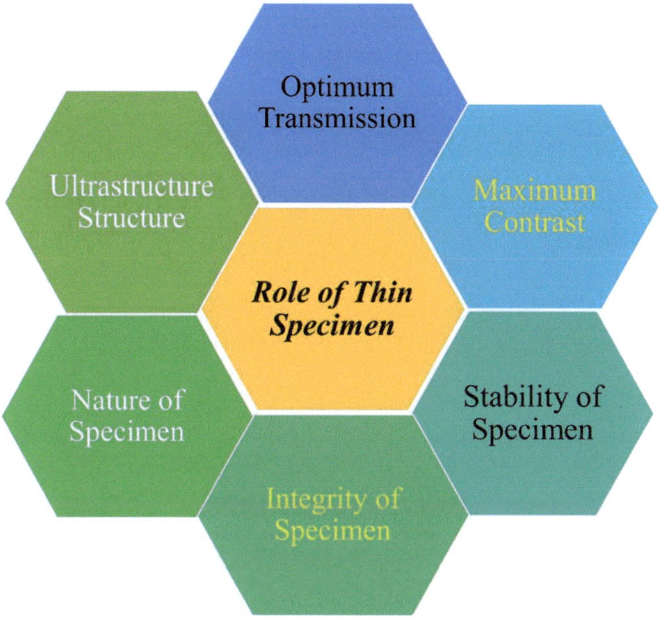

Fig. 3.1 Depicts the importance of thinning of specimen during TEM analysis

3.3.2 Do I Need Support for Specimen

Before loading of specimen for TEM analysis, we have to find out that whether our specimen is self-supporting nature or specimen need support during mounting on TEM grid. Self-supporting specimen must be adherent and stable with electron beam whereas grid of Cu or Au, Ni, etc., will be coated with thin support of carbon coating.

3.3.3 How Much Time Sectioning Will Take

Most of time, common question raised by TEM users, that in how much time to get results. We assume that a quality specimen preparation demand time from hours to days, as per nature of specimen. Normally, we will proceed with optimum drying, grinding, dispersion in appropriate solvent in case of powder samples. Further, suitable thin support-based grid like carbon coated copper grid will be used for drop casting of specimen. Sample like piece of metal or any other hard material, will be proceed with use of diamond saw for 3 mm diameter disk cutting, fine thinning on grinding wheel, dimpling of thin disk and ion milling for electron transparent specimen. Similarly, biological or any soft specimen will follow fixation, dehydration, embedding and infiltration with suitable epoxy, followed by ultramicrotomy and staining steps. Precise parameters related to thin sectioning of specimen can redesigned as per challenges faced during respecting sectioning and mounting on TEM grid.

3.4 Techniques of Thin Sectioning and Possible Trouble Shooting

In coming section, we are going to discuss about the different probable methods with respect to different samples for electron transparency requirement.

3.4.1 Thin Sectioning of Self Supported Bulk Sample

Nature of material for thin sectioning, will direct the selection of appropriate method. Material can be soft, hard, brittle, delicate, singe phase of composite etc.

3.4.2 Metals Thinning

Metal samples due to their ductile nature very much avoided with mechanical damage during their processing for TEM analysis. Initially, thin slices of < 200 μm thickness, will be desired with wafering saw or spark erosion-based setup [2].

3.4.3 Brittle Materials Like Ceramics

Material like ceramics which have brittle properties irrespective to their composition have well-defined cleavage plane. This can be proceeded with razor blade repeated cutting for electron transparency. Similarly, ultramicrotomy will also be utilized for thin slicing of such specimen. Otherwise, if we don't want cleavage-based cutting of specimen, we can proceed with technique like diamond wafering saw technique [2, 3].

3.4.4 Cutting into Disk Shape

Prior thin slicing of any ductile or brittle material, electron transparent thickness will be achieved with step called 'Coring'. If material under process for coring is compatible with mechanical damage, mechanical punch-based technique can be utilized. On the other side, if we want avoid any damage to specimen with process related effects, spark erosion, ultrasonic drilling and grinding drill etc., techniques will be preferred. Compatibility with standard size of TEM grid i.e. 3.05 mm, cutting tools are of hollow tube with internal diameter of ~ 3 mm. Further, the spark erosion coring technique deal for conducting sample with minimum mechanical process-oriented damage. Furthermore, the preference between ultrasonic drilling and grinding drilling process in ceramic or semiconductor specimen preparation depend upon the choice of drilling solvent. Above whole process operates with stress-based operation, mechanical damage to specimen can be minimized with protective layer coating on desired region of material. At later stage protective layer will be etched easily from specimen surface [2, 3].

3.4.5 Pre-thinning of Specimen

Current section deal with thinning of prepared disk (~ 3 mm) of prepared specimen into electron transparent thickness range without any damage to respective surface will be achieved by grinding and polishing of area under study. Thickness range at initial stage of specimen is roughly achieved in range of ~ 10 μm which further optimized to ~ 1 μm via dimpling technique. Further, mechanical polishing will be followed after dimpling. Dimpling process can also be performed with the impingement of chemical like hydrofluoric acid (HF) and nitric acid (HNO_3) in the desired disk area of specimen. Furthermore, the use of tripod polisher, will bring specified thickness area < 1 μm in less time and with precision [2, 3].

3.4.6 Fine Thinning of Disk with Electropolishing

This technique known for fine thinning of conducting metallic or alloys specimen without any mechanical damage. This mode will work at specific voltage which generate controlled current which lead anodic dissolution of specimen prepare smooth surface. The design of technique consists of single jet electrolyte reservoir as well double jet electrolyte-based jet electropolishing technique. Precision of the step will be achieved through manipulation in permutation and combination of electrolyte chemistry, stirring speed, jet incident speed on disk, applied voltage or polishing current combinations [3, 4].

3.4.7 Ion Milling

Ion milling techniques is also utilized in order to achieve the ultimate thin specimen for TEM analysis. Accelerating voltage in range of 4–6 kV, nature of ions (Ar, He or iodine), temperature of specimen (cold or hot milling), setup geometry etc., are the process related factors which need to optimize while preparing respective specimen. High angle incidence of ion beam, will be optimized w.r.t. level of beam penetration depth into specimen surface with minimum surface damage. In comparison to 15–25° incident angle of ion beam during thinning process, $< 5°$ angle will facilitate low ion implantation and lowest physical damage to specimen surface. Efficient cooling setup is the foremost requirement in ion milling setup in order to avoid overheating of specimen. In addition, ion beam temperature of specimen surface may also rise to 200 °C. As per nature and delicacy of specimen, help researchers to design ion milling experiment parameters like accelerating voltage, ion beam nature, geometry setup, cooling rate etc., in achieving flawless specimen surface for TEM analysis [2, 3].

3.4.8 Cross-Section Sectioning

Study of self-supporting specimen interfaces analysis is always challenging during TEM analysis due to similar direction of specimen interfaces with electron beam direction. In order to analyze the structural and chemical variation in specimen, appropriate direction of interfaces must be exposed to electron beam for desired imaging aspects. The monolayer or multilayer interface-based specimen, will be downscale in size size through ultrasonic drill. Epoxy used in fixing of specimen must be cured at controlled temperature and have sufficient compatibility in term of effective adhesion with secondary component. Final thinning of specimen will be performed with ion milling technique [2, 3, 5, 6] for precise sectioning of specimen.

Figure 3.2, shows about the different mechanical ways of TEM specimen preparation [6].

3.5 Specimen on Supported TEM Grid

3.5.1 Crushing and Grinding of Powder Sample

This is one of simplest, oldest and conventional technique in order to prepare bulk or nanomaterials sample for TEM analysis. Before proceeding with sample preparation, specimen must be in appropriately dried and stable form with electron beam. Sufficient amount of suspended material dispersion will be spread on the supported TEM grid. Minute presence of volatile or unstable content from specimen during beam

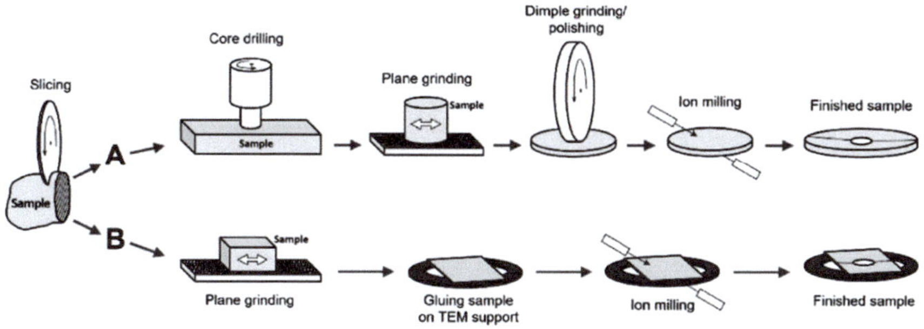

Fig. 3.2 Mechanical ways of TEM specimen preparation (Reprinted with permission from Whitmore et al. [6])

exposure during imaging, may deteriorate the level of TEM vacuum and downgrade the quality of imaging. TEM analyst has to encounter for differentiation between 'true aggregate' and 'formed aggregate' during imaging due to synthesis defects or drying artifacts etc. Further, the stabilization of colloidal suspension, will be improved through optimum addition of appropriate stabilizing agent like bovine serum albumin (BSA) etc., to control the steric hindrance and surface charge etc., parameters of synthesis. Challenge to achieve ideal dispersion of material under TEM analysis have risk of material aggregation to multiple layering during solvents drying and instability of specimen with electron beam exposure [2, 3, 7].

3.5.2 *Ultramicrotomy*

Ultramicrotomy is the composed of two words i.e. 'ultra + microtome' which means technique for very fine thin slicing of specimen. This technique equipped with a diamond or glass knife, used in fine sectioning (like < 100 nm) of specimen. Properly stabilized specimen embedded in suitable epoxy will be thin sliced for light microscopy study having thickness of < 0.1 mm whereas TEM analysis will be proceeded with < 100 nm thickness range. Use of different type of epoxies, embedded nanoparticles, cutting parameters, quality of glass knife, grid handling during lifting of thin slices from water surface to grid surface etc., are the ultramicrotomy related operational factors. All above stated factors need to be standardized and EM analysis approach for will vary from specimen to specimen [3, 7, 8]. Conclusively, according to biological, polymer, nanomaterial or fibrous nature of material for thin slicing, we have to change operational and processing parameters time to time as per requirement of study.

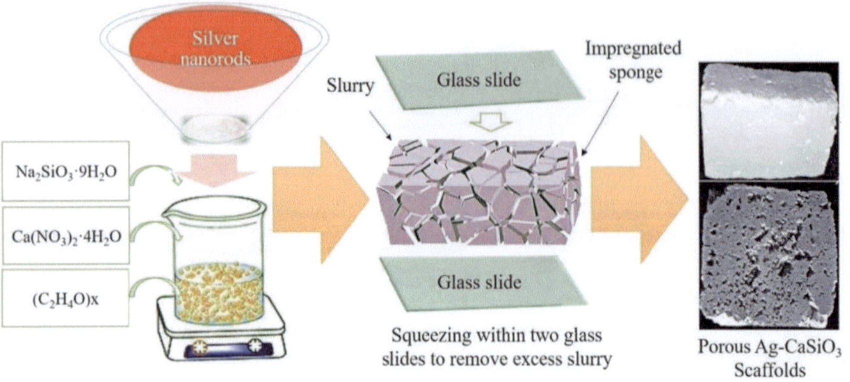

Fig. 3.3 Polymeric replica sponge-based synthesis of Ag–$CaSiO_3$ (Reproduced with permission from Pawan Kumar et al. [11] reference)

3.5.3 Replica Technique

Specimen which cannot be analyzed for surface texture or topography under TEM instrument directly, will be viewed indirectly through replicating the respective surface. Thin layer coating of material like carbon or metal, deposited on material surface need to study. Removal of underlying surface of specimen proceed with etching mechanism, followed by lifting of upper coated surface on TEM grid. Specifically, first step is to fix a polymer layer on specimen surface having good contact with specimen surface. The dissolution the underlying layer with suitable solvent facilitates the floating of respective replicated caron coated surface. Many times, replica of metal surface will be made directly with carbon coating on material surface. Whole procedure is subject to dissolution of metal part in suitable acid or solvent, lead to floating of coated surface on water surface [3, 9, 10].

Figure 3.3 shows the polymeric replica sponge-based synthesis of Ag-$CaSiO_3$ [11] whereas Fig. 3.4a, b shows the graphical overview of different type of replica representation [12].

3.5.4 Cleavage Based Technique

This is one of classical technique for thinning of specimen having weak interlayer interactions. Current method proceeds with fixing of double adhesive tape on both side of specimen bring electron transparent specimen surface through multiple scratches. Removal of glue from the specimen surface trend as a limitation factor in precise electron microscopy (EM) analysis. Cleavage of specimen get modified for precise thinning technique like small angle cleavage technique (SACT) for precise TEM analysis. Basically, cracking of specimen surface will be takes place through a

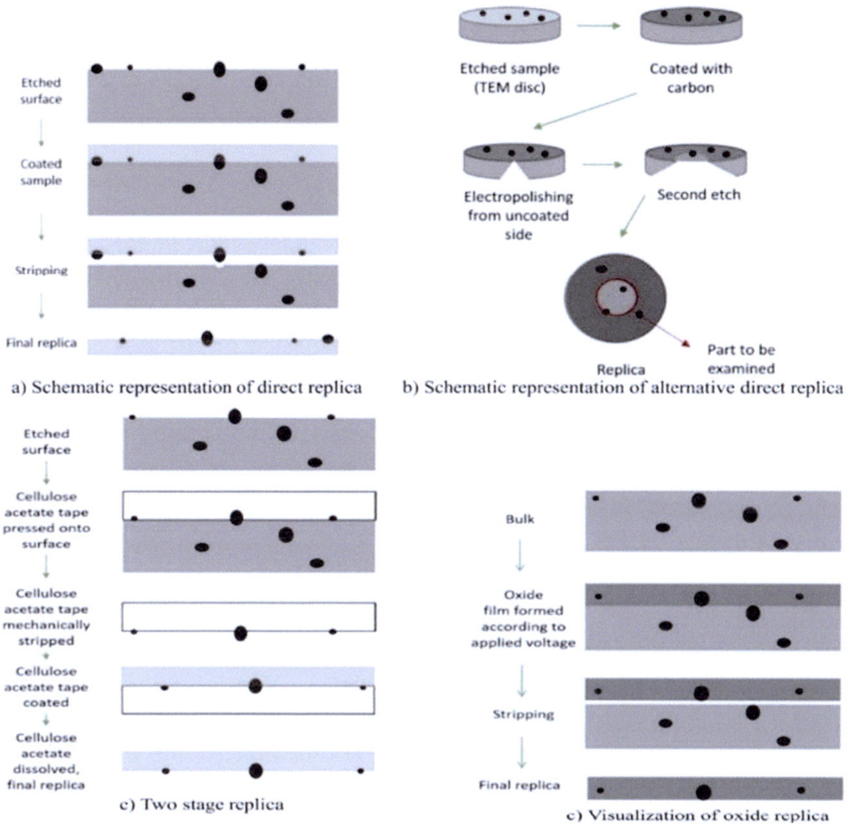

Fig. 3.4 Graphical overview of different replica techniques (Reproduced with permission from Rolinska et al. [12] reference)

plane which is not an actual fracture plane but is shallowly inclined to initial plane. The specimen having crystalline nature (thin layer of crystalline phase on silicon or glass substrate etc.), will be only preferred, due to its non-specific fracture plane behavior [3, 10, 13]. In addition, the electron transparent specimen behavior will be proceeded with technique like ion milling etc., for EM precise analysis.

3.5.5 90° Wedge Technique

This technique is meant for analysis of surfaces grown perpendicular on a parent plane. For example, GaAs will be preferably grown in (001) direction and easily cleaved in its perpendicular direction i.e. (110) and ($1\bar{1}0$) respectively. Mounting of specimen on the edge of the slot-based grid will be positioned with silver epoxy. Specific edge-based positioning of specimen followed by appropriate fine thinning with technique like FIB or ion milling etc. technique, prerequisite minimum tilting or troubleshooting for orientation of specimen during TEM imaging is observed [3, 14].

3.5.6 Lithography Technique

Under advance engineering area, microelectronics industry has high-rate demand of lithography technique in atomic structural imaging w.r.t. circuits failure investigations. With etching of desired region of specimen for TEM analysis, will be further bring in electron transparent range with ion milling or FIB techniques. Due to small area of exposure in specimen thinning process and further TEM confined beam diameter, have restricted the specimen imaging to small frame with limited titling of specimen [3, 15].

3.5.7 Chemical Etching Technique

This technique is work quiet similarly to that of lithography technique. The only difference is that present technique brings limited specimen portion into electron transparent. This technique mainly works with III–V compounds where a particular element presence acts as etch stop indication during surface thinning process. For example, during thinning of GaAs surface $Al_{1-x}Ga_xAs$ acts etch stop whereas boron implantation acts as barrier in case Si thin film thinning. The use of etch stop material during above chemical etching process, material like $Al_{1-x}Ga_xAs$, Si_3N_4 or boron implantation etc., will be used as a commercial support thin layer for other specimen analysis [3, 16].

3.5.8 Focus Ion Beam (FIB) Technique

FIB is one of precise, controlled and versatile technique for electron transparent specimen preparation. This technique known for controlled thickness and minimum damage to specimen structure under processing. FIB technique has inbuilt assembly in SEM having Gallium (Ga) ion gun will be exposed on specimen surface for milling process. Desired range of specimen thickness will be monitored and achieved with in-situ imaging monitoring device. In order to make artifacts free sliced surface, it will be polished at lower intensity of Ga ion exposure. In continuity before loading specimen into TEM machine, it must be cleaned with plasma cleaning. Finally, the electron transparent specimen, will be inserted in TEM machine for high resolution imaging and respective analysis [3, 16, 17].

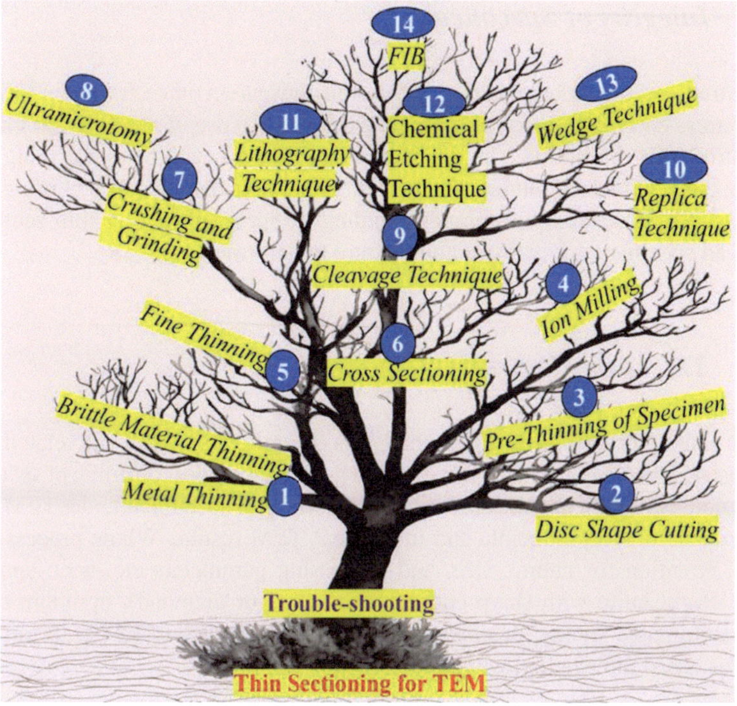

Fig. 3.5 Graphical tree depicting different specimen thinning techniques w.r.t. TEM analysis

From above discussion about different thin sectioning of different specimen for TEM analysis as shown in Fig. 3.5, we came to know about the requirements, experiment setup and working setup etc. Selection of suitable thinning technique will be depended on nature of specimen. The availability of suitable TEM facility with technical expertise on sample thinning and handling will be the most essential requirement in whole process.

3.6 Troubleshooting and Challenges During Thinning Process

As we are keen to learn about the different specimen preparation techniques according to type, properties of sample. More importantly, area of probable mistakes/artifacts induction with lack of expertise etc., bring incomplete and defected specimen preparation for TEM imaging. Here are some important points, which must be take care while performing specimen thinning:

3.6.1 Integrity of Specimen

Whole transforming thick specimen in electron transparent range, it will put specimen under stress and misaligned the original texture due to use of hard solvent like acid etc., during NPs dispersion. The use of technique like disc cutting or polishing or ion milling during precise thinning etc., during TEM specimen preparation bring many mechanical deformations. Improper handling of specimen during thin sectioning step, lead specimen original structure/texture to deformed state [18].

3.6.2 Thickness Control

As this chapter revolves around the thickness control of specimen and related ways, the most desirous requirement is precise and uniform thickness profiling of specimen. Due to non-availability of uniform thickness profiling of specimens under TEM study, will produce non-reproducible and in-efficient TEM results. Whole process needs special attention for nature, size, and processing parameters etc. w.r.t. specimen nature. Right knife with sharp cutting edge (glass or diamond), optimum cutting speed, automated slicing, precise mounting of thin slices on TEM grid, minimum wrinkles based thin slicing, will be ideally desired [19].

3.6.3 Beam Damage the Specimen

In order to get representative images of bulk specimen surface after miniaturization process for specimen, beam over exposure beam stress to specimen. In addition, we need to define the properties of beam as well specimen, so that unwanted beam stress will not be impacted on specimen. Specifically, beam diameter, type of filament source (Tungsten, LaB_6 or Field emission etc.), saturation of filament, beam current, spot size, biasing of filament, exposure time etc. are the properties which must be known and manipulated while performing precise TEM analysis with different modes [20, 21].

3.6.4 Artifacts from Embedding Process

Precise thin sectioning of specimen under slicing technique will be facilitated with appropriate size fixed in suitable embedding medium (epoxy etc.). The selection of embedding medium will depend upon the nature of specimen like biological or material science Due to non-compatibility between sample and support material (epoxy) during block preparation, bring damage to specimen externally as well internally. Furthermore, ineffective infiltration, non-uniform temperature condition with mixing species i.e. epoxies and specimen etc., bring inconsistent results. Specifically, the ratio of hardener and accelerator reagent used in block preparation, will decide the flexibility and strength features of specimen during nano-slicing process [22, 23].

3.6.5 Orientation of Specimen

The anticipated information from TEM specimen will be depend on cutting face of bulk sample in addition to its tilting and rotating options during EM imaging. For example, with random selection of animal or plant tissue specimen under TEM analysis, user is not sure about defined region of interest. Whereas, pre-defined and analyzed sample under suitable techniques like light microscopy, direct imaging analysis in more effective and precise manner. In context to orientation of specimen under TEM analysis, placement of specimen in epoxy for desired face interaction with electron beam, use of appropriate knife, strength of embedding media etc., factors, will affect position of specimen orientation w.r.t. desired specimen face [24].

3.6.6 Resolution Limit

The most talked but least in-sightly understood parameter by most of routine TEM users is term called 'Resolution'. Definition wise, smallest spacing at atomic scale between two atoms of specimen is termed as Resolution. During TEM analysis, lowest resolution of specimen has to optimize with electron transparent requirement of specimen, appropriate accelerating voltage of TEM w.r.t. nature of specimen, uniform specimen surface with minimum artifacts and most obvious experience of person preparing specimen and handling TEM [25].

3.6.7 Sample Size

One of most basic steps in TEM analysis, is specimen size which is to extracted from bulk respective bulk part. The restriction of specimen size limit during TEM analysis, will be depend on nature of sample (metal piece, animal tissue or powder etc.), specimen processing technique (ultramicrotomy, cryo-fixation, lithography, FIB etc.), self-supported or support supported specimen etc., conditions will vary specimen size w.r.t. standard TEM grid size i.e. ~ 3 mm diameter.

3.6.8 *Level of Expertise*

The whole process about which we are talking in current era of automations, TEM or EM imaging and respective analysis, revolves around the individual technical and scientific expertise. Before proceeding any specimen under processing technique or loading sample into TEM machine, user must need to know about essential factors related specimen as well about TEM instrumentation. Like what are precautions, limitation and strengths of specimen and TEM instrument, which need to take-care during respective analysis. Skilled sample processing with smooth TEM operation and precise interpretation of results, will save time having minimum damage to specimen [26, 27]. Figure 3.6, has demonstrated pictorially above discussed different challenges faced during thin specimen preparation TEM analysis.

Conclusively, idea to discuss appropriate sample size, processing, imaging and respective interpretation, is to make TEM user aware about unknown and known factors related to TEM imaging.

NOTE: Effective troubleshooting is essential in TEM thin sample preparation to overcome the challenges like thickness variation, artifacts etc.

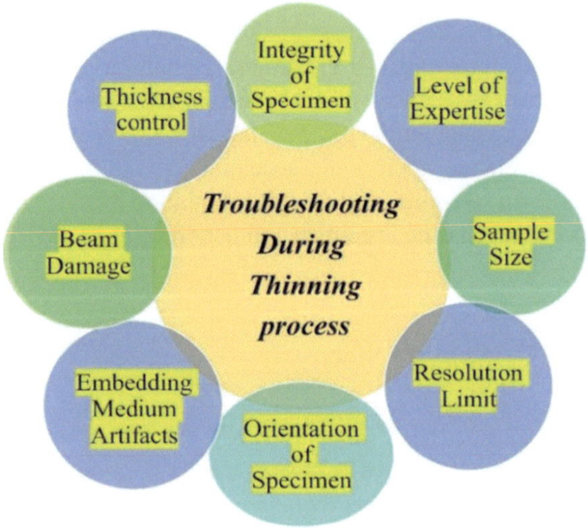

Fig. 3.6 Pictorial representation highlighting troubleshooting during specimen thinning process

3.7 Conclusion

In current chapter, we have described the complete detail about the thin specimen preparation of different categories of samples in a precise and conclusive manner. In addition to precise thinning of specimen, we have tried to familiarized readers about the role of specimen thinning in TEM imaging. Importance of specimen thinning will vary and need to redefined from sample to sample. Unless the specimen is prepared with inadequate pre and post EM related procedure, respective optimal results cannot be expected and obtained.

TEM technique will analyze the sample which is exposed to electron beam, irrespective to optimum sample preparation. There is always a major and minor changes has been desired and required in specimen preparation as per nature of specimen viz. metal to organic, biological to non-living etc. On one side, presence of water needs specialized care during its removal like dehydration procedure whereas hard material like metal piece etc., needs dominant thinning technique like FIB, electro-thinning etc. In both cases, major concern and focus is to bring specimen of precise thickness (~ 50–100 nm) from bulk state, will show representative area of specimen with minimum artifacts. Integrity of specimen after different processing steps, will be the main area of concern during different thinning procedure.

Conclusively, we have summarized about the different thin slicing techniques w.r.t. TEM analysis with their technical details, challenges and best possible troubleshooting. Main concern of current chapter is to equip every reader of this book aware and learned about do's and don't relate to EM sample processing with maximum insightful information from EM imaging process.

Declaration

Author declares that there is no personal or financial conflict of interest regarding publication of this chapter.

References

1. Madsen, L.D., Weaver, L., Jacobsen, S.N.: Influence of material properties on TEM specimen preparation of thin films. Microsc. Res. Tech. **36**(5), 354–361 (1997). https://doi.org/10.1002/(SICI)1097-0029(19970301)36:5%3c354::AID-JEMT2%3e3.0.CO;2-L
2. Rao, D.V.S., Muraleedharan, K., Humphreys, C.J.: TEM Specimen Preparation Techniques (2010)
3. Williams, D.B., Carter, C.B.: Transmission Electron Microscopy. Springer US, Boston (1996). https://doi.org/10.1007/978-1-4757-2519-3
4. Ma, L.: Comparison of different sample preparation techniques in TEM observation of microstructure of INCONEL Alloy 783 subjected to prolonged isothermal exposure. Micron **35**(4), 273–279 (2004). https://doi.org/10.1016/j.micron.2003.10.048
5. Bravman, J.C., Sinclair, R.: The preparation of cross-section specimens for transmission electron microscopy. J. Elec. Microsc. Tech. **1**(1), 53–61 (1984). https://doi.org/10.1002/jemt.1060010106

6. Whitmore, L.: A precision manual grinding tool for sample preparation. Ultramicroscopy **233**, 113436 (2022). https://doi.org/10.1016/j.ultramic.2021.113436
7. Dittmayer, C., Goebel, H.-H., Heppner, F.L., Stenzel, W., Bachmann, S.: Preparation of samples for large-scale automated electron microscopy of tissue and cell ultrastructure. Microsc. Microanal. **27**(4), 815–827 (2021). https://doi.org/10.1017/S1431927621011958
8. Zhang, H., Wang, C., Zhou, G.: Ultra-microtome for the preparation of TEM specimens from battery cathodes. Microsc. Microanal. **26**(5), 867–877 (2020). https://doi.org/10.1017/S1431927620024368
9. Rostamabadi, H., Falsafi, S.R., Jafari, S.M.: Transmission electron microscopy (TEM) of nanoencapsulated food ingredients. In: Characterization of Nanoencapsulated Food Ingredients. Elsevier (2020), pp. 53–82. https://doi.org/10.1016/B978-0-12-815667-4.00002-X
10. Kim, M.S., Kim, H.G.: Preparation and observation of an artifact-free Ge2Sb2Te5 TEM specimen by the small angle cleavage technique. Mater Charact **56**(3), 245–249 (2006). https://doi.org/10.1016/j.matchar.2005.11.020
11. Kumar, P., Dehiya, B.S., Sindhu, A., Kumar, R., Pruncu, C.I., Yadav, A.: Fabrication and characterization of silver nanorods incorporated calcium silicate scaffold using polymeric sponge replica technique. Mater. Des. **195**, 109026 (2020). https://doi.org/10.1016/j.matdes.2020.109026
12. Rolinska, M., Gustavsson, F., Hedström, P.: Revisiting the applications of the extraction replica sample preparation technique for analysis of precipitates in engineering alloys. Mater Charact **189**, 111978 (2022). https://doi.org/10.1016/j.matchar.2022.111978
13. McCaffrey, J.P.: Application of the small-angle cleavage technique to thickness measurement of TEM samples. Microsc. Res. Tech. **36**(5), 372–377 (1997). https://doi.org/10.1002/(SICI)1097-0029(19970301)36:5%3c372::AID-JEMT5%3e3.0.CO;2-N
14. Li, H., Salamanca-Riba, L.: The concept of high angle wedge polishing and thickness monitoring in TEM sample preparation. Ultramicroscopy **88**(3), 171–178 (2001). https://doi.org/10.1016/S0304-3991(01)00079-1
15. Sun, M., Tian, J., Chen, Q.: The studies on wet chemical etching via in situ liquid cell TEM. Ultramicroscopy **231**, 113271 (2021). https://doi.org/10.1016/j.ultramic.2021.113271
16. Wirth, R.: Focused ion beam (FIB) combined with SEM and TEM: advanced analytical tools for studies of chemical composition, microstructure and crystal structure in geomaterials on a nanometre scale. Chem. Geol. **261**(3–4), 217–229 (2009). https://doi.org/10.1016/j.chemgeo.2008.05.019
17. Stevie, F.A., Vartuli, C.B., Giannuzzi, L.A., Shofner, T.L., Brown, S.R., Rossie, B., Hillion, F., Mills, R.H., Antonell, M., Irwin, R.B., Purcell, B.M.: Application of focused ion beam lift-out specimen preparation to TEM, SEM, STEM, AES and SIMS analysis. Surf. Interface Anal. **31**(5), 345–351 (2001). https://doi.org/10.1002/sia.1063
18. Zhao, B., You, H., Miao, Q., Ding, W., Qian, N., Xu, J.: Surface integrity characterization of third-generation nickel-based single crystal blade tenons after ultrasonic vibration-assisted grinding. Chin. J. Aeronaut. S1000936124002656 (2024). https://doi.org/10.1016/j.cja.2024.07.010
19. Kang, S., Wang, D., Kübel, C., Mu, X.: Importance of TEM sample thickness for measuring strain fields. Ultramicroscopy **255**, 113844 (2024). https://doi.org/10.1016/j.ultramic.2023.113844
20. Egerton, R.F.: Mechanisms of radiation damage in beam-sensitive specimens, for TEM accelerating voltages between 10 and 300 kV. Microsc. Res. Techniq. **75**(11), 1550–1556 (2012). https://doi.org/10.1002/jemt.22099
21. Egerton, R.F., Li, P., Malac, M.: Radiation damage in the TEM and SEM. Micron **35**(6), 399–409 (2004). https://doi.org/10.1016/j.micron.2004.02.003
22. Carlemalm, E., Garavito, R.M., Villiger, W.: Resin development for electron microscopy and an analysis of embedding at low temperature*. J. Microsc. **126**(2), 123–143 (1982). https://doi.org/10.1111/j.1365-2818.1982.tb00362.x
23. Turner, E.M., Sapkota, K.R., Hatem, C., Lu, P., Wang, G.T., Jones, K.S.: Wet-chemical etching of FIB lift-out TEM lamellae for damage-free analysis of 3-D nanostructures. Ultramicroscopy **216**, 113049 (2020). https://doi.org/10.1016/j.ultramic.2020.113049

24. Viladot, D., Véron, M., Gemmi, M., Peiró, F., Portillo, J., Estradé, S., Mendoza, J., Llorca-Isern, N., Nicolopoulos, S.: Orientation and phase mapping in the transmission electron microscope using precession-assisted diffraction spot recognition: state-of-the-art results. J. Microsc. **252**(1), 23–34 (2013). https://doi.org/10.1111/jmi.12065
25. Egerton, R.F., Watanabe, M.: Spatial resolution in transmission electron microscopy. Micron **160**, 103304 (2022). https://doi.org/10.1016/j.micron.2022.103304
26. Chu, T., Zhou, L., Zhang, B., Xuan, F.-Z.: Accurate atomic scanning transmission electron microscopy analysis enabled by deep learning. Nano Res. **17**(4), 2971–2980 (2024). https://doi.org/10.1007/s12274-023-6104-1
27. Schubert, P.J., Saxena, R., Kornfeld, J.: DeepFocus: fast focus and astigmatism correction for electron microscopy. Nat. Commun. **15**(1), 948 (2024). https://doi.org/10.1038/s41467-024-45042-3

Chapter 4
TEM Sample Preparation for Powder and Liquid Formulations

The whole of science is nothing more than a refinement of everyday thinking
by ***Albert Einstein***

Abstract Analysis of every sample under TEM analysis require specific sample preparation protocol as per respective material properties. In current chapter, dedicatedly an attempt has been made w.r.t. TEM analysis of specimen belong to powder as well of liquid formulations. Systematic classification has been made for powder and liquid formulations/samples w.r.t. TEM and HRTEM instrument role in respective analysis. In order to achieve precise TEM analysis w.r.t. powder and liquid based samples, controlled synthesis conditions, insitu monitoring, uniform particle distribution with versatile and sustainable approach etc., will be immensely desired. In case of liquid formulation, properties of solvent like purity, density, dielectric constant, volatile nature, respective disposal etc., will be very much crucial and important in respective analysis. Recent chapter have also summarized about the role of ultrasonication, centrifugation, stabilizing agent, TEM grid drying validation etc. With the help of above-mentioned processes, different factor related to ideal imaging of specimen viz. suitable sample and grid selection, precise beam alignment with low dose imaging, balanced image contrast, tilt series acquisition etc., will be helpful in performing insightful imaging analysis. Further, the remediation-oriented approach towards different challenges during different modes on imaging with appropriate image processing also has been presented. Ultimately, the whole approach under current chapter will be focused in maintaining the integrity of sample with artefacts free surfaces for high quality ultrastructural imaging of liquid as well powder samples.

Keywords Liquid formulation · Solvent · Dispersion · Ultrasonication · High resolution TEM (HRTEM)

R. Singh, *Transmission Electron Microscopy Sample Preparation*,
https://doi.org/10.1007/978-3-031-82967-3_4

4.1 Introduction

The visualization, characterization and manipulation of material at nanoscale under nanotechnology arena, TEM technique will play a very decisive and innovative role. In addition to TEM basic analysis, high-resolution capabilities allow in revealing the shape and size etc., investigation at atomic-scale of different material-based nanomaterials for their insightful nanostructure analysis. Further, TEM facilitates with insightful information about crystal and lattice structure, defects and composition analysis by selected area electron diffraction (SAED), energy-dispersive-X-ray spectroscopy (EDS) or electron energy loss spectroscopy (EELS) etc. The quantitative analysis of material will update about the chemical composition and elemental distribution aspect, in addition to routine quality assessment. Further, with the help of TEM technique, visualization of physical or chemical interaction, aggregation, adsorption and surface modifications etc., phenomenon of NPs interaction with respective surfaces, interface become possible. Above stated explanations and mechanism can be applied in novel drug delivery, catalysis or any physical, chemical or life sciences applications of academic or industrial sector. In addition, TEM will also play crucial role in investigation of mechanical, electrical, optical and magnetic etc., properties of nanomaterials. Stated properties will be utilized in development of devices related to nano-mechanics, plasmonic, and magnetic properties-based requirements. With the help of in-situ and real time TEM imaging techniques, will be very helpful in guiding the nanofabrication systems in driving research arena towards innovated nanotechnology realm.

Ultimately, TEM can monitor actual and active role of catalyst through its quality capabilities, fundamentals understanding. The technological innovation and upgradation in electron microscopy instrumentation as well in application related process, can explore wide range of properties and application in scientific and industrial domains.

4.2 Nanomaterial (NM)

Any material which has at least one dimension in nanometer scale termed '*nanomaterial*'. Due to nanoscale dimension of material bring super activity due to high surface to area ratio, bring them most demanding in different sectors as per their specialization [1, 2]. The categorization among existing nanomaterials category is difficult as materials mostly similar features to each other with some differences. To make previse understanding material classification, we have tried to elaborate broadly nanomaterials into 'nanoparticles', 'nanostructures and 'nanocomposite' categories, which are explained as below.

4.2.1 Meaning of Nanoparticle (NP)

Nanoparticle are tiny particles of matter having at least one dimension in nanoscale, typically between 1 and 100 nm (nm). NPs are composed of various materials, including metals, semiconductors, polymers, ceramics or composite materials etc. NPs have unique and different properties than bulk counterpart due to high surface area to volume ratio and quantum effects bring their enhanced activity w.r.t. surroundings. NPs can be synthesized with different synthesis approaches and will exist in different forms like semiconductor, metals, ash, smoke, drug, polymer etc. This category will also include material like nanoclusters, nano-colloids, nanocrystal etc. category [1, 2].

In today's context NPs based formulations are present in our daily use items like toothpaste, medicine, soap, food, smartphone, cosmetics products etc., which broadly comes under nanotechnology, electronics, catalysis, or environment science etc., sectors.

4.2.2 Meaning of Nanostructures

The category of material having surface or internal structure is in nanoscale range. The atomic arrangements during growth of respective material bring their shape into nanowires, nanotubes, nanosheets, nanorods, nanoflowers etc. structures. The study of nanostructured materials gets importance due to their highly active electrical, optical, magnetic, mechanical or thermal features. Due to their high strength, flexible features and minimum concentration factors, bring them most demanding in food to medicine, textile to fashion or daily usage items to nanotechnology sectors very vigorously [1, 2].

4.2.3 Meaning of Nanocomposites

This the category of nanomaterial under which two or more different phases mixed together with at least one phase having nanoscale dimension. Current category of material exhibits mixture of nanoparticles or nanostructures with materials like polymer, ceramic or metals etc. Optimized synthesis between respective components brings construction of novel and efficient interfaces via strong bonding between active reacting species. Efficient nanocomposite brings improved strength, stiffness, toughness, durability, conductivity, flexibility etc. properties in comparison to material having inactive interface. There will be high demand in industrial manufacturing sectors for development of equipment or devices as per requirements, nanocomposite nanomaterial will play very important role [2].

4.3 Importance of Nanomaterial Analysis with TEM/ HRTEM

Nanomaterial analysis with TEM or HRTEM technique, has opens the doors towards new nanomaterial or device development w.r.t. different application [3]. In coming paragraph, an attempt has been made to summarize the importance of nanomaterials analysis.

4.3.1 Characterization of Size and Shape

The size dependent activity of any material, will be guided with the precise knowledge of respective material dimensions. The performance of any material during application, can perform very efficiently prior to characterization and analysis of material w.r.t. shape, size and elemental distribution aspect. With the help of abovementioned parameters, it will be very useful in optimization of synthesis conditions, reaction setup, operational parameters, and efficient application [2].

4.3.2 Visualization of Material's Structure at Nanoscale

TEM and HRTEM will helps in clear and close visualization of material's atomic structures. In addition to evaluation of material properties like shape and size, material crystal structure, defects, grain boundaries, surface properties and interfaces etc., will be in-sightly analysed for novel explanations. With the visual proof of structural properties in form of TEM or SEM images, respective material stability and failure mechanism, mechanical, optical, electrical and thermal etc., properties can be explained. Understanding and role of above stated properties in material growth and activity, will be utilized efficiently in device fabrication at large scale [2].

4.3.3 Advancement in Nanotechnology and Material Development

Fast growing nanotechnology and material development manifestation, will only be understood and functionalized through sophisticated instrumentation technologies. TEM is dominant tool in testing and analysis of materials with growing technologies for their enhanced performances, functionality and sustainability aspect. Research and development conducted with the help of TEM techniques for different nanomaterial analysis, will contributes in respective major breakthrough in area viz. nanoelectronics, nanomedicine, renewable energy or environmental remediation research.

This approach will widely cater for solution of global challenges for ultimately improving the quality of life [2].

The objective of explaining importance of nanomaterials analysis under TEM/HRTEM is to make readers of book aware about answer of question like: *Why we want to study our material under TEM/HRTEM* or *how the analysis of material under TEM/HRTEM takes place.*

NOTE: TEM technique will not only be used in observing the materials but it will be helpful in exploring insightful aspects of materials essential for innovation and development.

4.4 Basics of TEM and HRTEM

4.4.1 About TEM

TEM is the technique which utilizes the transmitted electrons through specimen for analysing shape and size of respective material. This is also known for high contrast imaging as differential contrast generated with specimen due to variable thickness and density profile of specimen. Under diffraction mode, TEM will utilize the scattered electron which give information about the crystal structure and specimen orientation. Normally, TEM will give black and white two-dimension (2D) images, which with the help of three-dimension (3D) tomography attachment can be converted into 3D representation. TEM will be widely used in scientific fields such as material science, life science, environment science and nanotechnology science for investigating the morphology, contrast elaboration, and composition analysis. Figure 4.1, has demonstrated the schematic and actual picture of 120 kV TEM at department of CIL/SAIF, Panjab University Chandigarh, India.

4.4.2 About HRTEM

High Resolution TEM simply means analysis of material at atomic scale, obviously have very fine resolution i.e. of atomic size. Advanced electron optics with minimum aberration based electromagnetic lenses, will differentiate HRTEM from TEM. HRTEM atomic scale resolution capabilities will differentiate it from conventional TEM. Detection ability of phase change of transmitted electron in HRTEM, will make it a capable tool in analysing and explaining about crystal structure, diffraction imaging, defects and various interfaces for different materials. Figure 4.2a, has

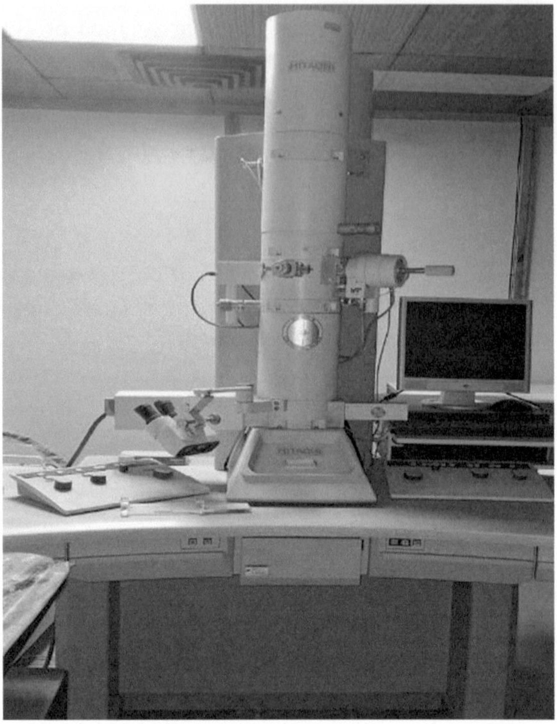

Fig. 4.1 Picture of TEM 120 kV (Hitachi H7500) installed at Department of CIL/SAIF, Panjab University, Chandigarh (TEM image represented with courtesy of TEM Lab, CIL/SAIF, Panjab University, Chandigarh)

depicted the visualization of HRTEM 200 kV LaB_6 at department of CIL/SAIF, Panjab University, Chandigarh, whereas Fig. 4.2b shows the schematic representation of different sections detail in HRTEM.

Majorly, TEM will information about the shape and size with contrast differentiation in contrast to HRTEM credits with atomic scale imaging of same specimen having high resolution structural imaging with transmitted electron.

4.4.3 Importance of HRTEM Over TEM

There is no question of TEM inferiority or HRTEM superiority or vice versa even, both EM instrumentation have their own importance during sample analysis as per their capabilities. Researchers who are interested only in assessment of shape and size information or want to scrutinize specimen for high end EM analysis, normally analyse specimen under TEM. In addition, any experienced microscopist-material scientist/researcher, will not prefer for HRTEM analysis directly. With the prior analysis of material under normal TEM (120 kV accelerating voltage), as per qualitative and quantitative study of specimen, will direct for further analysis plan. Many times,

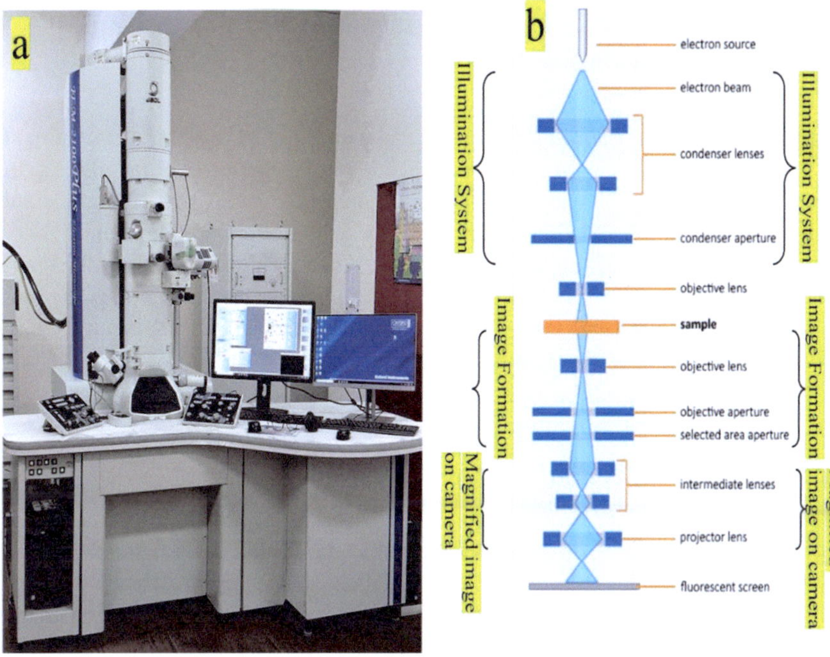

Fig. 4.2 **a** Picture of HRTEM 200 kV (JEOL 2100 PLUS) installed at Department of CIL/SAIF, Panjab University, Chandigarh, **b** Schematic diagram of TEM working and principle (HRTEM image represented with courtesy of HRTEM Lab, CIL/SAIF, Panjab University, Chandigarh)

on the basis of TEM results, user need to re-design their synthesis setup or conditions or even experiment also, to get desired results.

In addition to morphological information of specimen under HRTEM, high resolution mode will visualize the atomic arrangements, lattice fringes and defects aspect of respective specimen. On other contrast, TEM cannot underestimate w.r.t. capabilities, as it is known for high contrast imaging which is ideally essential in imaging of biological or low-density specimen like polymer, emulsions etc. Specifically, with prior study of material under TEM, respective identification of structural purity and evaluation of defects level in specimen will be predicted and investigated by HRTEM (200 kV or 300 kV instrumentation) technique. Both TEM and HRTEM techniques, have their own credibility of scientific information/data as per their capabilities, which can be utilized and interpreted as per different research objectives.

4.5 Factors Affecting Quality Analysis of Powder or Liquid Based Formulation

When we report any extraordinary or poor results under TEM or HRTEM instrument, it is not solely ruled by electron microscope, but there is the series of factors responsible. The factors responsible in revealing research objective, start from grade and purity of used reagents and chemicals, synthesis setup, preservation and purification of final product, ideal dispersion condition like nature of solvent, ultrasonication, TEM grid drying conditions or ideal imaging parameters etc. In coming paragraph, we have tried best to explain every step very minutely and carefully to ensure quality performance of TEM or HRTEM imaging.

4.5.1 Synthesis Method

"How good the recipe of food has been made in the kitchen with help of different ingredients, will decide the taste and flavour of dish". On same line, when we want to analyse any material specimen under TEM/HRTEM, it must be prepared, guided and optimized by appropriate synthesis method and related operational parameters. Ultimately, with efficient synthesis conditions, the shape, size, crystal structure, defects etc. information will be in-sightly determined. Level of controlled and precise reaction conditions/environment like temperature, pressure, dispersion, ultrasonication etc. conditions with compatibility of reacting species with each other, will propagate towards uniform nanomaterial synthesis. Nanomaterial synthesis method like precipitation method, emulsion, sol–gel, hydrothermal or chemical vapor deposition etc., credits with specialized efficient operational properties w.r.t. different synthesis conditions of nanomaterials [4, 5]. Following conditions will be desired from any synthesis method w.r.t. TEM/HRTEM analysis.

4.5.2 Controlled and Homogenous Particle Size Synthesis

It is desirous from any synthesis method to produce controlled shape and size NPs having homogenous size distribution. The uniformity of specimen's smallest entities i.e. particle size and shape, will enhance the optical, catalytic, thermal, electrical or mechanical etc., properties based application mechanism [4, 5]

4.5.3 High Purity Specimen

The most obvious expectation from any synthesis method is to produce high purity, impurity and debris free yield. Nature of sample crystallinity or amorphous nature, will enhance or downgrade the stability, reactivity, sensitivity etc., features during various applications with respective material. Purified form of specimen will be very much helpful during TEM/HRTEM imaging, due to presence of minimum foreign contamination and interference [4, 5].

4.5.4 Sustainable Conditions

Sustainable conditions of any material synthesis will include its eco-friendly aspects, use of green resources, use of non-toxic precursors etc., which bring minimum hazard to environment, human as well to electron microscope during their analysis [3, 5].

4.5.5 Versatility and Adaptability

Any synthesis method must have adaptive perspective for use of variable material system and fabrication techniques. The features of adaptability and versatility nature of synthesis method will make it efficient during application in real conditions [4, 5].

4.5.6 In-Situ Characterization and Monitoring

The inbuilt ability of material to grow and generate themselves of millions of times, face as a challenge to ensure their controlled growth with homogeneity issue. Real time and in-situ capabilities monitoring of material growth analysis, will be help amazingly to control respective material growth and unexplored mechanism insights. Techniques such as in-situ EM setup, diffraction mode, correlative light electron microscopy (CLEM) etc., will provide idea about growth kinetics, phase transformation etc., which ultimately become helpful in designing the final product novel properties as per desired application [4, 5].

Figure 4.3, has depicted the role of synthesis method in quality material TEM/HRTEM analysis.

With the help of appropriate synthesis method for material growth as per requirement of applications, will become a dominating factor towards fabrication of novel material for efficient devices.

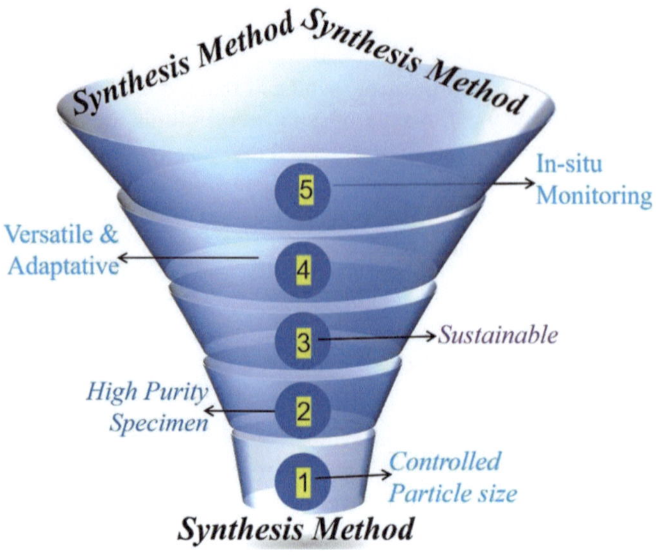

Fig. 4.3 Pictorial representation of showing role of material synthesis method in TEM analysis

4.5.7 Role of Dispersion Solvent

As current section deals with ideal characterization of any powder or liquid based formulation under TEM/HRTEM technique, respective material stable and homogeneous dispersion is very much desirous. In addition to stable and uniform dispersion of material in solution form, maximum transferring of dispersed component onto TEM grid is also an area of optimization and a challenge. Due to variable compatibility of the nanoparticles with different solvents as well with support surface of TEM grid, will affect variable dispersibility, extent of aggregation and interaction behavior with grid surface. Due to polar nature of solvents like water and ethanol, will be preferred in dispersion of hydrophilic materials whereas non-polar solvents like hexane, toluene will be preferred in dispersion of hydrophobic material [6, 7]. In coming paragraph, few factors have been disclosed related to dispersion of material w.r.t. TEM/HRTEM analysis.

4.5.7.1 Purity of Solvent

The solvent used in dispersion of material must be of having minimum background signal generation and interference ability for TEM/HRTEM and EDS analysis. Low level of impurities in solvent, reduces the risk of contamination and artifacts generation during solvent drying, minimum hindrance of image background due to grid support surface during imaging etc., during acquisition of electron microscope (EM) imaging [5–7].

4.5.7.2 Low Electron Density Solvents

Solvent used in dispersion of material under TEM/HRTEM study must have feature of minimum electron absorption and background scattering. The excess of stated features during EM analysis, will degrade the contrast as well the high-resolution aspect of imaging of specimen. Low density solvent like ethanol, water etc. will be preferred in comparison to high density solvent like heavy metal stain etc. More importantly, low density requirement of solvent, compatibility, toxicity, safety, residue content etc. factor must be considered while choosing respective solvent for dispersion of specimen [5–7].

4.5.7.3 Non-reactive w.r.t. Specimen

Solvent preferred for dispersion of specimen under TEM/HRTEM analysis, must be non-reactive with material to avoid any chemical reaction or any other alteration. The over-reactivity of solvent with material under EM analysis, may bring alteration in morphology, composition or structure. Ultimately, solvent must be of such physical and chemical behavior, that it will protect and maintain the integrity of specimen during dispersion and analysis of sample under EM analysis [5–7].

4.5.7.4 High Dielectric Constant

Solvent with high dielectric constant behavior have ability to disperse material or any charged material with electrostatic stabilization mechanism. Minimum aggregation and maximum dispersion features have been observed with use of high dielectric solvents like water, dimethyl sulfoxide (DMSO), ethanol, acetonitrile etc. [5–7]. Although, EM analysis w.r.t. stated solvent with material under study, need to standardize and validate to get reproducible and repeatable results.

4.5.7.5 Volatile

Ideally, solvent used in TEM specimen drop casting in grid, high volatility nature like chloroform solvent, must be preferred irrespective to its toxicity, reactivity and safety features. Due to rapid drying approach of solvent used in material dispersion, minimum artifacts and quality specimen preparation will be obtained for TEM/HRTEM analysis [5–7].

4.5.7.6 Solvent Inertness w.r.t. TEM Grid and Support Film

Any solvent of polar or non-polar properties, its non-reactive behavior with TEM grid (copper, nickel, molybdenum or gold etc.) and support film (carbon, collodion, formvar etc.) is desired during TEM/HRTEM analysis. The reactivity of solvent with grid may bring generation of secondary phase on grid surface which may deteriorate the basic transmission of electron. Additionally, non-compatibility between TEM grid support surface and solvent used in dispersion step, bring damage of support surface, or thick layer deposition during grid drying. Intactness of TEM grid support surface and optimum solvent deposition (layer must be electron transparent) will bring quality high resolution imaging, high contrast and compositional analysis [5–7].

4.5.7.7 Handling and Disposal

The solvent used in dispersion of material for TEM analysis, properties such as flammability, storage and disposal etc. must be taken care. The utmost concern of any laboratory work will start and close with follow of certain guidelines, which will maintain the health hygiene, safety and obviously at the end the quality work performance [5–7].

All above stated factors related to importance of solvent in material dispersion and other related factors has been depicted in Fig. 4.4.

Conclusively, current section has explained about the role of solvent utilized in ideal dispersion of material for TEM analysis, its non-reactivity, compatibility, low density, volatile etc. features, which will play a very crucial role in achieving proposed research goals.

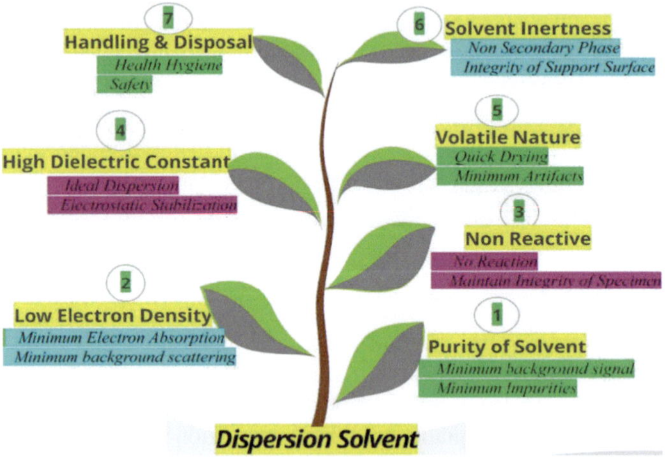

Fig. 4.4 The factors related to solvent used in dispersion of material for TEM analysis

4.5.8 *Role of Ultrasonication*

Ideal imaging through TEM/HRTEM technique of any material under study, will be only achieved with standardization and validation of different operational parameters related to respective precise sample preparation protocol. On same line, uniform dispersion of powder or liquid sample, will be achieved through use of optimum frequency (ultrasound) agitation energy (~ 20 Hz to 40 kHz) for material in most appropriate liquid medium [5–7]. In coming paragraph, factors related to ideal dispersion of material have been summarized w.r.t. perfect EM imaging analysis.

4.5.8.1 Breaking of Agglomerates and Aggregates

Due to multiple compositional variations in different synthesis processes, Vander-Waal and electrostatic forces etc., get activated, lead to un-desired agglomeration and aggregation behavior of materials entities under interest like particles or sheets or rods etc., at nanoscale. According to strength and stability of material (polymer, metal or non-metal etc.) under study, confined ultrasonication energy, will disrupt the probable aggregates and agglomerates. Fundamentally, formation and collapse of cavitation bubble has been proceeded around the agglomerates/aggregate, via mechanical energy felicitation of ultrasound energy input, bring dispersion of targeted entities [5–7]. Figure 4.5a–f, have clearly shows differentiation between aggregated and non-aggregated as prepared flame spray pyrolysis (FSP)-TiO_2 and sintered at different temperature (400, 600, 800 °C) particles under suitable processing techniques [8].

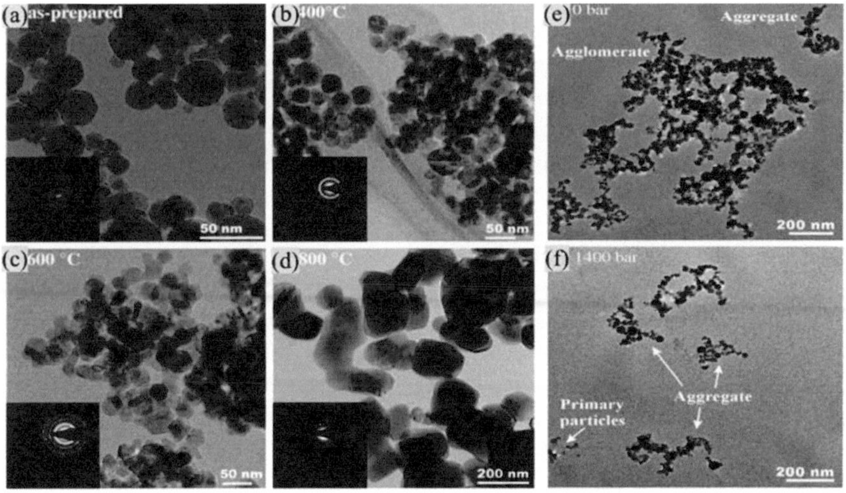

Fig. 4.5 **a** As prepared through flame spray pyrolysis (FSP)-TiO_2, sintered at **b** 400 °C, **c** 600 °C, **d** 800 °C, **e** as prepared nanoparticles, **f** dispersion at 1400 bar (Reprinted with permission from Teleki et al. [8])

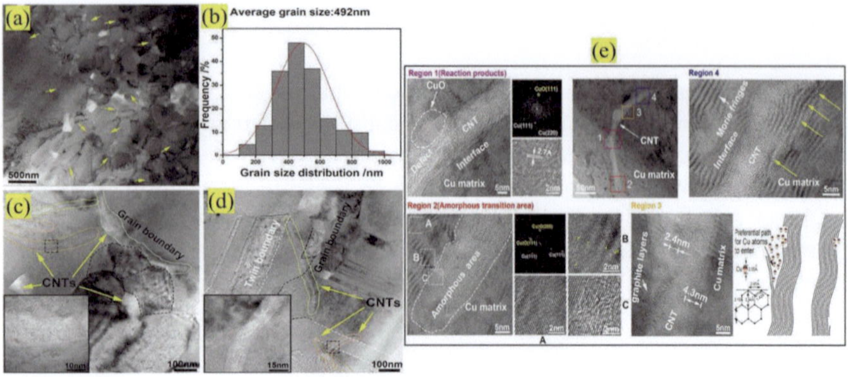

Fig. 4.6 Cu-CNTs/Cu composite TEM observation for **a** shows dispersion of CNT in Cu matrix, **b** grain size after sintering, **c** different distribution pattern of CNT in Cu matrix; **e** AT-CNT/Cu composite region 1 shows interfacial products, region 2 shows amorphous area, region 3 shows defects on CNTs and region 4 shows Morie fringes at interface zone (Reprinted with permission from Chen et al. [9])

4.5.8.2 Enhanced Uniform Dispersion

Uniform dispersion of material inside solvent, will be ensure with homogenous deposition of material on TEM grid for observation. The optimum dispersion conditions will bring representative shape, size and respective distribution of material on TEM grid, as which was actually prepared in lab. Proper dispersion of specimen, TEM analysis will be protected from any misleading interpretation due to clustering and uneven particle distribution [5–7]. Figure 4.6 demonstrates the Cu-CNTs/Cu composite TEM observation for dispersion of CNT in Cu matrix (a), whereas grain size after sintering, and different distribution pattern of CNT in Cu matrix has been shown in Fig. 4.6c, d. Further, AT-CNT/Cu composite depicted from region 1 about interfacial products followed by region 2 for amorphous area whereas region 3 and region 4 shows defects on CNTs and Morie fringes at interface zone respectively [9].

4.5.8.3 Preventing Sedimentation

During the most of time due to instability of specimen in solvent, stable dispersion cannot be achieved. The optimized ultrasonication conditions like frequency of sonication, time of ultrasonication etc., bring particles agitated for long time. This will help and guide the material to deposit or settle on TEM grid uniformly, bring quality analysis under TEM [5–7]. Figure 4.7 shows image of sedimented (Fig. 4.7a, b) and well dispersed suspension (Fig. 4.7c, e), which will directly affect the uniform deposition of particles on grid support surface.

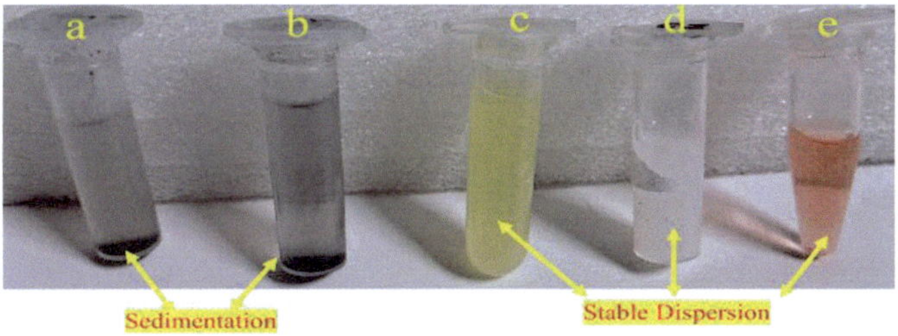

Fig. 4.7 **a–b** NPs Sedimented dispersion, **c–e** NPs Ideal dispersion respectively

4.5.8.4 Material Washed Surface

Due to complex reaction conditions including use of multiple chemical or reagents during synthesis process, bring adsorption or attachment of many contaminants on active material surface. This will mislead and degrade the TEM analysis and overall efficiency of material as well precise interpretation of data. The defined ultrasonication energy oriented mechanical agitation and cavitation effect will dislodge the impurities from material surface, followed by subsequent washing steps with inert solvents. This will bring the specimen surface active and efficient during active participation in suitable application [5–7]. Mohan et al. [10] reported the morphology of ~ 25 nm size silver nanoparticles in zoom and full view in deionized water. Under Fig. 4.8a, TEM image demonstrated silver nanoparticles zoomed view having clean surface-based NPs with spherical shape without any presence of secondary phase. Further, respective specimen full area view shows mono-dispersion of NPs having minimum aggregation [10].

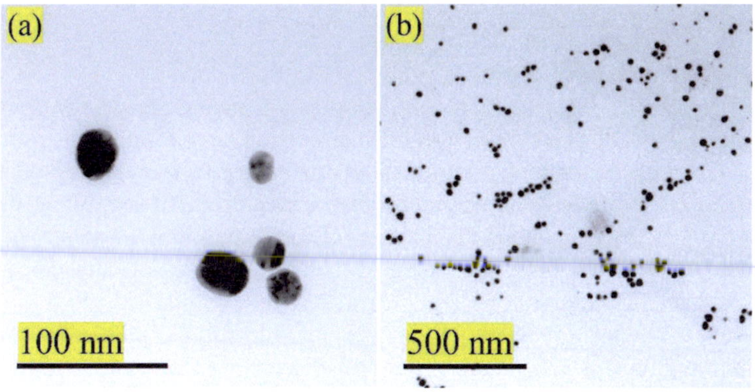

Fig. 4.8 Silver nanoparticles dispersion in deionized water, **a** zoomed view of nanoparticles showing mostly NPs spherical shape (having 25 nm size), **b** full view respective area shows mono-dispersed silver NPs having minimum aggregation (Reprinted with permission from Mohan et al. [10] under open access)

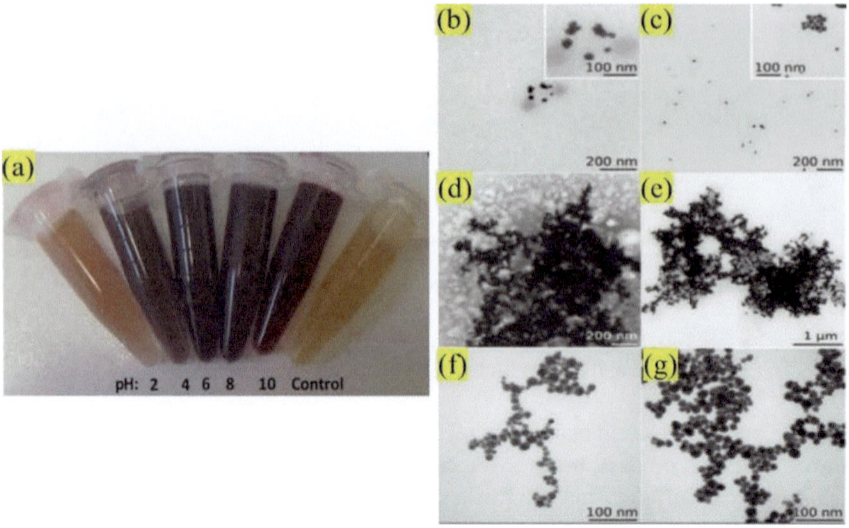

Fig. 4.9 **a** Mycelium free supernatant w.r.t. different pH values, **b** unwashed sample at pH2 (image at 200 nm), **c** washed sample at pH6, **d–e** washed sample at pH2, **f–g** washed sample at pH10. Scale bar of image **b**, **c** and **d** is 200 nm, **e** image at 1 μm whereas image **e–f** at 100 nm (Reprinted with permission from Pourali et al. [11] under open access)

In similar study, Fig. 4.9a–g shows the effect of washing on the physical appearance of nanomaterial solution through TEM analysis. Figure 4.9a shows the color appearance change of mycelium free supernatant at different pH values. Further, with the effect of pH condition of synthesized Au NPs at pH = 2, 6, and 10 (Fig. 4.9b–g, optimally washed specimen at pH = 10 shows polydisperse specimeñ [11].

4.5.8.5 Temperature Control

During ultrasonication process of specimen dispersion, monitoring and control over solution temperature and time is important in order to prevent sample degradation or overheating effects. Solution temperature must be in controlled during ultrasonication of material in order to maintain the integrity of specimen [5–7].

Under Fig. 4.10, we have demonstrated the role and need of ultrasonication in TEM specimen preparation.

Overall, optimum use of ultrasonication mode in sample preparation through minimum agglomerates/aggregates, uniform dispersion, minimum sedimentation and contamination free material surface, temperature control etc. features towards representative TEM imaging.

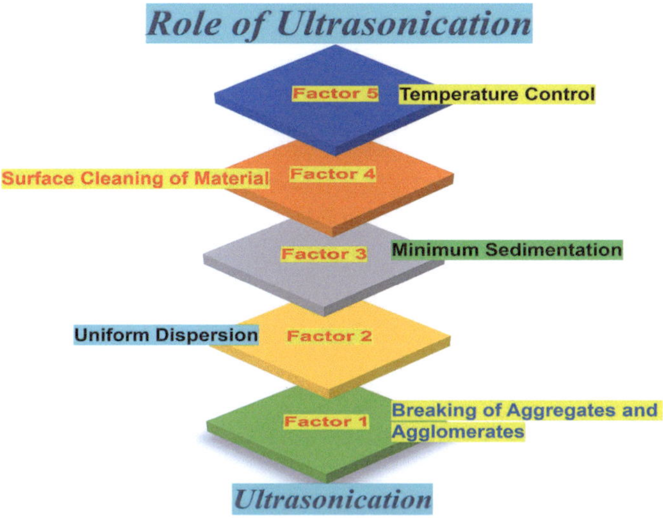

Fig. 4.10 The role and need of ultrasonication in TEM specimen preparation

4.5.9 Effect of Centrifugation

Purification and separation of material of interest from unwanted component at final stage of product, can be achieved by centrifugation technique. Primarily, with appropriate centrifugation condition like rotation speed, solution concentration, type of solvent etc., facilitates removal of debris, contaminants from bulk solution. In addition, the localization suspended material from supernatant or sedimented form of material according to shape, size and density, will be isolated and analyzed as per requirement study. For example, isolation of NPs having size < 10 nm or isolation of DNA or RNA from original existing state etc., will be achieved through appropriate centrifuge instrumentation like micro-ultracentrifuge at appropriate condition [12, 13]. Figure 4.11, shows the effect of centrifugation on collection of material at the bottom of container.

Similar explanation of effect of centrifugation and respective NPs distribution has been presented under Fig. 4.12c–g [12]. Figure 4.12a, b shows Au NPs appearance before and after centrifugation at 25,000 rpm. Broadly w.r.t Fig. 4.12b different gradient solution position different size range distribution has been depicted (Fig. 4.12c–g). Figure 4.12h shows red color histogram in upper section via uncentrifuged NPs presence in comparison to centrifuge gradient solution of same NPs distribution.

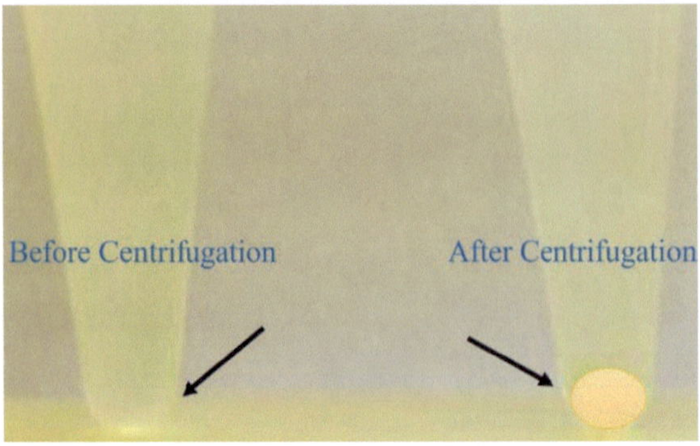

Fig. 4.11 Pictorial representation of pellet formation of scattered particles in solution after centrifugation

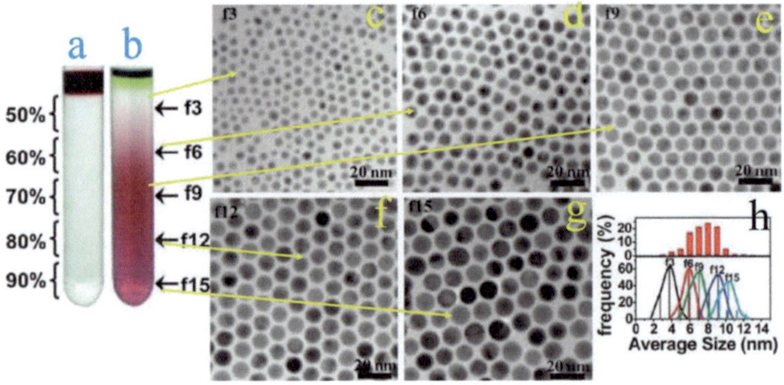

Fig. 4.12 **a** Digital image of centrifuge tube with Au NPs before centrifugation, **b** centrifuge tube after separation at 25,000 rpm for 12 min and TEM images of different separated suspension of Au NPs w.r.t. size as shown from **c–g** respectively (Adapted with permission from Bai et al. [12] under open access)

4.6 Stabilizing Agent During Grid Preparation

The challenge of material or nanomaterial dispersion and adhesion on grid supporting surface can be enhanced with presence of suitable stabilizing agent. Presence of optimum amount of stabilizing agent like surfactant or polymer etc., will prevent the aggregations of NPs and enhance their deposition on grid surface. Commonly, polyvinyl alcohol (PVA), Tween 20, and sodium dodecyl sulfate (SDS) etc., will be helpful in uniform deposition of respective material with minimum artifacts dominated EM imaging. The selection of appropriate stabilizing agent will be guided with factors such as nature of material or NPs size, surface structure, compatibility and reactive behavior etc. [14].

In coming paragraph, an attempt has been made regarding the role and use of stabilizing agent in material dispersion for TEM grid preparation.

4.6.1 Prevention of Aggregation

Solution-based formulation will face challenges to control the aggregation of respective active entities (nanomaterial or bulk material etc.). The use of non-reactive stabilizing agent during synthesis plan at appropriate conditions, will make it's a thin layer around the respective material surface which will minimize the interparticle interaction. This will be very helpful in maintaining the dispersion stability with uniform deposition of material on grid support surface [14, 15]. Under one related study, authors have elaborated about the role of optimum concentration of bovine serum albumin (BSA) on the dispersion of Au NPs as shown in Fig. 4.13a–c.

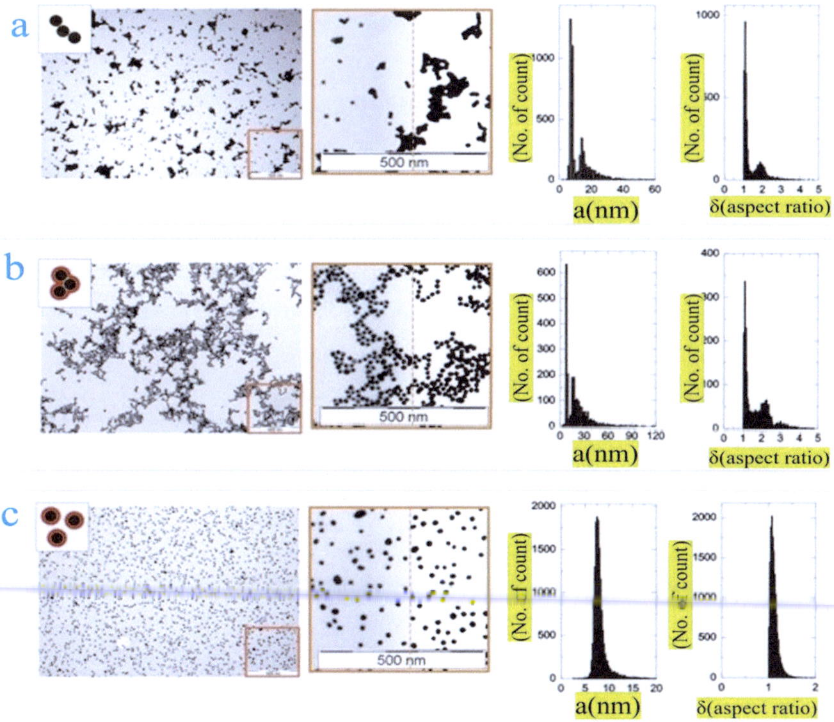

Fig. 4.13 TEM micrographs with drop cast of Au nanoparticles. **a** without bovine serum albumin (BSA), **b** With BSA below optimal concentration, **c** with optimal concentration (middle images), **a** aggregation due to Vander Waal forces, **b** aggregation due to protein bridging, **c** stable dispersion due to BSA shield Scale bar: **a** 500 nm, **b** 500 nm, **c** 500 nm (Adapted with permission from Michen et al. [14] under open access)

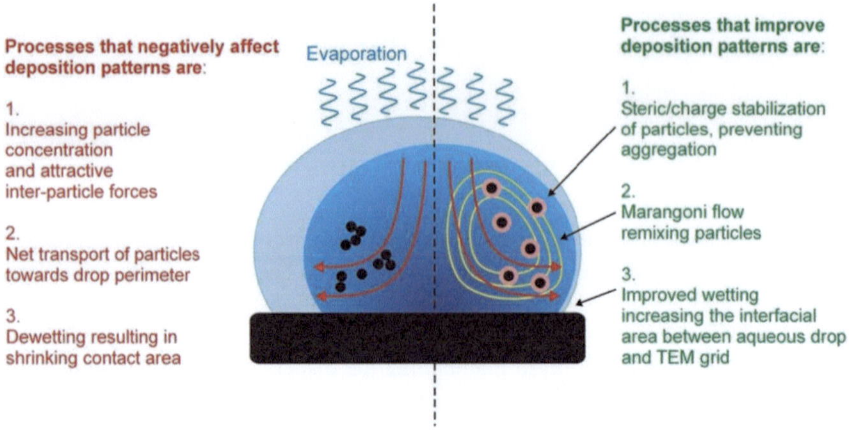

Fig. 4.14 Illustration of an aqueous drop and the dominant processes influencing the deposition pattern of suspended particles onto a TEM grid surface. Red shows effect of coffee ring effect whereas yellow lines show flow introduced by the Marangoni flow [14] [Adapted with permission from Benjamin Michen et al. [14] under open access]

4.6.2 Minimum De-Wetting Behavior

Addition of stabilizing agent during dispersion of material during TEM grid preparation, will reduce the surface tension property of respective formulation. This will ultimately lead to hydrophilic behavior of suspension having maximum deposition of nanomaterial on support surface to form respective material thin layer via solvent controlled drying mechanism [14, 15].

4.6.3 Controlled Drying

Guest stabilizing agent presence will influence the drying kinetics of nanomaterial suspension with controlled rate of solvent evaporation and minimized drying dominated artifacts. The controlled solvent drying and active content deposition behavior bring uniformly monolayer formation of active phase on grid support surface. Figure 4.14, has highlighted the possible negative and positive factors related to solvent droplet drying from dispersion solution during TEM grid preparation [14].

4.6.4 Improved Dispersion Stability

Incorporation of optimize guest stabilizing agent during nanomaterial synthesis plan will contribute in improvement of behavior like electrostatic stabilization and steric hindrance etc., between respective nanoparticles. Homogenous distribution of nanomaterial will be observed in respective TEM as well in all other related observations. In addition, optimum content of stabilizing agent into respective formulation brings minimum sedimentation of respective material of solution for long time. Specifically, on the basis of polarity of nanomaterial surface will direct to choose the nature of stabilizing agent like non-ionic surfactant (e.g., Tween, Triton X etc.), anionic surfactant (e.g. sodium dodecyl sulfate etc.), cationic surfactant (e.g., certytrimethyl ammonium bromide etc.), polymeric stabilizer (e.g., polyvinylpyrrolidone, polyethylene glycol etc.) [7, 14, 15].

4.6.5 Low Electron Density Features

In addition to guest stabilizing active role in dispersion of NPs, it also must have minimum electron absorption ability which bring minimum interference and background signal during TEM observation.

Figure 4.15, shows the pictorial representation of role of stabilizing agent in TEM specimen preparation and observations.

From above section, we came to know about the different factors related to use of stabilizing agent and their direct and indirect impact on the homogenous dispersion, TEM grid drying mechanism as well in ideal process of imaging.

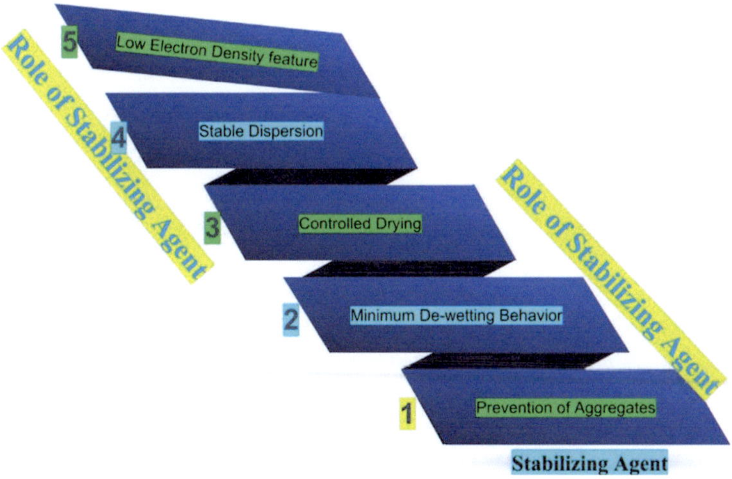

Fig. 4.15 Depicted the probable outcome with use of appropriate stabilizing agent in TEM specimen preparation

4.7 TEM Grid Drying Validation

In coming section, we have dedicatedly explained about do's and don't focus onto TEM grid drying behavior and its optimization. Validated and minutely understood solution drying mechanism which is to be deposited on TEM grid support surface, will protect specimen from drying artifacts with reproducible TEM imaging data [5, 14].

4.7.1 Sample Deposition

Before explaining about the grid drying mechanism, it is important to mention about the best ways to deposit the material on TEM grid surface uniformly. The deposition of material on TEM grid is felicitated with drop casting, spin coating or vacuum filtration etc. methods. It will be decided and planned on the basis of nature of specimen as well on the solvent properties.

4.7.2 Controlled Solvent Removal

The optimized solvent evaporation at optimum concentration of active material will induce minimum drying effect-oriented artifacts. The factors such as temperature, pressure, humidity, airflow etc., are the factors which influence the drying mechanism directly and indirectly. It is essential to optimize and validate the drying process for reproducible TEM results with minimum specimen damage [2, 14]. Under similar work authors has studied about the effect of weight loss of particle under vacuum and desiccant presence.

4.7.3 Preventing Edge Effect Mechanism

Due to accumulation of nanomaterial at the edges of grid due to "coffee ring effect" also known as "Edge effect", came as a challenge for material scientist during TEM analysis. The non-uniform distribution of materials on TEM grid, will be proceed with tilting of the grid during drying, use of edge repelling coating or use of controlled drying chambers etc. This will present as the novel approaches towards ideal grid drying with uniform nanomaterial deposition for TEM imaging. Above statement related mechanism has been depicted under Fig. 4.16a, b [16].

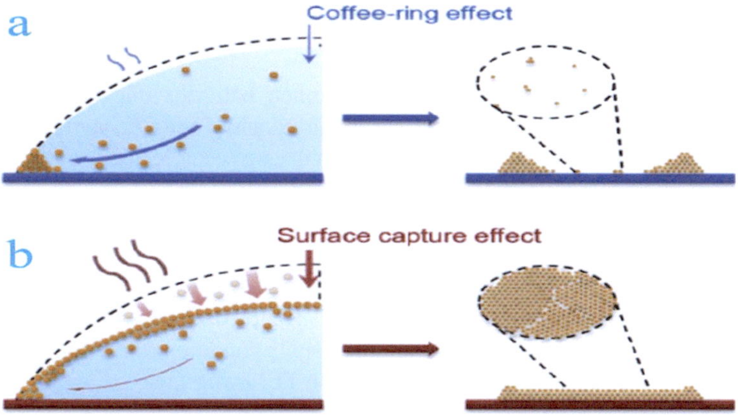

Fig. 4.16 **a** representation of coffee ring effect of NPs, **b** raised temperature bring uniform dispersion of particles on TEM grid during drying (Adapted with permission from Li et al. [16] under open access)

4.7.4 *Optimized Surface Tension*

The forceful drying mechanism of TEM grid, will bring extra stress and artifacts on the specimen morphology behavior. Use of appropriate solvent and guest stabilizing agent will direct the controlled drying mechanism via optimized surface tension behavior. This will lead to uniform and artifacts free distribution and observation of material during TEM analysis [4, 17]. Figure 4.17, demonstrated the effect of surface tension behavior w.r.t. water and ethanol-based dispersion droplet on TEM grid surface.

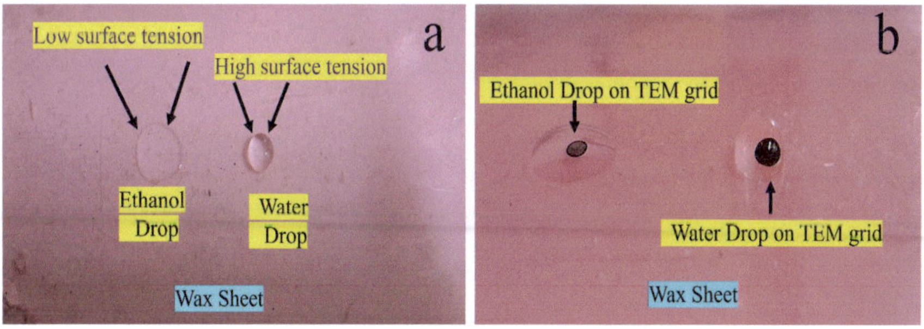

Fig. 4.17 **a** Visual picture shows droplet shape of ethanol and water-based droplet, **b** view of ethanol and water droplet on carbon coated TEM grid

4.7.5 Monitoring of Drying Process

It is more preferred to monitor dried specimen behavior under some optical microscopy or in-situ techniques for specimen insight drying behavior. With this step user can understand about solvent uniform drying scenario and accordingly can change or reschedule the whole process or experiment again.

Figure 4.18, Illustrated below the different factors related TEM grid drying for its analysis under TEM.

Through optimization of TEM grid drying behavior, we must get ensured about maximum removal of solvent from specimen during grid drying mechanism. This will be very helpful in achieving high resolution imaging conditions through maintaining ideal vacuum and operational conditions during TEM working.

4.8 Ideal Imaging

High quality TEM imaging of materials will be observed with prior optimization of different imaging parameters like contrast, resolution and signal to noise ratio etc. Instrumental factors such as beam energy, beam alignment, aperture size, stigmatism, and defocus setting etc., are very important in respective modes of TEM operations. In addition, without precise specimen preparation including optimum specimen thickness, electron dose and beam induced specimen artifacts etc., factors must be controlled to obtain presentable and actual TEM results with maintaining the

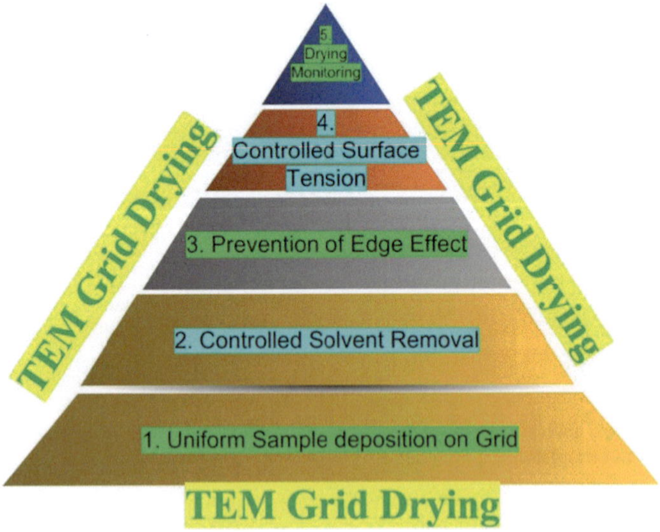

Fig. 4.18 Illustration of different factors related TEM grid drying

specimen integrity. With the sufficient knowledge and experience of TEM operation, one can extract the valuable and informative morphological and structural information from specimen under study prior to its precise preparation. This will be really useful in understanding the respective material properties towards efficient use in related applications. In coming paragraph, factors related to quality imaging process has been summarized.

4.8.1 Sample Preparation

Specialized sample preparation of specimen is required in order to produce best representative TEM images with maintaining the integrity of specimen. Use of appropriate solvent, dispersion condition, ultrasonication, solution concentration, staining, conditioning of material before preparing TEM grid etc., are the factors related to sample preparation which will improve the probability of TEM quality analysis.

4.8.2 Grid Selection

Selection of appropriate TEM grid will impact the TEM analysis up to a great extent. The nature of TEM grid stability and support as per its body material (Cu, Ni, Au or Carbon etc.), support layer (carbon, holey carbon, formvar, collodion etc.), grid mesh size (100, 200, 300 or 400 mesh etc.), mesh shape (square, spherical, hexagonal etc.), will impact directly uniform particles distribution with optimum contrast achievement during TEM imaging. Figure 4.19, demonstrated the visuals of different type and design of TEM grid and respective support films.

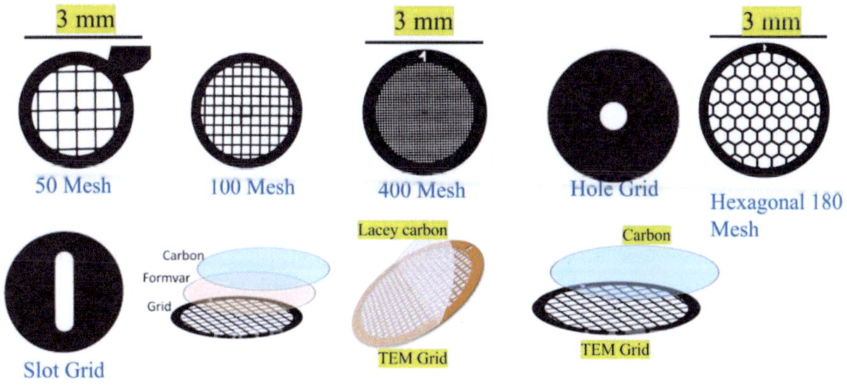

Fig. 4.19 Demonstration of different type of TEM grid design with different support on grid

Grid material will also impact the background interference and mechanical stability factors during live. The electron transparent support material (carbon, holey carbon, formvar, collodion etc.) on grid one face, will enhance the TEM image contrast, sample adhesion having minimum artifacts during imaging. In addition, small mesh size grid has chances of individual particles high resolution imaging with low background interference whereas large size mesh grid will face challenge of clustering and aggregation behaviors.

4.8.3 Beam Alignment

Unless the electron beam travel symmetrically without specimen in TEM column, until we cannot proceed for normal or advance imaging. We must have to ensure optimum setting of beam alignment related parameters like emission of electron beam, beam-centric position of condenser and objective aperture, wobbler setting, spot size alignment with beam, condenser and objective lens stigmatism correction, optimal beam convergence and focus etc. settings [18].

4.8.4 Optimal Staining

Any low-density material (emulsion, polymer etc.) visualization under TEM may demand exposure of high-density heavy metal (uranyl acetate, phosphotungstic acid, ammonium molybdate etc.) exposure, to make its data more informative and interpretable. Effect of staining behaviour with RuO_4 on the visualization of poly (hydroxy ethyl acrylate)-b-poly(styrene)($PHEA_x$-b-PS_y) particles has been demonstrated in Fig. 4.20a–d where x and y are the degree of polymerization of respective block [19]. Figure 4.20a–b shows the collapse of lyophilic layer of $PHEA_x$-b-PS_y upon air drying lead to misinterpreted TEM imaging. Figure 4.20c–d shows positive staining images highlighting the boundaries of $PHEA_x$-b-PS_y polymer particles whereas Fig. 4.20e–f highlighted more better structure and preservation under negative staining with uranyl acetate [19].

Positive and negative staining procedure, will chose as per nature of stain and type of information expected from specimen. Staining procedure will improve the contrast and image quality very drastically. There is immense need of detailed standardization for different staining protocols at their different concentration without hampering the imaging detail of specimen irrespective to nature and type of specimen [20].

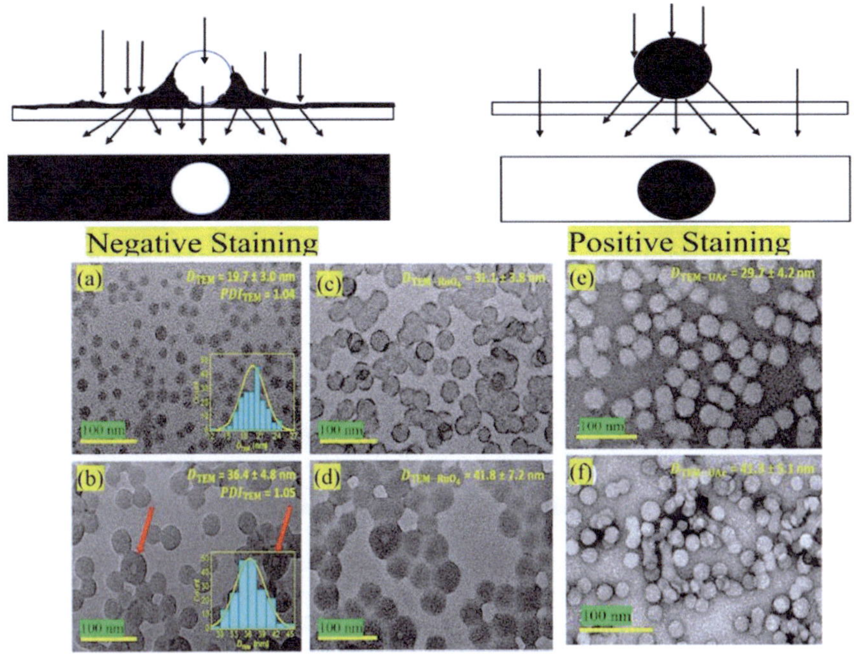

Fig. 4.20 **a** Unstained conventional TEM image of $PHEA_{85}$-b-PS_{130}, **b** $PHEA_{23}$-b-PS_{130} highlighting vesicular structure, **c** positive stain EM images of $PHEA_{85}$-b-PS_{130} and **d** $PHEA_{23}$-b-PS_{130}, **e** negative stain EM images of $PHEA_{23}$-b-PS_{130} respectively (Reprinted with permission from Tkachenko et al. [19] under open access)

4.8.5 Use of Objective Aperture (OA)

Quality imaging of specimen under TEM will be further improved with use of objective aperture. Ability of OA spatial filtering bring optimal convergence angle, which will restrict the unwanted signal, improve depth of focus, enhance the image contrast and resolution of specimen under observation [5]. Improved signal to noise ratio, minimized unwanted signal like inelastic scattering or multiple scattering and controlled thickness plane of specimen w.r.t. focus plane etc., are the factors will be felicitated by use of OA during TEM imaging as per nature of specimen.

4.8.6 Defocus Adjustment

Intentional misalignment of TEM from perfect focus, during imaging referred as defocus setting. This is related to improve the insight features of specimen. With the help of defocus adjustment, amplitude and phase contrast of specimen will be further tuned towards finer morphological and structural information of specimen. Defocus mode of operation will compensate the lens aberration factor to its best limit towards best resolution imaging. Further, with appropriate defocus setting in phase contrast mode, TEM microscopist can tune final signal for enhanced phase shift between scattered and un-scattered electron bring excellent visualization of area under study [21].

4.8.7 Electron Dose Optimization

Nature of specimen having low density behavior like polymer, emulsion, organic formulations etc., need optimized electron beam exposure during TEM imaging. The electron dose optimization (low dose) will bring balance between contrast and specimen damage. Reduction in electron beam intensity with lower beam current or low accelerating voltage bring decrease in number of electrons hitting specimen surface, finally protecting it from damage. Further, for example the use of short beam exposure time like 3 s or 4 s to 10 s or more and the application of beam blanker during TEM imaging, facilitate minimum beam damage to specimen. In addition, high sensitivity TEM detector feature of capturing low number electron signal during beam interaction with specimen, will also contribute in low dose imaging [21].

Mittelberger et al. [22] presented low dose imaging of gold nanoparticles at 3000 e/A^2. Figure 4.21a shows the image of NPs on carbon support surface whereas Fig. 4.21b shows line profile from carbon film and figure (c) demonstrate the respective line profile from NP surface. Poor line profile of NPs surface due to scattering strength, carbon surface profile shows better individual sharp peaks of electron positions, presented best representation of low dose imaging. Figure 4.21, has depicted the role of optimum electron dose on SW CNT imaging [22].

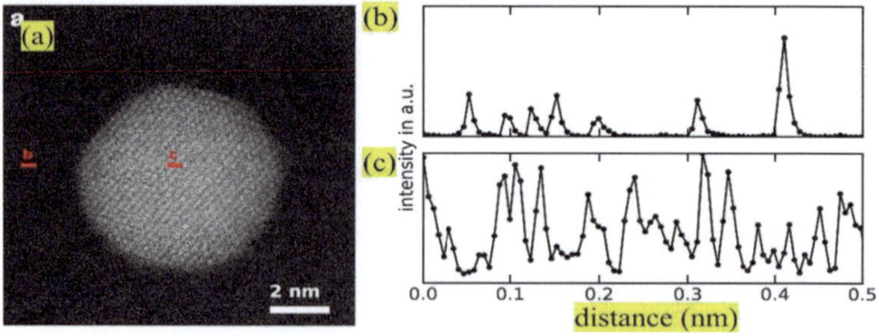

Fig. 4.21 **a** Low dose image of gold NPs lying on amorphous carbon support, **b** line profile of carbon film, **c** line profile of gold NPs (individual electron impact not visible) (Adapted with permission from Mittelberger et al. [22])

4.8.8 Tilt Series Acquisition

TEM normally provide 2-dimensional (2D) image of specimen which have actually three-dimensional boundaries. 3D tomography mode of TEM operation, capture the specificized specimen position at different tilting angles, enables the reconstruction of 3D model of specimen. This will open many unseen morphological aspects of specimen imaging for researchers [23].

4.8.9 Use of Beam Blanker

One of challenge while analyzing specimen under TEM is with over exposure of electron beam on specimen surface. This leads to specimen damage or artifacts generation related undesired effects. The use of beam blanker during TEM imaging, will provide minimum potential damage to specimen, lowest noise and capturing of fast changing dynamic processes of specimen with high resolution.

4.8.10 High Resolution (HR) and Diffraction Imaging

In addition to conventional TEM imaging which is governed by amplitude contrast imaging, phase contrast imaging brings additional high-resolution imaging. Amplitude contrast relies on detection of amplitude contrast which sensitive to variation in electron density whereas phase contrast governed by detection of transmitted electron phase change w.r.t. un-scattered electrons. HR mode will bring deep elaboration about microstructure, defects, interfaces and phase transformation of material category belong to metal, non-metal, semiconductor or biological specimen. Ene et al. [24] demonstrated the qualitative and quantitative analysis w.r.t. crystal structure, growth orientation, defect's locations etc., in GaN/AIN/Si heterostructures as shown in Fig. 4.22a–d. Minimum lattice mismatch through buffer AIN layer between heterojunction of GaN and Si has been observed (GaN700/Si-AIN/GaN interface) through high resolution imaging at atomic scale, in comparison to other samples. Uniform crystal structure orientation has been observed by SAED images of respective specimen in inset images of Fig. 4.22d [24].

4.8.11 Bright Field and Dark Field Imaging

Bright field (BF) imaging deals with transmitted electrons in comparison to dark field (DF) and high angle annular DF (HAADF) imaging which deals with diffracted electrons as shown in Fig. 4.23 [25]. Under DF imaging mode of TEM, contrast

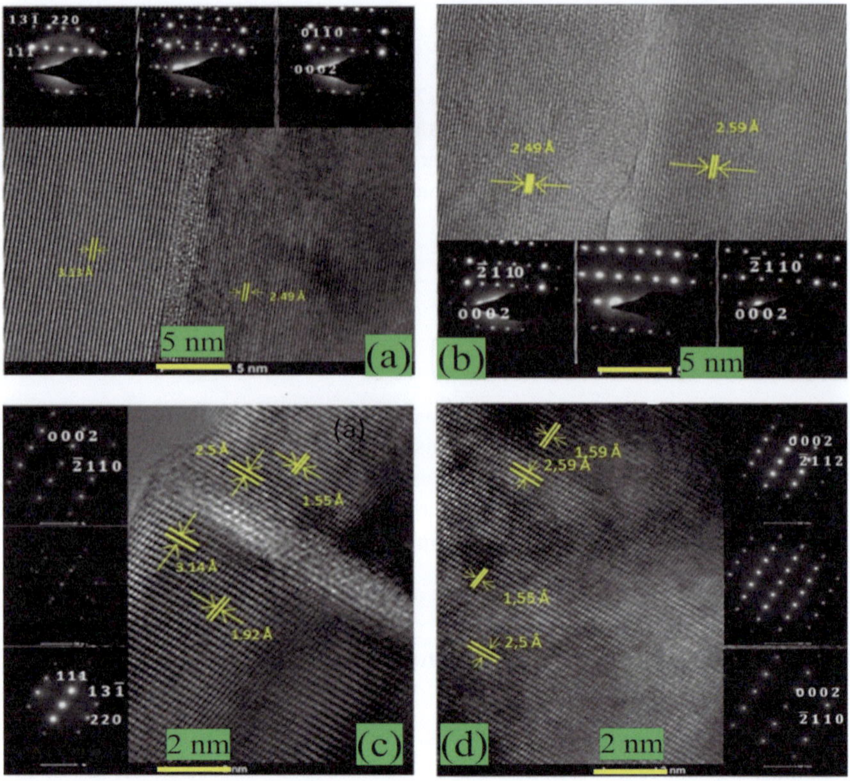

Fig. 4.22 HRTEM images with SAED micrograph showing atomic planes with diffraction images for **a** GaN300/Si–Si/AIN interface, **b** GaN300/Si-AIN/GaN, **c** GaN700/Si–Si/AIN, **d** GaN700/Si-AIN/GaN interface (Adapted with permission from Ene et al. [24] under open access)

enhancement due to mass, thickness, orientation and composition of specimen can be imaged depending on specification and capabilities of TEM. Dedicate defects analysis of crystalline nanomaterial including dislocation, grain boundaries or stacking faults etc., features, can also be reported more precisely via phase contrast imaging under HAADF mode.

Loos et al. [27] reported carbon black (CB)/polymer nanocomposite imaging under BF-STEM and HAADF-STEM as shown in Fig. 4.24a–f. BF-STEM images from Fig. 4.24b–d shows the dark particles (CB) contrast in polymer matric, whereas HAADF-STEM measure inelastic scattering at 200 nm camera length highlights proper location CB NPs inside the polymer matrix.

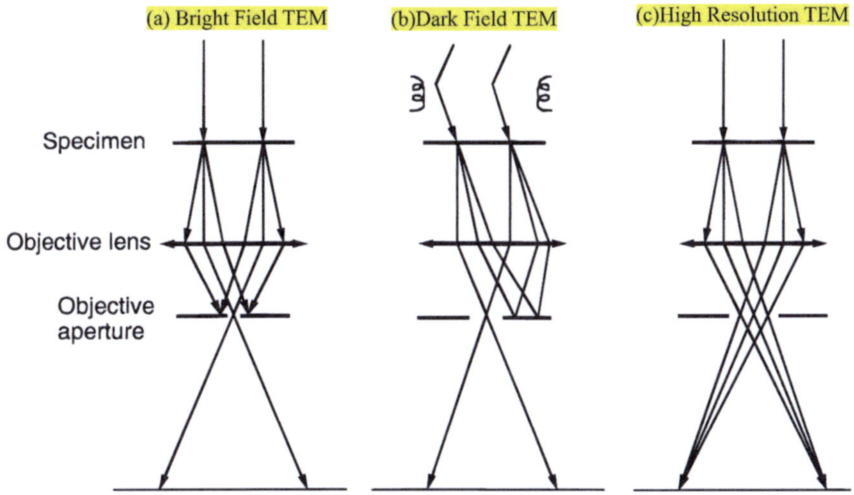

Fig. 4.23 Working of bright filed (BF), dark field (DF) and High-resolution TEM mode of operation has been demonstrated (Reprinted with permission Wang et al. [26] under open access)

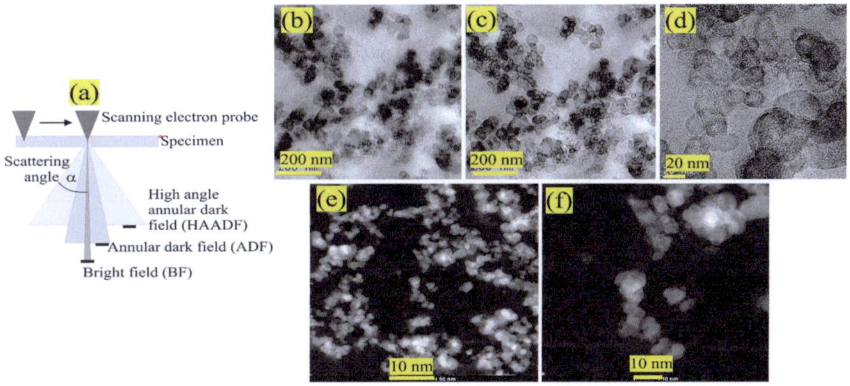

Fig. 4.24 **a** Ray diagram showing working STEM, **b** conventional TEM (CTEM) of conductive CB/polymer nanocomposite for, **b** in focus, **c** – 5 μm defocus, **d** – 1 μm defocus, in HAADF-STEM modes images of CB/polymer nanocomposite at **e** low magnification, **f** high magnification, with camera length of 200 nm (Adapted with permission from Loos et al. [27] under open access)

4.8.12 *Image Processing*

Image processing techniques which get utilized in TEM image processing will be depend upon the specifications of particular software installed with system under usage. Generally, with image processing software, noise reduction of image will be ensured with median filtering, gaussian filtering or wavelet denoising in order to maintain and highlight the finer detail of images. Further, the contrast adjustment of

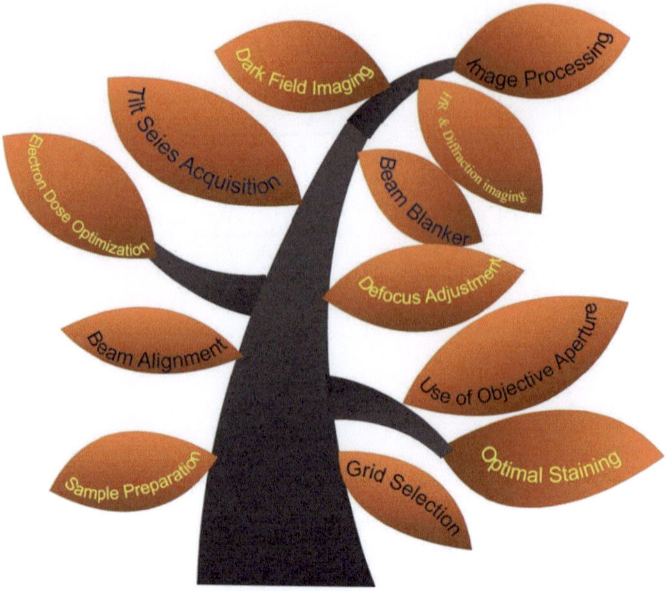

Fig. 4.25 Pictorial tree having branches showing factor affecting and improving ideal imaging

captured images will be felicitated with histogram equalization or contrast stretching towards informative imaging. Detail of particle tracking w.r.t. TEM analysis, will be felicitated by available software for algorithms of particle detection, tracking the region of interest (ROI) and quantification of materials study for dynamics behavior. Advanced image processing techniques will utilize the machine learning or artificial intelligence-based technologies for automatic particles detection, faster image capturing and accurate image analysis [28].

Figure 4.25, has shown in tree form about the different factors affecting and improving the processes of ideal imaging.

With implementation of above stated factors related to quality synthesis of nanomaterial, followed by analysis under TEM/HRTEM techniques, bring novel imaging outcomes explaining functional behavior of material under study. The optimization of appropriate synthesis method, dispersion conditions, grid selection, drop-casting, grid-drying, grid preservation and quality imaging with appropriate image processing etc., bring excellent visualization of functional behavior of material under study results into excellent respective interpretation.

NOTE: TEM imaging is not just about the capturing of images, but it is a systematic approach dealing with quality sample preparation steps, conditioning of EM to quality imaging with their precise interpretation as per pre or post defined objectives.

4.9 Conclusion

The actual morphological and textural analysis of material will be reported with updated module of TEM/HRTEM techniques. The application of the high-end TEM/HRTEM instrumentation with standardized specimen preparation protocol, will play major role in quality analysis of specimen. Initially, detail about broad category of different type of samples viz. nanoparticles, nanocomposite etc., material has been explained. Further, the importance of TEM/HRTEM analysis w.r.t. morphological, structural, and high-resolution analysis for novel material development has been explained.

As chapter specifically deals with EM imaging analysis of powder and liquid formulations, we have summarized detail w.r.t. pre and post conditions related to detail processing and respective do's and don't. For example, appropriate synthesis method must have controlled shape, size, high specimen purity, in-situ monitoring features. Similarly, ideal dispersion of powder sample will be felicitated by use of appropriate solvent at optimum conditions. This will include solvent high purity, low density, non-reactive, volatile, easy to handle and disposal etc. Challenge of agglomeration and aggregation behavior of specimen in solution state, will be countered with ultrasonication of specimen dispersion with appropriate solvent. Further, the use of suitable stabilizing agent during specimen dispersion with controlled grid drying procedures will improve EM imaging quality. Before performing precise TEM imaging analysis, users must need to optimize factors viz. quality sample preparation, grid selection, beam alignment, optimal staining, electron dose optimization, tilt series acquisition, use of beam blanker and bright field or dark field imaging etc. Finally, current chapter present simple, easy and precise sample preparation and different mode guided TEM insightful analysis.

Declaration

Author declares that there is no personal or financial conflict of interest regarding publication of this chapter.

References

1. Baer, D.R., Engelhard, M.H., Johnson, G.E., Laskin, J., Lai, J., Mueller, K., Munusamy, P., Thevuthasan, S., Wang, H., Washton, N., Elder, A., Baisch, B.L., Karakoti, A., Kuchibhatla, S.V.N.T., Moon, D.: Surface characterization of nanomaterials and nanoparticles: important needs and challenging opportunities. J. Vac. Sci. Technol., A: Vac., Surf. Films **31**(5), 050820 (2013). https://doi.org/10.1116/1.4818423
2. Baer, D.R., Amonette, J.E., Engelhard, M.H., Gaspar, D.J., Karakoti, A.S., Kuchibhatla, S., Nachimuthu, P., Nurmi, J.T., Qiang, Y., Sarathy, V., Seal, S., Sharma, A., Tratnyek, P.G., Wang, C.-M.: Characterization challenges for nanomaterials. Surf. Interface Anal. **40**(3–4), 529–537 (2008). https://doi.org/10.1002/sia.2726
3. Golberg, D., Costa, P.M.F.J., Wang, M., Wei, X., Tang, D., Xu, Z., Huang, Y., Gautam, U.K., Liu, B., Zeng, H., Kawamoto, N., Zhi, C., Mitome, M., Bando, Y.: Nanomaterial engineering

and property studies in a transmission electron microscope. Adv. Mater. **24**(2), 177–194 (2012). https://doi.org/10.1002/adma.201102579

4. Jain, S., Naveen, K., Muhammad, T., Sapana, G.: Nanoparticle synthesis, characterization and applications. In: The Impact of Nanoparticles on Agriculture and Soil Nanomaterial-Plant Interactions 13–40 (2023). https://doi.org/10.1016/B978-0-323-91703-2.00007-5
5. Ayache, J., Beaunier, L., Boumendil, J., Ehret, G., Laub, D.: Sample Preparation Handbook for Transmission Electron Microscopy. Springer, New York (2010). https://doi.org/10.1007/978-0-387-98182-6.
6. Muller, F., Peukert, W., Polke, R., Stenger, F.: Dispersing nanoparticles in liquids. Int. J. Miner. Process. **74**, S31–S41 (2004). https://doi.org/10.1016/j.minpro.2004.07.023
7. Naguyen, V.S., Rouxel, D., Hadji, R., Vincent, B., Fort, Y.: Effect of ultrasonication and dispersion stability on the cluster size of alumina nanoscale particles in aqueous solutions. Ultrason. Sonochem. **18**(1), 382–388 (2011). https://doi.org/10.1016/j.ultsonch.2010.07.003
8. Teleki, A., Wengeler, R., Wengeler, L., Nirschl, H., Pratsinis, S.E.: Distinguishing between aggregates and agglomerates of flame-made TiO_2 by high-pressure dispersion. Powder Technol. **181**(3), 292–300 (2008). https://doi.org/10.1016/j.powtec.2007.05.016
9. Chen, X., Tao, J., Yi, J., Liu, Y., Bao, R., Li, C., Tan, S., You, X.: Enhancing the strength of carbon nanotubes reinforced copper matrix composites by optimizing the interface structure and dispersion uniformity. Diam. Relat. Mater. **88**, 74–84 (2018). https://doi.org/10.1016/j.diamond.2018.06.026
10. Mohan, S., Princz, J., Ormeci, B., DeRosa, M.C.: Morphological transformation of silver nanoparticles from commercial products: modeling from product incorporation, weathering through use scenarios, and leaching into wastewater. Nanomaterials **9**(9), 1258 (2019). https://doi.org/10.3390/nano9091258
11. Pourali, P., Benada, O., Pátek, M., Neuhöferová, E., Dzmitruk, V., Benson, V.: Response of biological gold nanoparticles to different pH values: Is it possible to prepare both negatively and positively charged nanoparticles? Appl. Sci. **11**(23), 11559 (2021). https://doi.org/10.3390/app112311559
12. Bai, L., Ma, X., Liu, J., Sun, X., Zhao, D., Evans, D.G.: Rapid separation and purification of nanoparticles in organic density gradients. J. Am. Chem. Soc. **132**(7), 2333–2337 (2010). https://doi.org/10.1021/ja908971d
13. O'Neill, A., Khan, U., Coleman, J.N.: Preparation of high concentration dispersions of exfoliated MoS_2 with increased flake size. Chem. Mater. **24**(12), 2414–2421 (2012). https://doi.org/10.1021/cm301515z
14. Michen, B., Geers, C., Vanhecke, D., Endes, C., Rothen-Rutishauser, B., Balog, S., Petri-Fink, A.: Avoiding drying-artifacts in transmission electron microscopy: characterizing the size and colloidal state of nanoparticles. Sci. Rep. **5**(1), 9793 (2015). https://doi.org/10.1038/srep09793
15. Mandzy, N., Grulke, E., Drufel, T.: Breakage of TiO_2 agglomerates in electrostatically stabilized aqueous dispersions. Powder Technol. **160**(2), 121–126 (2005). https://doi.org/10.1016/j.powtec.2005.08.020
16. Li, Y., Yang, Q., Li, M., Song, Y.: Rate-dependent interface capture beyond the coffee-ring effect. Sci. Rep. **6**(1), 24628 (2016). https://doi.org/10.1038/srep24628
17. Hu, Z.S., Dong, J.X., Chen, G.X.: Replacing solvent drying technique for nanometer particle preparation. J. Colloid Interface Sci. **208**(2), 367–372 (1998). https://doi.org/10.1006/jcis.1998.5551
18. Rodenburg, J.M.: Understanding transmission electron microscope alignment: a tutorial. Microsc. Anal. 9–12 (2004)
19. Tkachenko, V., Vidal, L., Josien, L., Schmutz, M., Poly, J., Chemtob, A.: Characterizing the Core-Shell Architecture of Block Copolymer Nanoparticles with Electron Microscopy: A Multi-Technique Approach (2020)
20. Franken, L.E., Boekema, E.J., Stuart, M.C.A.: Transmission electron microscopy as a tool for the characterization of soft materials: application and interpretation. Adv. Sci. **4**(5), 1600476 (2017). https://doi.org/10.1002/advs.201600476

21. Williams, D.B., Carter, C.B.: Transmission Electron Microscopy: A Textbook for Materials Science, 2nd edn. Springer, New York (2008)
22. Mittelberger, A., Kramberger, C., Meyer, J.C.: Software electron counting for low-dose scanning transmission electron microscopy. Ultramicroscopy **188**, 1–7 (2018). https://doi.org/10.1016/j.ultramic.2018.02.005
23. Hutchings, J., Zanetti, G.: Fine details in complex environments: the power of cryo-electron tomography. Biochem. Soc. Trans. **46**(4), 807–816 (2018). https://doi.org/10.1042/BST20170351
24. Ene, V.L., Dinescu, D., Djourelov, N., Zai, I., Vasile, B.S., Serban, A.B., Leca, V., Andronescu, E.: Defect structure determination of GaN films in GaN/AlN/Si heterostructures by HR-TEM, XRD, and slow positrons experiments. Nanomaterials **10**(2), 197 (2020). https://doi.org/10.3390/nano10020197
25. Klein, N.D., Hurley, K.R., Feng, Z.V., Haynes, C.L.: Dark field transmission electron microscopy as a tool for identifying inorganic nanoparticles in biological matrices. Anal. Chem. **87**(8), 4356–4362 (2015). https://doi.org/10.1021/acs.analchem.5b00124
26. Wang, Z.L.: Transmission electron microscopy of shape-controlled nanocrystals and their assemblies. J. Phys. Chem. B **104**(6), 1153–1175 (2000). https://doi.org/10.1021/jp993593c
27. Loos, J., Sourty, E., Lu, K., De With, G., Bavel, S.: Imaging polymer systems with high-angle annular dark field scanning transmission electron microscopy (HAADF−STEM). Macromolecules **42**(7), 2581–2586 (2009). https://doi.org/10.1021/ma8026589
28. Lam, J., Katti, P., Biete, M., Mungai, M., AshShareef, S., Neikirk, K., Garza Lopez, E., Vue, Z., Christensen, T.A., Beasley, H.K., Rodman, T.A., Murray, S.A., Salisbury, J.L., Glancy, B., Shao, J., Pereira, R.O., Abel, E.D., Hinton, A.: A universal approach to analyzing transmission electron microscopy with image. J. Cells **10**(9), 2177 (2021). https://doi.org/10.3390/cells10092177

Chapter 5
Sample Preparation for Soft Matters (Non Biological) and Biological Samples

Foundation of preparing sample for TEM analysis is to achieve balance between specimen thinness for electron transparent nature and preservation of specimen original structure and composition
by ***Jeanne Ayache***

Abstract This chapter dedicatedly addresses requirements related to sample preparation and analysis of specimen belong to soft matter and biological samples through TEM technique. Chapter begins with overview of stated samples classification w.r.t. TEM analysis. Most importantly, importance of fixation with detail of different type of fixative, their properties, dehydration, embedding medium, block preparation followed by ultrathin sectioning have discussed. During ultrathin sectioning and precise handling w.r.t. their transferring onto grid surface, staining and respective storage etc., also has been mentioned in detail w.r.t. precise TEM imaging. In addition, challenges w.r.t. soft and biological sample preparation and imaging has been discussed with optimization towards ideal imaging. Ultimately, current chapter will equip researchers/scientist with extraordinary skills, technical expertise during soft and biological sample consistent and authentic TEM imaging database.

Keywords Soft matter · Dehydration · Embedding medium · Ultrathin section · Technical skills

5.1 Introduction

The water-based basic structure of soft material like gel, hydrogel, liquid crystal, colloids etc. and biological species like animal or plant tissues etc., emerge as a most delicate category to analyse under electron microscopy. In this respect, realistic and easy sample preparation, will be desired in maintaining the integrity of specimen from conventional and high-resolution TEM imaging. Flexible approach will be followed while working with process of sample preparation as per their nature and properties.

R. Singh, *Transmission Electron Microscopy Sample Preparation*,
https://doi.org/10.1007/978-3-031-82967-3_5

TEM sample preparation of soft and biological materials, is not only need scientific temper, but more of an art, need precision and accuracy with complete knowledge of material. One of basic challenge for researcher in preparing specimen from bulk specimen is in extracting best representative specimen. Before selection and execution of any protocol in specimen preparation, respective physical, chemical aspect of material must be duly studied.

Specifically, stabilization of specimen while extracting from parent source, fixation is the crucial step. Further, the gradient dehydration series will proceed for gentle removal of water from specimen. In order to produce thin slices of specimen with the help of knife face must be performed in contamination and vibration free environment. In continuation, the optimized sample analysis will be achieved with appropriate image processing and interpretation of respective data. Moreover, low temperature-based specimen synthesis, will also be analysed as per requirement of sample.

Current chapter deals with most of minor and major challenges related to soft and biological specimen preparation, which is most essential during accurate imaging.

5.2 Soft Material (Non-biological)

The materials which can be easily deformed or distort under mechanical or thermal stress classified as soft material. Broadly different colloids, gel, granular material, polymer etc., material can be classified under this category. Due to their delicate mechanical, thermal, optical, electrical and rheological properties, respective materials applications in different sectors such as healthcare, electronics, cosmetics or paint industry, can be utilized [1].

5.2.1 Types of Soft Material

5.2.1.1 Polymer

This is the category of soft material comprised of building blocks of repeating of smallest unit called monomer. Broadly polymer will be classified under two sections, in which first section comprise of synthetic polymer like polyethylene, polystyrene etc., whereas second category named biopolymer which includes different protein, DNA or polysaccharides etc. In order to understand the morphological and structural investigation of material under the category, TEM/HRTEM analysis become very important [2].

5.2.1.2 Hydrogel

Hydrogel deals with network of polymer chain and have ability of retaining large amount of water. Due to easy biodegradability, hydrophilicity, super-absorbency, softness etc. features, current material become most demanding in different biomedical application. This will include their applications in fabrication of contact lenses, bone cement for orthopaedics, wound dressing or self-healing material etc. The presence of water as the structure of hydrogel material, poses major challenge to achieve nearly similar image of processed specimen, under TEM/HRTEM through proper stabilization of respective samples [3].

5.2.1.3 Lipids

Lipid are the category of organic compound which are non-polar in nature and are soluble in organic solvent and insoluble in water. The chemical structure of molecules under this category includes fatty acids, hormones, phospholipids, sterols, terpenes etc. These are responsible for different functions in human as well in animals' metabolism. The multifunctional role and control of lipids on our health, extend importance of respective analysis under TEM/HRTEM. Stability of respective samples under electron beam is always a challenge during EM analysis [4, 5].

5.2.1.4 Surfactant

Surfactants are the category of compounds which will lower the surface tension between two mixed phases which may be two liquids or a liquid and a gas or a liquid and a solid. These are commonly used as a detergents, emulsifier and foaming agent etc., during different chemical reactions or synthesis processes. Commonly, removal of any oil or dirt-based contamination from any surface, solubilization of hydrophobic drug in aqueous media or as a self-assembly vehicle etc., applications. On the basis of respective material properties and applications, directed imaging analysis through TEM/HRTEM technique [6].

5.2.1.5 Colloids

This is category of material in which particles will exist in dispersed state of continuous medium. The size of particles may vary from nanometre to micrometre as per nature of sample. Colloids will be used as thickening agent in different industrial applications such as lubricants, lotions, toothpaste formation etc. Food colloids contain hydro-colloid nature which provide thickening, gelling, emulsifying and stabilizing features. Due to wide variety of applications in stated areas, respective materials morphological and structural investigation with TEM/HRTEM, become important and demanding to develop novel formulations [7].

5.2.1.6 Food Materials

Different food products namely dairy products (like milk, cheese etc.), fruit, vegetables etc., are very much important in present time due to their high demand and challenge of maintaining high quality and purity. Due to presence of water as the major component of food as the part of structure, respective analysis under electron microscopy is very crucial with optimized sample preparation. Visualization of nearly same imaging information of respective source during TEM analysis is very much expected [8].

5.2.1.7 Liquid Crystal (LC)

Liquid crystal is the state of matter whose properties lies between liquid and solid phases. Orientational and positional order are the two factors related to arrangements of LC. Due to unique dual phase properties, LC material will be utilized in wide range of application in different display devices of mobile, television, solar cell, photonics devices, photovoltaic cell devices etc. During development phase of different novel materials, related structural defects and nanoscale orientation growth etc., will be monitored with the help of TEM/HRTEM technique precisely [9, 10].

Detail of above stated soft material has been depicted diagramically under Fig. 5.1.

With the classification of soft materials, from their nature and properties, researchers/EM users, can pin-pointly plan for precise preparation and respective EM analysis.

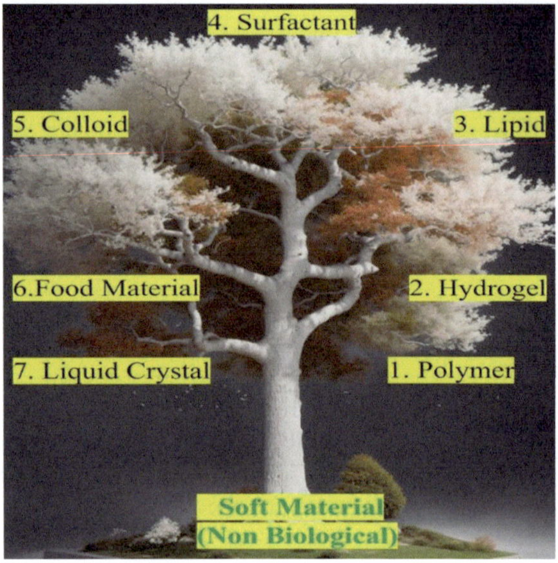

Fig. 5.1 Pictorial representation of probable type of soft material which can be analysed under TEM

NOTE: Selection of appropriate sample preparation approach for biological/soft materials for accurate TEM analysis, will be guided through pre-classification of specimen.

5.3 Biological Material and Their Types

Biological material describes under wide range of matters belong to living organism and their affiliates. Current category of material belongs to biology, zoology, medicine, biotechnology related areas. Biological material includes study of cells, tissues, extracellular matrices, bacteria, viruses and different biomaterials analysis under TEM. Ultimately, with the understanding of different biological processes in respective areas, improvement in quality of healthcare, agriculture sector, can be achieved [11]. Current category will cover following material as mention below.

5.3.1 Cells

Cell is the basic structural, biological and functional unit of all living organisms for their living processes. Due to limited dimension visualization under light microscope, respective analysis under TEM become very common and important. Challenges with cells isolation from main tissue/specimen, respective drying protocol, preservation for long time and imaging under EM, need to optimize w.r.t. nature of sample [12].

5.3.2 Tissues

Group of many cells that perform specific function for living species termed as Tissue. It is also known as cellular organizational structure which exist between cell and organ system. Broadly four types of tissues will exit namely connective, epithelial, muscle and nervous tissue. Optimized tissue specimen preparation after extraction from specific organ, is always a challenging and need further expertise w.r.t. TEM analysis [12].

5.3.3 Extracellular Matrices

The study and discussion on different biological material is incomplete without studying about properties and features of extracellular matrices. It is composed of collagens, proteoglycan, elastin, cell binding glycoprotein-based network. This will be further responsible for providing support, communication platform in cells and growth environment. The stabilization of extracellular matrix of any organ tissue is very crucial and important in order to understand and analyse the cellular system of any living species under EM [12, 13].

5.3.4 Virus

It is sub-microscopic non-living infectious agent which will replicate only in living cells of organism. It is composed of genetic material i. e. DNA and RNA, surrounded by protein coat called capsid. Virus will infect host cell first and extend the infection in animals, humans or in plants also. Horrible form of virus named 'COVID' infection faced by world in 2020, is known from younger to old generation globally. Due to severe challenge to humanity with spreading of infectious virus, analysis under TEM become very much genuine and demanding to explore and control their adverse actions for future [12, 14].

5.3.5 Exosomes

This is the category of extracellular vesicles released by cells which contain protein, nucleic acid, and other biomolecules. They are specifically contributing in different cellular communications, immunity response etc., and also involved in biomedical research and diagnostic applications. Respective material analysis while defining the state of existence of respective material, EM techniques will play very crucial role [12, 15].

5.3.6 Bacteria

Bacteria are the single thin cell walled organism without distinctive nucleus having plasma membrane. Different bacteria based on their shape like Rod (Escherichia Coli), spiral (spirillum volutans), spherical (Streptococcus pneumoniae), comma-shaped (Vibrio cholerae) etc., will exist around us. Respective material characteristics behaviour study like reproduction, cellular arrangement, evolution and adaptation, metabolism etc., will be analysed and understand through EM techniques very closely and authentically [12, 16].

5.3.7 *Biological Fluid*

Biological fluid is classified as the liquid part in body of any living organism. The most common fluids present in living body are blood, saliva, urine, semen, mucus, tears, gastric juices etc. As, all these fluids are the integral part of any living organism, their slight imbalance in body will create huge problem in individual healthy existence [12, 17]. Root causes of biological fluid imbalance with side effect on other organelles during life span, will be very closely monitored and analysed under EM techniques viz. TEM, SEM etc.

In order to make summarized representation of different types of biological material suitable for TEM analysis are placed at Fig. 5.2a–g.

5.4 Role of Water in Soft as Well Biological Material

Life on earth or on any planet of the universe, cannot be imagined and evolved without water. Water universal properties such as polar nature, high heat capacity, high heat of vaporization, high surface tension etc., stand it as the base of different form of life on earth. For example, polar nature of water brings unique solvation and complex formation via hydrogen bonding. High heat capacity feature provides stability of biological structure and environment via controlled heat regulation mechanism. Dissipation of excess of heat in living organism proceed with the process of

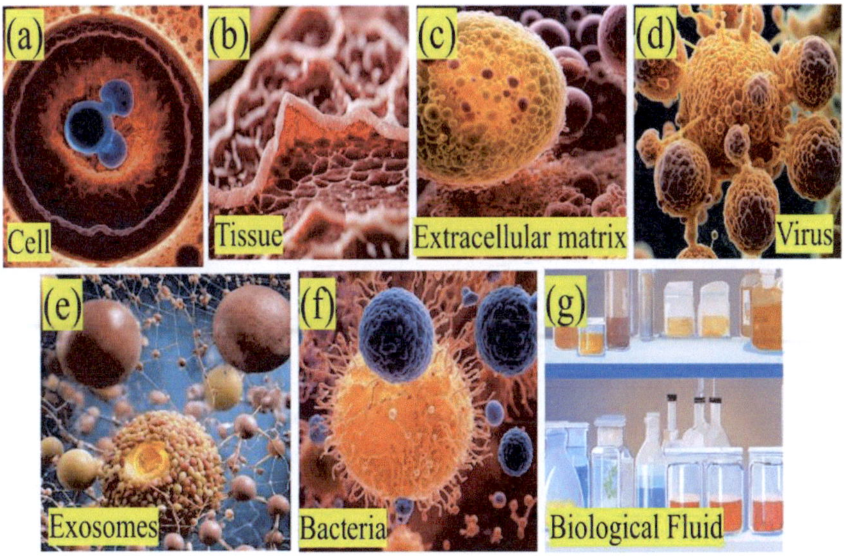

Fig. 5.2 Schematic representation **a** cells, **b** tissue, **c** extracellular matrix, **d** virus, **e** exosomes, **f** bacteria, **g** biological fluid, of biological material

evaporation whereas the feature of high surface tension facilitates the capillary action and flow of water inside any organism during their life. Basis of different processes like photosynthesis, cellular respiration, aquatic life, cellular structure etc., will work for the creation and stability of different living processes [18].

Through current section, our readers must get aware about the water properties and importance w.r.t. physiology of living organism. For analysis of any living specimen under EM techniques, while stabilizing the specimen it needs to fix first, followed by gradient dehydration through validated protocol as per nature of sample. Specific protocols will sensitively designed w.r.t. stabilization of specimen physiology with maintaining respective chemical structures. Role of optimize fixation, controlled dehydration, ultramicrotomy (if required) for cellular structure visualization under EM (SEM or TEM) techniques, will be required.

NOTE: Careful removal of water is the indispensable criteria to maintain the structural integrity of biological samples, especially during em analysis.

Our ultimate aim to study soft and biological specimen through EM (SEM/TEM) techniques is to understand the physiology mechanism of biological species with and without in any condition of infection/disease. This approach will lead to develop novel metabolic physiological behaviour database of living species in accurate and reliable manner.

5.5 Possible Ways for TEM Sample Preparation

With earlier discussion about the soft and biological materials types and nature, we are now very much aware about the probable sample preparation precaution w.r.t. TEM analysis. We have explained about the TEM sample preparation w.r.t. soft specimen (other than life science samples) and biological specimen.

Within soft and biological specimen categorization, many times it is difficult to have similar approach for their preparation. For example, polymer, emulsion or gel-based etc., specimen may or may not needed fixation, dehydration, slicing conditions/protocols in comparison to any biological specimen like plant or animal tissue, bacteria, virus etc. [19]. The selection and usage of specialized chemicals like fixative, dehydrating agent, embedding media, drying conditions etc., will be depend upon the nature of specimen in term of water content, chemical structure and stability and storage conditions requirements.

5.5.1 Need and Usage of Chemical Fixation

5.5.1.1 Fixative and Usage

Fixative are the chemicals which used in preservation and stabilization of living or protein-lipid-water-based samples, making suitable for EM analysis. Fixative will work for stability and maintenance of cellular structure of specimen via crosslinking ability between different present proteins and other biomolecules, just after its extraction from parent tissue/source. Commonly, glutaraldehyde, formaldehyde, paraformaldehyde, osmium tetroxide, karnovsky's fixative will be used in respective sample preparation procedure. Chemical crosslinking probable reaction of glutaraldehyde and osmium tetroxide bonding with protein and lipid molecule during fixation protocol has been depicted in Fig. 5.3a, b, respectively.

Specifically, glutaraldehyde, formaldehyde and paraformaldehyde etc., will bind the protein part of specimen via covalent bond cross links between amino acid groups as shown in Fig. 5.3a. Whereas, osmium tetroxide is utilized in stabilization of lipid and protein component of specimen (Fig. 5.3b). Further, the usage of above fixatives as individually or in combination (karnovsky's fixative) or in variable concentrations, fixation time, fixation temperature etc., will be decided as per nature of specimen and requirement of study. Any sample under study like plant (stem, root, leaf etc.) or human/animal organs (tissue, kidney, lungs, brain etc.) or delicate sample like gel, polymer etc., will need standardized and validated fixation procedure for TEM analysis [20–22].

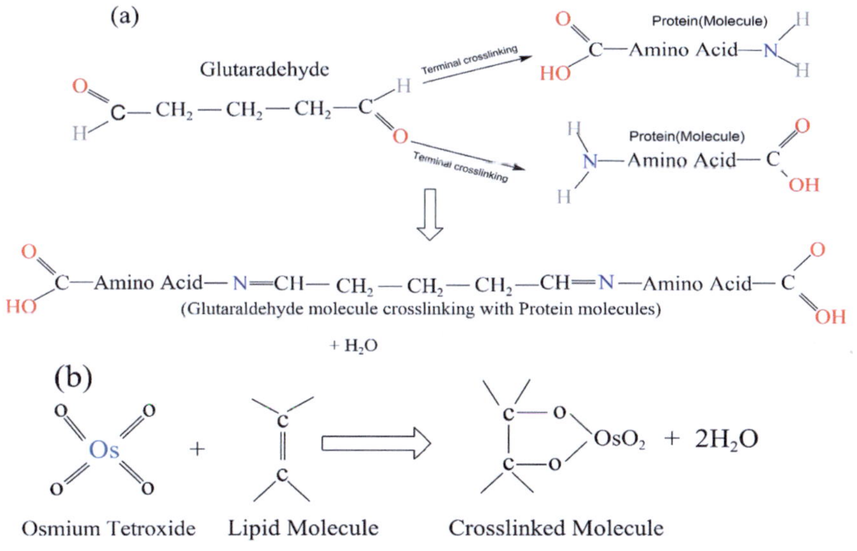

Fig. 5.3 Structural representation of **a** probable glutaraldehyde bonding with protein molecule, **b** osmium tetroxide bonding with lipids molecule, during fixation protocol respectively

5.5.1.2 Fixation for Soft Materials (Other Than Biological)

Generally, the fixation procedure, will be followed to provide support and stability for specimen structure to be analysed any EM technique. The level of water in any polymer, gel, emulsion, lipid-based specimen, will direct for need for fixation process w.r.t. stabilization and drying requirements of respective specimen. For example, polymer like polystyrene (PS) which get easily dissolved in suitable solvent or liposomes having bilayer membrane structure or isolated plasma cell membrane or respective fragments, need not fixation procedure to follow. Whereas sample like agarose gel may need fixation, dehydration steps, due to presence of delicate components [23–25].

5.5.1.3 Fixation for Biological Materials (Living Species)

The working and structure physiology of any living species will depend on its water network. The most essential requirement of any biological specimen for TEM analysis, is start from stabilizing the basic structure through fixation. According to initial source of specimen like plant, animal tissue or organ etc., will direct for selection criteria of fixative, its concentration and timings conditions etc.

Due to basic structural difference in cellular composition, and physiological process between plant and animal species, we need to apply different fixation protocol during their specimen preparation for TEM analysis. For example, the presence of rigid cell wall in plant tissues, large vacuole, chloroplast and pigment structure, high water content, interference of secondary metabolites like phenolics, terpenoids etc., will make plant specimen largely different from animal-based tissues. Furthermore, the absence of cell wall in animal tissues, presence of extracellular matrix, wide variety of cellular and sub cellular system, preservation of lipid rich structure and higher enzymatic activity etc., suggest animal-based tissues or organs fixation procedure different in comparison to plant specimen. The individual and combination ratio of above stated fixatives viz. glutaraldehyde, formaldehyde, paraformaldehyde, osmium tetroxide, karnovsky's etc., will be utilized as per nature, type, size, composition of sample [23–26].

5.5.2 *Dehydration Step*

The foremost objective of water-based sample preparation process w.r.t. EM analysis, is to replace structural water of specimen through suitable dehydrating agent, subsequent to fixation step. Effectiveness of dehydration solvent in terms of minimum shrinkage, lower vapor pressure, electron transparent nature, toxicity, safety with cost factors etc., are the key factors which need to assessed and maintained at optimal conditions towards efficient specimen preparation. Commonly, solvent like ethanol,

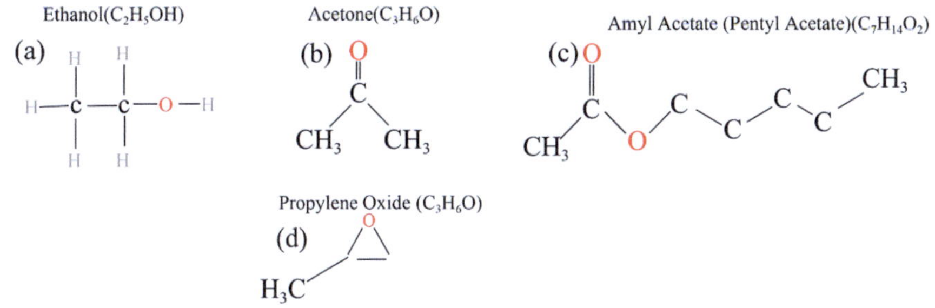

Fig. 5.4 Chemical structures of **a** ethanol, **b** acetone, **c** Amyl acetate, **d** propylene oxide, dehydrating agents

acetone, amyl acetate, and propylene oxide etc., will be used for dehydration process, whose respective chemical structure has been demonstrated in Fig. 5.4a–d.

Miscibility feature of above solvents with water in the specimen presence, direct its active role in replacement of water. Replacement or substitution of water will be proceeded with increasing concentration of dehydration solvent (like 30, 50, 60, 70, 80, 90, 100% ethanol) [23–27].

In comparison to ethanol and acetone, later have quick water removal/replacement ability, toxicity and handling issues etc. This may lead to shrinkage of specimen and complication to user health as compared to former. In addition to ethanol or acetone non-compatibility with some specific specimen, propylene oxide's low vapor pressure feature, has advantage for specimen's dehydration process. In addition, supporting interaction of dehydration solvent with epoxy, its electron transparent nature, minimum background noise etc. will be desired towards ideal TEM imaging.

Finally, the choice of dehydrating agents during dehydration of water from soft or biological specimen, will depend on the nature of specimen, desired rate of dehydration or embedding media compatibility etc., will decide its usage and outcomes during sample preparation and TEM imaging stage [23–25].

5.5.3 Embedding Medium and Block Preparation

Specimen under visualization for TEM analysis, need holding support while performing slicing of respective specimen. The features of embedding medium will bring direct and indirect effects on specimen behaviour w.r.t. specimen structure preservation, sectioning quality and contrastful imaging. Ideally, a most suitable embedding medium have sufficient compatibility, structure preservation, optimum rigidity with flexibility and stability, optimum contrast, low temperature embedding block hardening conditions, post embedding treatments w.r.t. quality specimen slicing and informative imaging [23–25, 28]. Figure 5.5a, b shows images of Araldite resin CY212 kit include BDMA, DDSA from TAAB company and PON 812 epoxy resin kit with DDSA, NMA, DMP-30 from SP1-CHEM, respectively.

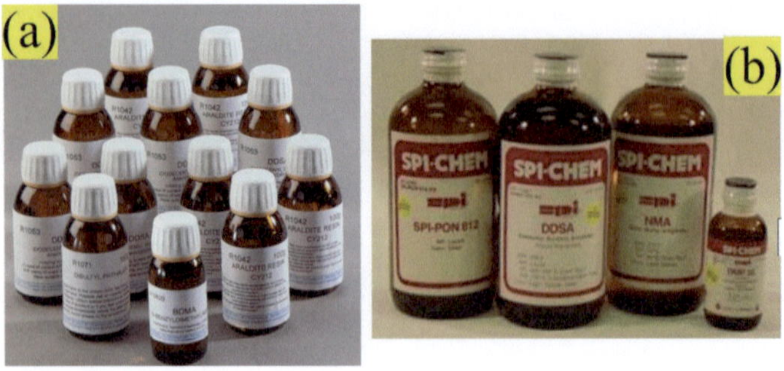

Fig. 5.5 Images of **a** Araldite resin CY212 kit include BDMA, DDSA from TAAB company, **b** PON 812 epoxy resin kit with DDSA, NMA, DMP-30 from SP1-CHEM, respectively

The compatibility of embedding medium w.r.t specimen is expected in term of preservation of specimen overall integrity. It is expected that any plant or animal or soft specimen, which is to embedded with suitable epoxy must have minimum shrinkage and artefacts effects on specimen surface. The rigidity of block during polymerization and stability for specimen via embedding media, will provide a backup support from beam damage and deformation during live imaging. The surrounding support of epoxy with thin specimen slice must be beam supportive with stable and non-interfering during final TEM imaging. In addition to well-known conditions w.r.t. contrast enhancement of specimen like staining or use of objective aperture, embedding medium have also major impact on TEM imaging. Further, uniform mixing of embedding medium components like resin, accelerator, hardener and curing conditions like time, temperature, polymerization conditions etc., must have also lowest or minimum artefacts and deformation development chances during respective process. Moreover, during ultrathin sectioning in range of ~ (50–200) nm of specimen as per nature of specimen, sections uniformity and stability behaviour will be expected, again controlled and decided by epoxy behaviour. The post embedding conditions of thin specimen slices like staining and immunolabelling etc., must be have minimum interference with embedding media, otherwise it will create noise and interference in high contrast imaging [23–25, 28].

Mainly, embedding resin used in embedding process for block preparation are paraffin wax, epoxy resin or acrylic resin etc. Stated resins will be utilized in different specimens (plant or animal or soft specimen) block preparation as per their nature and requirement of study.

For example, paraffin wax low electron density and low contrast features, restrict its use only in light microscopy (LM) analysis and have limited preference for TEM analysis. Whereas epoxy resin has uniform polymerization, low shrinkage, stability with light, heat, oxygen or electron beam exposure, compatibility with specimen specimen etc., conditions will support its use in specimen preparation. Spurr's resin, EMbed 812 (hardness ratio can be modified with ratio of DDSA: MNA with accelerator like DMP-30, BDMA etc.), Araldite, Durcupan etc., are some specific epoxy resins, which will also be used during respective process of block preparation. Whole process of embedding must be performed in efficient fuming hood as due to high viscosity and prolonged exposure of above resins by users, may have adverse impact on their health [23–25, 27, 28].

In addition, the acrylic resin which includes L R Gold, LR white, Lowicryl resins, will be specifically utilized in immunocytochemistry analysis. They will also be preferred in large section cutting, staining compatibility and UV polymerization. Parallelly, uneven polymerization, high shrinkage tendency, low stability with e-beam and difficulty in small size sectioning, during TEM sample preparation have restricted their use in limited specimen's analysis. In conclusion, out of epoxy and acrylic resin, anyone can be preferred as per requirement of study. If we want high contrast, superior mechanical features with stability aspect of embedding, epoxy resin will be preferred. Whereas, if we want a shorter processing time (fast polymerization), lower toxicity, fine ultrastructure preservation features during the process, we go with the use of acrylic resin. Epoxy resin's long curing time, toxicity whereas acrylic resin's lower contrast, low mechanical strength behaviour stands parallelly as their limitations and strengths [23–25].

5.5.4 Ultramicrotomy and Sectioning

5.5.4.1 Working and Principle

Analysis of any thick or bulk specimen internal structure at atomic scale (nanoscale) under TEM, will be processed by ultramicrotome instrument in thickness range from ~ 20 to 150 nm. Major challenge of inhomogeneous specimen during SEM imaging, will be controlled and optimized to a great extent through its ultrathin sectioning. In current chapter, specifically we are going to discuss about the biological and soft specimen ultra-thin sectioning procedure. Although, ultramicrotomy technique also have wide capabilities in specimen processing belong to material science field also [23–25, 29, 30].

Figure 5.6a shows the digital panel of ultramicrotome for smooth its operation whereas Fig. 5.6b displays the photo of Ultramicrotome Leica UC7, installed at Department of CIL/SAIF, Panjab University Chandigarh.

The EM imaging of any thick specimen under TEM or 3D reconstruction tomography etc., respective specimen ultrathin sectioning is pre-requisite condition. Thin slices of specimen must be electron transparent nature with stable behaviour under electron beam exposure. Optimum thickness of specimen under TEM analysis will be required for ideal electron beam transmission with adherent behaviour with electron beam during quality imaging [23–25].

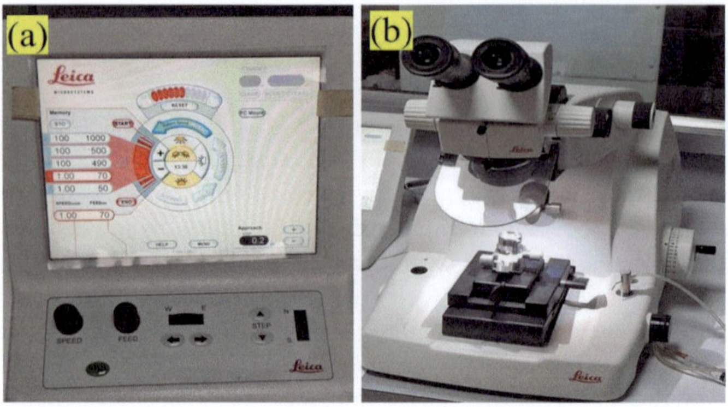

Fig. 5.6 **a** Digital screen of Ultramicrotome for smooth operation, **b** image of Ultramicrotome Leica UC7, installed at Department of CIL/SAIF, Panjab University Chandigarh (Ultramicrotome Leica UC7 image represented with courtesy of HRTEM Lab, CIL/SAIF, Panjab University, Chandigarh)

5.5.4.2 Requirement for Thin Sectioning

To make the optimal encounter between specimen sections with TEM electron beam, certain crucial steps related to sample processing and with operation of ultra-microtome need to discussed and followed, are stated as:

Specimen Embedding in Suitable Resin

In order to process the ultrathin sectioning of specimen for TEM analysis, respective specimen must be processed with optimized fixation and dehydration steps. In continuation, as per nature of specimen and size range ~ (1–3) mm or better, suitable resin will be used for infiltration, embedding process [23–25]. Figure 5.7, shows (a) different shape blocks for embedding process, (b) silicon embedded mould having 21 flat empty cavities Type B, (c) specimen with embedded block (specimen with black contrast), (d) specimen embedded block mounted for trimming process, respectively [29].

Knief Selection and Adjustments

Minimum artefacts and stress-free ultrathin sectioning of specimen, will be attained with appropriate knife i.e. glass knife or diamond knife. In case of glass knife, we have to proceed always with freshly prepared glass knife through knife maker (as shown in Figs. 5.8 and 5.9) to ensure minimum contamination w.r.t. knife cutting edge surface (Fig. 5.10a, b). Whereas in case of diamond knife, its pre-fixed cutting face must be properly cleaned and stored in suitable box to avoid any chances of contamination as shown in Fig. 5.10c. The proper aligned, positioned and adjusted

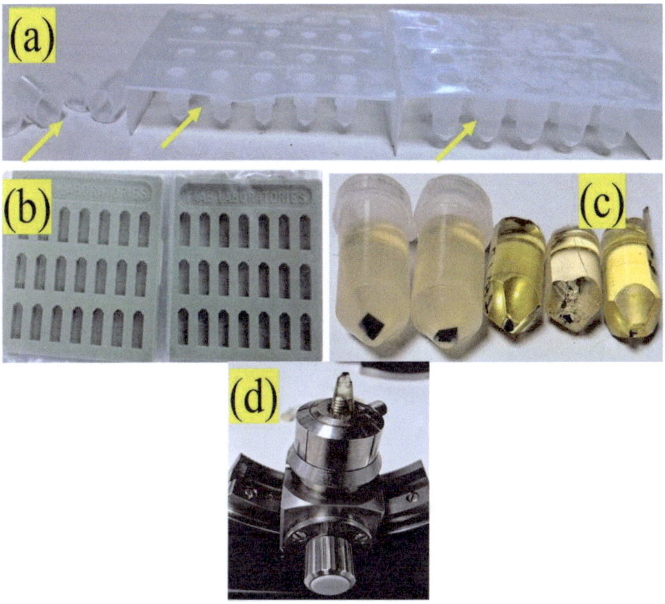

Fig. 5.7 **a** Different shape blocks for embedding process, **b** silicon embedded mould, **c** embedded block with specimen (having black contrast), **d** specimen with embedded block for trimming process, respectively (Represented images presented with courtesy of HRTEM Lab, CIL/SAIF, Panjab University, Chandigarh)

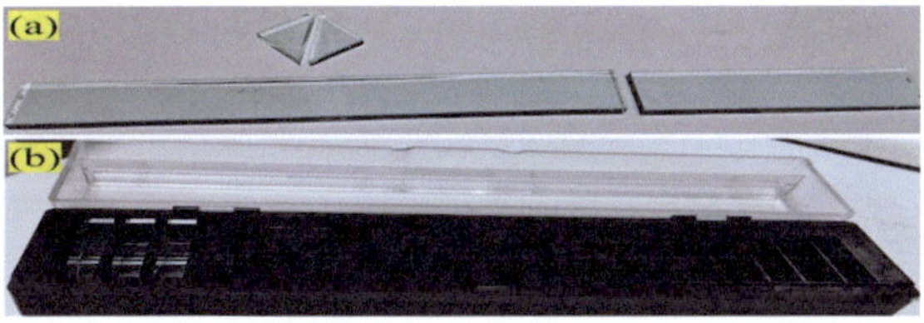

Fig. 5.8 **a** Glass strip used in knife formation, **b** storage box for glass knife preservation (Represented images presented with courtesy of HRTEM Lab, CIL/SAIF, Panjab University, Chandigarh)

knife boat must be made while cutting procedure of respective specimen for smooth and uniform sectioning as per manual of ultramicrotome operation and requirement of specimen [23–25, 28, 30]. Obviously, research team efforts and technical expertise behind the whole process have major contribution in whole process. Figures 5.8, 5.9, 5.10 has depicted in detail about the visual of glass and diamond knife formation, water boat design, impact of knife on specimen surface respectively. Figure 5.11a, b demonstrated the effect of blunt knife cutting face and debris during thin slicing of specimen under study.

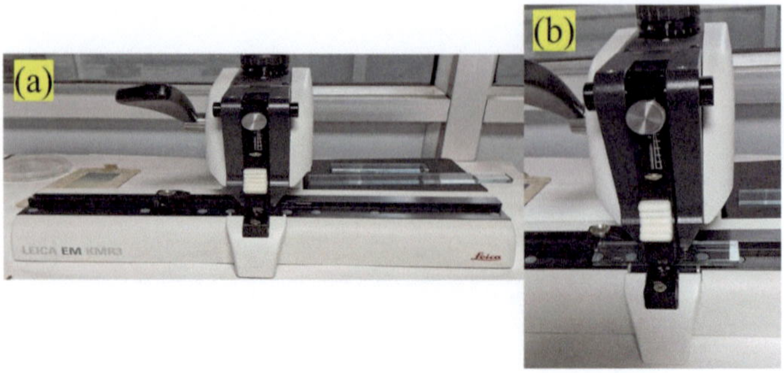

Fig. 5.9 **a** Glass knife Maker Leica EM KMR3, **b** zoom view of cutting panel of knife maker (Represented images presented with courtesy of HRTEM Lab, CIL/SAIF, Panjab University, Chandigarh)

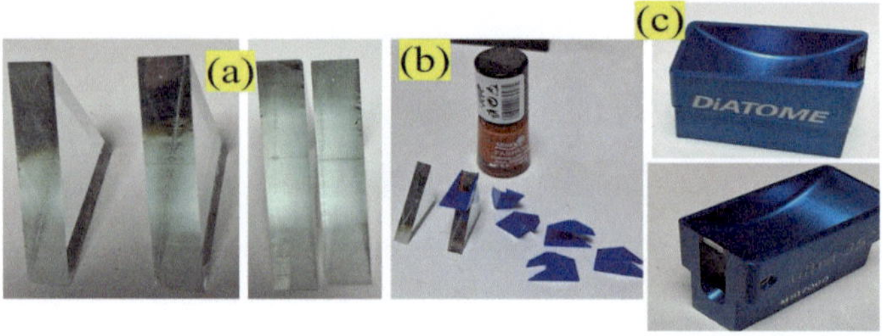

Fig. 5.10 **a** Image of glass knife having upper edge for cutting process, **b** water boat with glass knife design for sectioning process, **c** readymade Diamond knife having auto fitted water boat for sectioning process (Represented images presented with courtesy of HRTEM Lab, CIL/SAIF, Panjab University, Chandigarh)

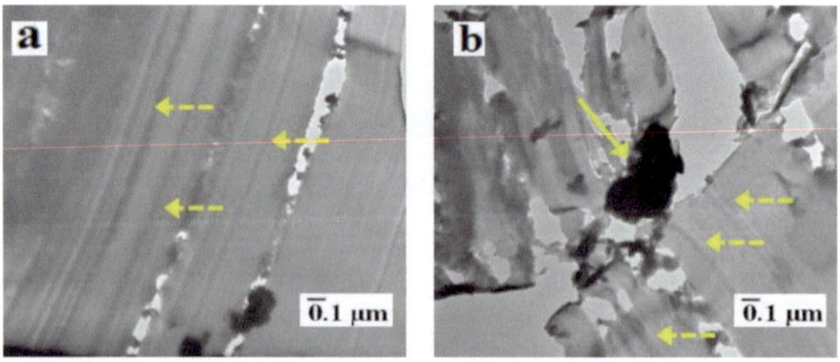

Fig. 5.11 **a** TEM micrograph shows a knife marks with dotted arrow, **b** wear debris with arrow and knife marks with dotted arrow (Reprinted with permission from Manikandan et al. [31] under open access)

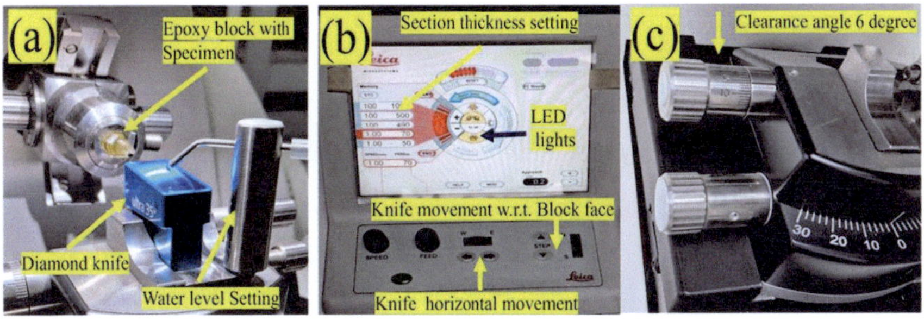

Fig. 5.12 **a** Positioning of Specimen block with knife cutting face, **b** setting and detail of different cutting parameters on ultramicrotome screen, **c** knife holder having aligned clearance angle while sectioning, respectively (Represented images presented with courtesy of HRTEM Lab, CIL/SAIF, Panjab University, Chandigarh)

Sectioning Parameters

Before ultrathin sectioning of specimen, the proper positioning/orientation of specimen w.r.t. specimen holding arm in ultra-microtome instrument, appropriate position of water boat w.r.t. knife, vibration free room, dust free environment etc., condition immensely required and must be fulfilled. The preferred slicing direction of specimen face will be ensured as per required component analysis through TEM. Optimum trimming of epoxy must be performed to expose the specimen surface from embedded block in order to achieve smooth sectioning of desired area. In addition, the optimum level of distilled water must be filled in water boat w.r.t. cutting face of glass or diamond knife, to ensure the smooth floating of thin slicing on liquid surface whose detail is shown in Fig. 5.12a. The cutting speed, cutting angle and specimen thickness (as shown in Fig. 5.12b, c etc., conditions must be adjusted as per requirement of specimen during live processing with as per available ultramicrotome model [28, 29]. Further, Fig. 5.13a, b demonstrate about view of specimen cutting arm control wheel and specimen colour reflection on water surface having different slices thickness range.

Ultrathin Collection and Mounting on TEM Grid

Whole process of ultrathin sectioning of specimen will be performed under vibration free environment. Appropriate thin sections lifting process from water surface of water boat will be ensured with the help of EM loop set or fine tweezer or fine tip brush etc. The lifting and mounting of specimen ultrathin slice ideally on TEM grid have to optimize for its twisting, folding and overlapping of thin sections. There is always a minute chances of human or process error during handling of thin slices floating on water surface, which will be minimized w.r.t. individual expertise and practice. In-built auto-mode for precise ultrathin slicing must be preferred in comparison to manual mode to ensure minimum artifacts during

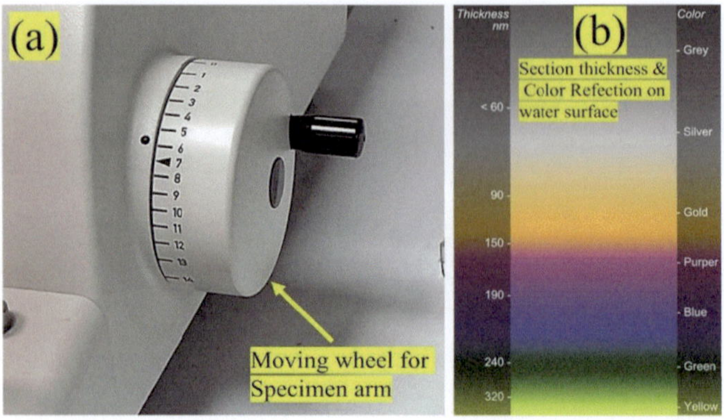

Fig. 5.13 **a** Moving wheel for movement of specimen arm while sectioning, **b** visual of colour contrast of specimen section on knife water surface (Represented images presented with courtesy of HRTEM Lab, CIL/SAIF, Panjab University, Chandigarh)

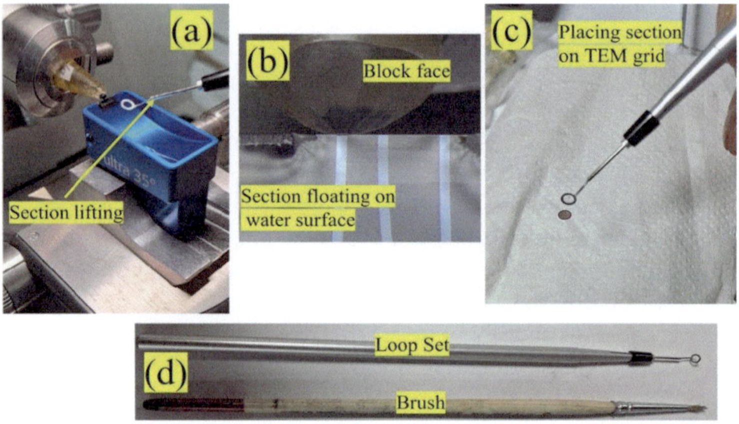

Fig. 5.14 **a** Lifting of sectioning from water boat surface, **b** view of specimen section on water surface, **c** placement of lifted ultrathin section on TEM grid, **d** tool used in handling of ultrathin section (Represented images presented with courtesy of HRTEM Lab, CIL/SAIF, Panjab University, Chandigarh)

cutting process [30]. Figure 5.14a–d shows, different steps related to cutting, handling, and placing the ultrathin specimen section on appropriate TEM grid.

In-Process Monitoring

In order to save time, energy and to enhance the efficiency of whole sectioning process, respective specimens thick section (~1–5 μm) must be monitored under light or stereo microscope, before ultrathin slicing. The precise knife edge outcomes

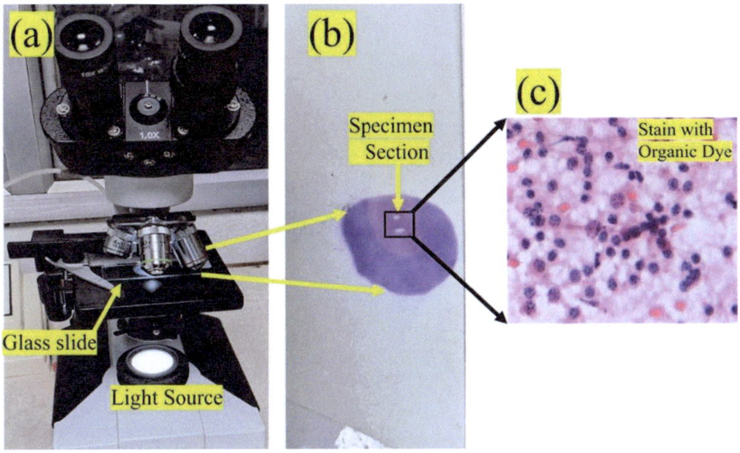

Fig. 5.15 **a** Image of light Microscope (LM), **b** suitable specimen thickness ~ (1–5) μm for LM study, **c** LM view of thin biological section, respectively (Represented images presented with courtesy of HRTEM Lab, CIL/SAIF, Panjab University, Chandigarh)

in terms of epoxy slicing, clear visualization of specimen components, integrity of specimen etc., will be the utmost requirement and need to monitored cautiously during whole cutting [23–25]. Figure 5.15a–c, shows the in process monitoring of sectioning of specimen under LM technique.

As ultramicrotomy is a precise mechanical ultrathin specimen slicing technique, through which quality imaging aspect of specimen can be improved via contrast enhancement with staining or immunogold labelling etc. This will be very much helpful in reproducibility and consistency of TEM results with prior to sample preparation for desired imaging prospective. In order to ensure desired visualization of organelles in biological or soft samples under TEM analysis, prior light microscopy (LM) guided appropriate staining with organic dye viz. toluidine dyes etc., will be essentially required in order to enhance the accuracy of final analysis under TEM [30].

Storage and Preservation

The uncontrolled storage conditions of prepared TEM grids lead to contamination and damage of respective grids. Ideally, we have to prefer with the viewing of specimen grids within time after slicing and staining procedure. Although, due to some unavoidable reasons, their storage need to do at clean appropriate storage boxes (as shown in Fig. 5.16) with protected environment from heat, moisture or dust etc. [23–25].

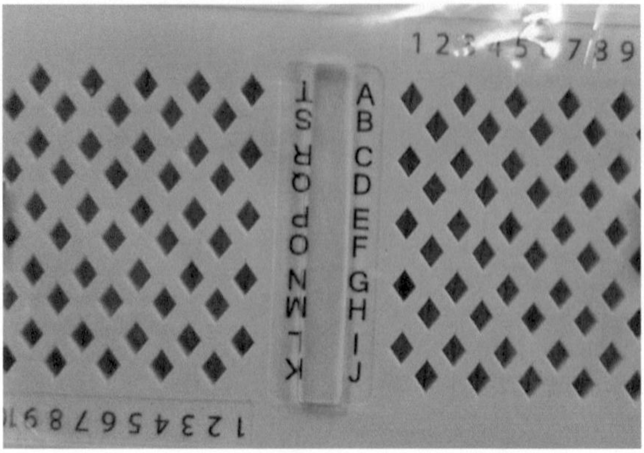

Fig. 5.16 Grid preservation box (Represented images presented with courtesy of HRTEM Lab, CIL/SAIF, Panjab University, Chandigarh)

In summary, ultramicrotomy is a versatile technique in ultrathin slicing of various samples belong to various disciplines viz. zoology, biology, nanotechnology or materials science etc. The respective specimen appropriate processing through optimized fixation, dehydration, embedding, infiltration and ultra-thin slicing as per requirement and nature of sample, will credits insightful imaging of any specimen under TEM study.

5.5.5 Staining Procedure

Staining procedure will be applied with those materials having low density led low contrast. Low contrast visualization in TEM images, is least informative due to least distinguish between respective components specially in case of multicellular tissue parts like kidney, lungs etc. Broadly, positive and negative staining will be used in different biological specimen as per their nature, properties and expected information. Normally, uranyl acetate, lead citrate, ammonium molybdate, phosphotungstic acid (PTA) etc., appropriate concentration and pH, will be used in respective procedure [24, 32].

5.5.5.1 Positive Staining

looseness-1Staining which binds or adhere with specimen surface against the background. Current staining procedure will bind the structures like cell wall, flagella or low-density nanoparticles etc., which lead respective components informative visibility under TEM analysis. Further, positive staining pH sensitive aspect will be useful in highlighting specific organelles components via affinity of uranium ion towards nucleic acid, membranes etc. Normally, uranyl acetate will work in pH range from 4.5 to 5.5 in respective mechanism. Whereas lead citrate stain work at alkaline

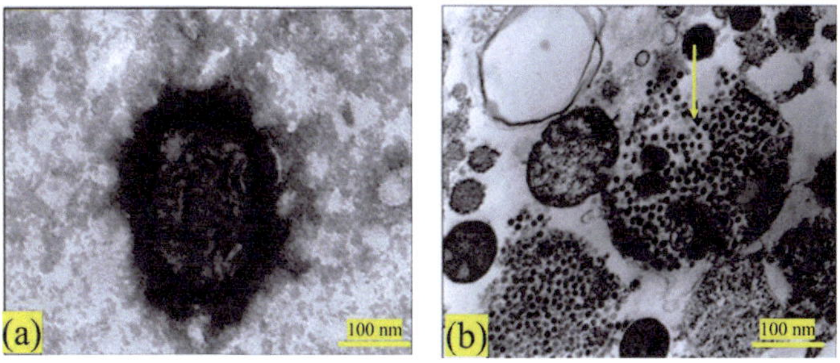

Fig. 5.17 **a** Negative stained image of orthopox virus with 2% phosphotungstic acid, **b** positive stained Dengue virus particles (shown by arrow) with lead citrate and uranyl acetate (Adapted with permission from Vieira et al. [34] under CC BY 4.0)

pH = 7.4–7.6, with binding of lead ion with protein rich structure of specimen. Both types of staining procedure will bring high contrast induction during TEM imaging process [32].

5.5.5.2 Negative Staining

Negative staining deals with visualization of material which are normally difficult to stain directly their surface, follow interaction with background surface. Different types of viruses, protein and macromolecule's etc., structure will have clear visibility during negative staining procedure. Normally, PTA will be used in pH range from 5.0 to 8.0, depending upon the nature and properties of specimen under TEM study [32, 33].

In related work, Debora Ferrira Barreto Vieira et al. [34] reported clear demonstration of negative and positive staining effect on the visualization of orthopox and dengue virus under Fig. 5.17a, b, respectively.

5.5.5.3 Precautions During Staining

There are following precautionary ways for optimal staining of specimen w.r.t. TEM analysis.

Background Noise and Optimum Staining

Due to over concentration of stain solution, bring deposition of stain debris on TEM grid, will lead to background interference during TEM imaging. Well filtered and clean stain solution must be used. Figure 5.18a–f shows, negative stained TEM imaging (a) anthrax PA63 protective antigen, (b) fiber produced from Alzheimer

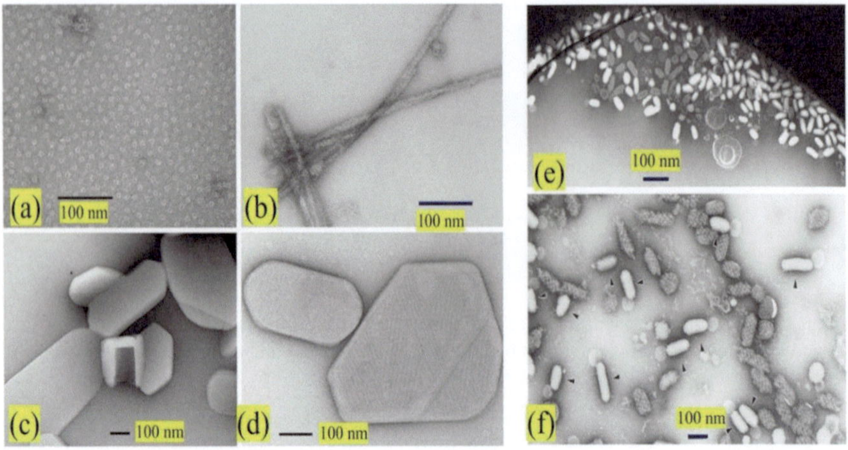

Fig. 5.18 Negative stained TEM imaging, **a** anthrax PA63 protective antigen, **b** fiber produced from Alzheimer amyloid beta peptide, **c** cholesterol microcrystal with cochleate cylinder, **d** cholesterol microcrystal bound with polylysin domain, (stained with 2% uranyl acetate), **e** clustered microneme from sporozoites of parasites cryptosporidium parvum, **f** comparison between damaged and undamaged microneme at higher magnification (5% ammonium molybdate and 0.1% trehalose (pH = 7) respectively (Reprinted with permission from De Carlo et al. [33])

amyloid beta peptide, (c) cholesterol microcrystal with cochleate cylinder, (d) cholesterol microcrystal bound with polylysin domain, (stained with 2% uranyl acetate), (e) clustered microneme from sporozoites of parasites cryptosporidium parvum, (f) comparison between damaged and undamaged microneme at higher magnification has been summarized. Specifically, Fig. 5.18f shows clustered microneme negative stained image from sporozoites of parasites cryptosporidium parvum with 5% ammonium molybdate and 0.1% trehalose (pH = 7) having noisy background. Whereas anthrax PA63 protective antigen, amyloid beta peptide, cholesterol microcrystal with cochleate cylinder species staining through 2% uranyl acetate has shown crisp clear surrounding background, in addition different informative imaging details [33].

Uneven Staining Through Stain Precipitation

The variation in contrast and visibility of unicellular or multicellular structure of biological specimen, may be observed due to uneven staining. Non-uniform stain solution led to uneven distribution and improper stain penetration on TEM grid w.r.t. specimen. For example, stain like lead citrate prone to precipitation behaviour bring unwanted precipitates on specimen surface bring poor quality and misleading imaging. In addition, multiple rinsing of specimen grids with suitable solvent for removal of excess of stain will be required before respective analysis under TEM.

Risk to Specimen Integrity

The over-concentrated, unsuitable pH, prolonged staining time, improper sample handling etc., factors will lead to harsh conditioning bring damage to specimen integrity. The specimen integrity will be maintained through delicate sample preparation and respective imaging under TEM.

Addressing above stated challenges and ideal procedure related to staining during TEM analysis, bring minimum artefacts, high quality imaging having repeatable and reproducible TEM results.

5.5.6 *TEM Imaging*

Ideal TEM analysis needs to followed with validated or inhouse standardized protocol or parameters in respective imaging analysis. In comparison to non-living material analysis, biological or soft specimen need special care and expertise while performing respective analysis. The optimization for high contrast at appropriate accelerating voltage, beam current with well aligned EM system via appropriate staining procedure is the upmost requirement during TEM analysis [32]. Figure 5.19a, b shows operating panel image of JEOL 2100 Plus HRTEM installed at CIL/SAIF, Panjab University, Chandigarh with instrument complete vacuum status, respectively.

Further, Fig. 5.20 comprised of (a) column image of JEOL 2100 Plus directing numerous mechanical aperture positions and Fig. 5.20b–f shows both TEM (left side and right-side from centre position of TEM) operation panels, respectively.

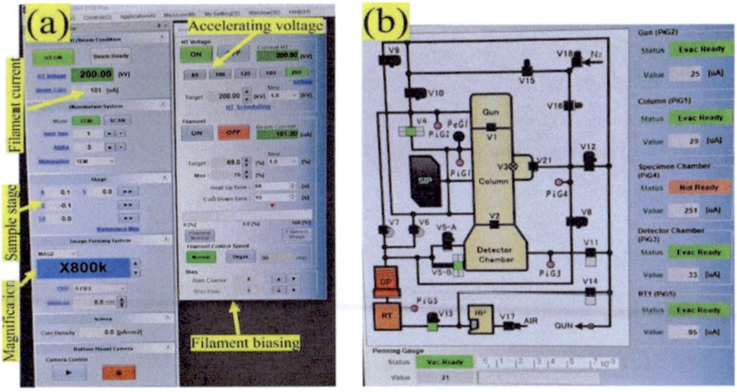

Fig. 5.19 **a** Operating panel of JEOL 2100 Plus HRTEM at CIL/SAIF, Panjab University, Chandigarh, **b** instrument vacuum working status, respectively (Represented images presented with courtesy of HRTEM Lab, CIL/SAIF, Panjab University, Chandigarh)

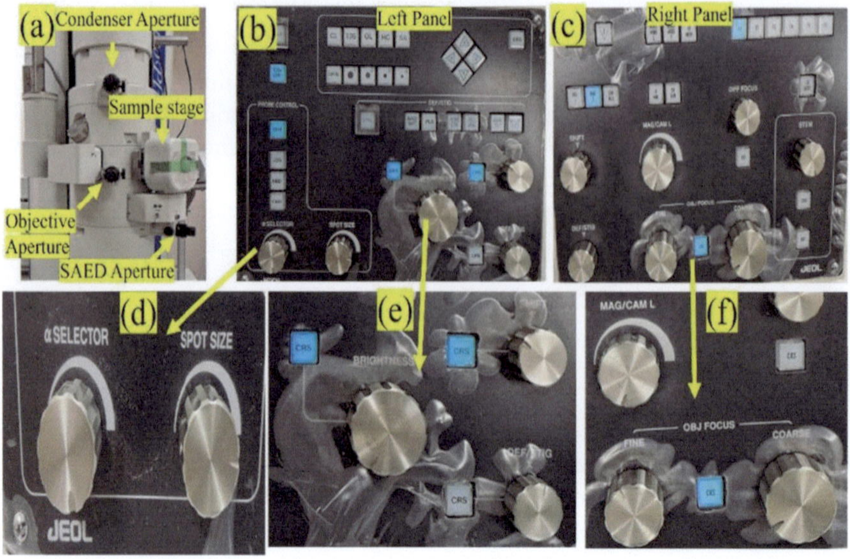

Fig. 5.20 **a** Column image of JEOL 2100 Plus, **b** left side operation panel, **c** right side operation panel, **d–f** zoom view respective panels important knobs (Represented images presented with courtesy of HRTEM Lab, CIL/SAIF, Panjab University, Chandigarh)

With the optimum use of above demonstrated operational parameter as shown in Figs. 5.19 and 5.20. Figure 5.21a–e has demonstrated precise and informative analysis LoVo-S(sensitive) and LoVo-R (resistant) mitochondria analysis with Doxorubicin antibiotic drug under TEM has been demonstrated [35]. LoVo-S specimen shows irregular nucleus with dissolved chromatin having overlapping of some related components. In contrast to LoVo-S, LoVo-R specimen shows roundish mitochondria with dispersed chromatin and regular nucleus are more in regular shape with modest cristolysis. Mean area evaluation for mitochondria species shows higher values for LoVo-R sample in comparison to other specimen has been observed and respective detail is demonstrated in Fig. 5.21e.

NOTE: Advance understanding of prone areas of errors w.r.t. sample preparation, processing, TEM imaging and respective interpretation etc., will be minimized with careful proceedings.

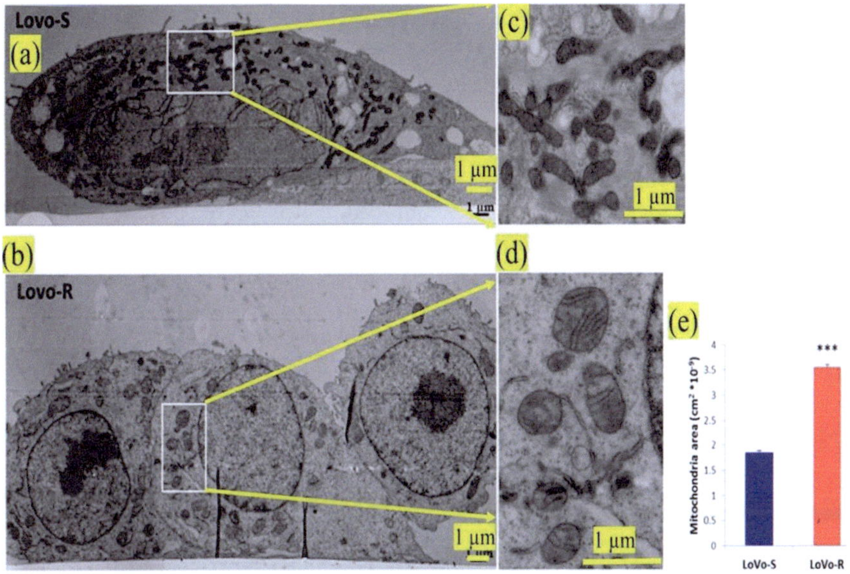

Fig. 5.21 Ultrastructure analysis of cell cultured in 2D monolayer by electron microscopy for **a**, **c** LoVo-S(sensitive) mitochondria with specific area enlarged view, whereas, **b**, **d** shows LoVo-R (resistant) mitochondria with specific area enlarged view, **e** mitochondria area for above samples (Reprinted with permission from Moscheni et al. [35] under open access)

5.5.7 Protocol for Soft and Biological Specimen Preparation

Under current section, we are going to discuss about the soft and biological specimen processing via direct drop casting or chemical fixation methodology [32]. Although, in coming chapter we will specifically be discussed about cryo-based (low temperature) sample preparation procedure of respective sample for TEM analysis.

(a) **Direct Drop Casting**: Direct dispersed soft specimens without fixation (depending on the stability of sample and properties) drop casted on TEM grid can be utilized for TEM imaging purpose. If staining is required, follow steps at current Sect. 5.5.5. Dry respective TEM grid at least for 24 h before viewing under TEM.
(b) **Fixation**: Under this approach samples like hydrogel, lipids, biological specimen (tissue etc.) etc., which are unstable under vacuum, will need to stabilized appropriately via fixed with primary fixative (2–4% glutaraldehyde in buffer) followed by secondary fixative (osmium tetroxide = 1–2% in buffer) for ~ (1–5) hrs as per nature of samples. Just to fixation step, follow the optimum washing steps in buffer or water as per requirement.
(c) **Dehydration**: Complete fixation step of specimen, need to follow the dehydration serial steps with acetone or ethanol from 50% (10–15 min. exposure), 70%

(10–15 min), 80% (10–15 min), 90% (10–15 min) to 100% (10–15 min). *(Refer Sect. 5.5.2 for more detail).*

(d) **Use of exchanging solvent**: Use exchanging solvent like (propylene oxide etc.) to replace dehydrating solvent, so that effective infiltration with epoxy or resin can be achieved.

(e) **Infiltration and Embedding**: The freshly prepared resin (Araldite or Epon 812 etc.), will be used in infiltration and embedding process of specimen after step (d). Appropriate size of specimen i.e. 1–2 mm or powder form, will be place at cutting face of epoxy block. No air bubbles must be present during block preparation. (*Refer Sect. 5.5.3 for detail*)

(f) **Sectioning**: *Refer Sect. 5.5.4 for detail.*

(g) **Staining**: If specimen under TEM observation will not show sufficient contrast, it will be stained with appropriate heavy metal salt like uranyl acetate, lead citrate, ammonium molybdate, phosphotungstic acid as per requirement. Properly filtered stain drops on dental wax will be faced by specimen grid for 5–10 min as per nature of sample and requirement of study, followed by grid washing with water or buffer. (*Refer Sect. 5.5.5 for detail*).

(h) **TEM Imaging**: Prepared grid of biological and non-biological soft samples will be viewed under TEM at 80–200 kV accelerating voltage as per requirement of contrast and high-resolution requirement.

5.6 Challenges w.r.t. Specimen Preparation and TEM Imaging

In current chapter, we have discussed about the sample preparation of biological and soft specimen with the help of chemical processing and ultramicrotomy. Although, specimen which needs specialized low temperature preparations and EM analysis, will be discussed in next chapters.

In current chapter, due to sensitivity of biological and soft specimen w.r.t. EM analysis, whole approach will revolve around the maintaining integrity of specimen and insightful TEM. There are following basic points which must be aware and taken care by researcher while dealing with respective specimen analysis under EM techniques.

5.6.1 Fixation and Dehydration

Fixation and dehydration are the two steps which will be followed to stabilize and replace water content from any biological and non-biological (soft) samples. Both steps may lead to disrupt the integrity of sample, bring distorted structure and morphology, if proceed without standardization. Standardized and validated processing parameters in fixation and dehydration process like type and nature of fixative, time and concentration of fixative, nature of dehydration agent etc., w.r.t. nature of specimen, must be followed to achieve quality imaging [30, 32].

5.6.2 *Embedding and Thinning of Specimen*

Due to delicacy of biological and soft specimen, embedding medium may lead to stress and disrupt the integrity of specimen during the embedding and infiltration procedure. Appropriate hardness of prepared block must be supportive towards stability and integrity of embedded specimen. In addition, appropriate conditioning related to ultra-microtomy technique viz. perfect knife, desired specimen orientation, optimum trimming, minimum shrinkage and folding of specimen section on grid, and cutting speed etc., will be desired during whole process [24, 32].

5.6.3 *Low Contrast and Beam Damage*

Low density features of specimen under TEM analysis, will be always be challenging in order to interpret the specific phenomenon or mechanism. Over and under exposure of e-beam during TEM analysis, come up with issue of specimen damage and low contrast imaging. Suitable accelerating voltage, use of suitable objective aperture, appropriate staining, optimize beam exposure etc., will credit TEM imaging with informative insights [19, 24].

Overall, optimization of above discussed challenges w.r.t. sample preparation, imaging, interpretation etc., will present TEM imaging as novel outcomes-based electron microscopy techniques.

5.7 Conclusion

With the study and understanding about the nature and properties of biological and non-biological (soft materials) materials, readers and researchers get aware about the precise and accurate TEM analysis. With the detail classification about the soft material (non-biological) and biological specimen, readers became mindful about do's and don't during respective sample preparation. More specifically, water has been found the one of major structural and basic part of biological species (plant, animal tissues etc.) and non-biological species (polymer, protein, lipids, hydrogel etc.). In order to protect the integrity of specimen through suitable sample preparation protocol via appropriate fixation and dehydration w.r.t. structural stabilization and gentle substitution/replacement of water with suitable dehydrating solvent can be performed.

We have also discussed about the embedding resin in providing hard support for processes specimen for ultrathin-sectioning with ultramicrotomy. Furthermore, during ultramicrotomy for ultrathin sectioning, specimen must have minimum shrinkage/folds for specimen sections, negligible artefacts etc. Parallelly, optimization for sharp knife edge, stable water boat with optimum water level, aligned specimen face w.r.t. knife edge, precise lifting of ultrathin section on TEM grid, suitable staining etc., essentially required. Above stated whole process need to handle and follow with care, patience and expertise. Specifically, staining procedure is also useful in improving the low contrast challenge during TEM imaging. Positive or negative staining etc., will be applied for specimen conditioning will be decided as per unicellular, multicellular nature or desired information from specimen.

In the end, with the challenges and possible solutions w.r.t. biological and soft specimen analysis for TEM analysis, optimization in fixation, dehydration, embedding, electron transparent stable sections, has been proposed. Ultimately, with standardized specimen preparation and imaging protocols w.r.t. TEM analysis, bring repeatable and reproducible results for novel innovations.

Declaration

Author declares that there is no personal or financial conflict of interest regarding publication of this chapter.

References

1. Franken, L.E., Boekema, E.J., Stuart, M.C.A.: Transmission electron microscopy as a tool for the characterization of soft materials: application and interpretation. Adv. Sci. **4**(5), 1600476 (2017). https://doi.org/10.1002/advs.201600476
2. Libera, M.R., Egerton, R.F.: Advances in the transmission electron microscopy of polymers. Polym. Rev. **50**(3), 321–339 (2010). https://doi.org/10.1080/15583724.2010.493256
3. Kiyama, R., Yoshida, M., Nonoyama, T., Sedlačík, T., Jinnai, H., Kurokawa, T., Nakajima, T., Gong, J.P.: Nanoscale TEM imaging of hydrogel network architecture. Adv. Mater. **35**(1), 2208902 (2023). https://doi.org/10.1002/adma.202208902
4. Tiwari, S., Kumar, V., Randhawa, S., Verma, S.K.: Preparation and characterization of extracellular vesicles. Am. J. Rep. Immunol. **85**(2), e13367 (2021). https://doi.org/10.1111/aji.13367
5. Bello, V., Mattei, G., Mazzoldi, P., Vivenza, N., Gasco, P., Idee, J.M., Robic, C., Borsella, E.: Transmission electron microscopy of lipid vesicles for drug delivery: comparison between positive and negative staining. Microsc. Microanal. **16**(4), 456–461 (2010). https://doi.org/10.1017/S1431927610093645
6. Yin, H., Lei, S., Zhu, S., Huang, J., Ye, J.: Micelle-to-vesicle transition induced by organic additives in catanionic surfactant systems. Chem. A Eur. J. **12**(10), 2825–2835 (2006). https://doi.org/10.1002/chem.200501053
7. Kim, B.H., Yang, J., Lee, D., Choi, B.K., Hyeon, T., Park, J.: Liquid-phase transmission electron microscopy for studying colloidal inorganic nanoparticles. Adv. Mater. **30**(4), 1703316 (2018). https://doi.org/10.1002/adma.201703316
8. Dudkiewicz, A., Tiede, K., Loeschner, K., Jensen, L.H.S., Jensen, E., Wierzbicki, R., Boxall, A.B.A., Molhave, K.: Characterization of nanomaterials in food by electron microscopy. TrAC, Trends Anal. Chem. **30**(1), 28–43 (2011). https://doi.org/10.1016/j.trac.2010.10.007

9. Wu, D., Zhang, Y., Yang, H., Wei, A., Zhang, Y., Mensah, A., Yin, R., Lv, P., Feng, Q., Wei, Q.: Scalable functionalized liquid crystal elastomer fiber soft actuators with multi-stimulus responses and photoelectric conversion. Mater. Horiz. **10**(7), 2587–2598 (2023). https://doi.org/10.1039/D3MH00336A
10. Szebeni, J., Kiss, B., Bozó, T., Turjeman, K., Levi-Kalisman, Y., Barenholz, Y., Kellermayer, M.: Insights into the structure of comirnaty Covid-19 vaccine: a theory on soft, partially bilayer-covered nanoparticles with hydrogen bond-stabilized mRNA–lipid complexes. ACS Nano **17**(14), 13147–13157 (2023). https://doi.org/10.1021/acsnano.2c11904
11. Meyers, M.A., Chen, P.-Y., Lopez, M.I., Seki, Y., Lin, A.Y.M.: Biological materials: a materials science approach. J. Mech. Behav. Biomed. Mater. **4**(5), 626–657 (2011). https://doi.org/10.1016/j.jmbbm.2010.08.005
12. Jiang, L., Yuan, X., Pan, Y., Liang, J., Zeng, G., Wu, Z., Wang, H.: Doping of graphitic carbon nitride for photocatalysis: a review. Appl. Catal. B **217**, 388–406 (2017). https://doi.org/10.1016/j.apcatb.2017.06.003
13. Hama, R., Reinhardt, J.W., Ulziibayar, A., Watanabe, T., Kelly, J., Shinoka, T.: Recent tissue engineering approaches to mimicking the extracellular matrix structure for skin regeneration. Biomimetics **8**(1), 130 (2023). https://doi.org/10.3390/biomimetics8010130
14. Hou, P., Wang, X., Wang, H., Wang, T., Yu, Z., Xu, C., Zhao, Y., Wang, W., Zhao, Y., Chu, F., Chang, H., Zhu, H., Lu, J., Zhang, F., Liang, X., Li, X., Wang, S., Gao, Y., He, H.: The ORF7a protein of SARS-CoV-2 initiates autophagy and limits autophagosome-lysosome fusion via degradation of SNAP29 to promote virus replication. Autophagy **19**(2), 551–569 (2023). https://doi.org/10.1080/15548627.2022.2084686
15. Zhou, M., Weber, S.R., Zhao, Y., Chen, H., Sundstrom, J.M.: Methods for exosome isolation and characterization. In: Exosomes. Elsevier (2020), pp. 23–38. https://doi.org/10.1016/B978-0-12-816053-4.00002-X
16. Jiao, S., Lu, Y.: Soil pH and temperature regulate assembly processes of abundant and rare bacterial communities in agricultural ecosystems. Environ. Microbiol. **22**(3), 1052–1065 (2020). https://doi.org/10.1111/1462-2920.14815
17. Bhanderi, D., Lakhani, P., Modi, C.K.: Graphitic carbon nitride (g-C 3 N 4) as an emerging photocatalyst for sustainable environmental applications: a comprehensive review. RSC Sustain. **2**(2), 265–287 (2024). https://doi.org/10.1039/D3SU00382E
18. Ball, P.: Water as an active constituent in cell biology. Chem. Rev. **108**(1), 74–108 (2008). https://doi.org/10.1021/cr068037a
19. Trépout, S., Bastin, P., Marco, S.: Preparation and observation of thick biological samples by scanning transmission electron tomography. JoVE **121**, 55215 (2017). https://doi.org/10.3791/55215
20. Zeller, R.: Fixation, embedding, and sectioning of tissues, embryos, and single cells. Curr. Protocol. Molec. Biol. 14.1.1–14.1.8 (1989)
21. Eltoum, I., Fredenburgh, J., Myers, R.B., Grizzle, W.E.: Introduction to the Theory and Practice of Fixation of Tissues.
22. Wilson, S.M., Bacic, A.: Preparation of plant cells for transmission electron microscopy to optimize immunogold labeling of carbohydrate and protein epitopes. Nat. Protoc. **7**(9), 1716–1727 (2012). https://doi.org/10.1038/nprot.2012.096
23. Dykstra, M.J.: Biological Electron Microscopy: Theory, Techniques, and Troubleshooting. Springer US, Boston (1992). https://doi.org/10.1007/978-1-4684-0010-6
24. Luo, Z.: A Practical Guide to Transmission Electron Microscopy: Fundamentals, 1st edn. Momentum Press, New York (2016).
25. Bozzola, J.J., Russell, L.D.: Electron Microscopy, Principle and Techniques for Biologists, 2nd edn.
26. Mielańczyk, Ł., Matysiak, N., Klymenko, O., Wojnicz, R.: Transmission electron microscopy of biological samples. In: Maaz, K. (Ed.) The Transmission Electron Microscope - Theory and Applications. InTech (2015). https://doi.org/10.5772/60680
27. Neikirk, K., Vue, Z., Katti, P., Rodriguez, B.I., Omer, S., Shao, J., Christensen, T., Garza Lopez, E., Marshall, A., Palavicino-Maggio, C.B., Ponce, J., Alghanem, A.F., Vang, L., Barongan, T.,

Beasley, H.K., Rodman, T., Stephens, D., Mungai, M., Correia, M., Exil, V., Damo, S., Murray, S.A., Crabtree, A., Glancy, B., Pereira, R.O., Abel, E.D., Hinton, A.O.: Systematic transmission electron microscopy-based identification and 3D reconstruction of cellular degradation machinery. Advanced Biology **7**(6), 2200221 (2023). https://doi.org/10.1002/adbi.202200221

28. Hinton, A., Katti, P., Christensen, T.A., Mungai, M., Shao, J., Zhang, L., Trushin, S., Alghanem, A., Jaspersen, A., Geroux, R.E., Neikirk, K., Biete, M., Lopez, E.G., Shao, B., Vue, Z., Vang, L., Beasley, H.K., Marshall, A.G., Stephens, D., Damo, S., Ponce, J., Bleck, C.K.E., Hicsasmaz, I., Murray, S.A., Edmonds, R.A.C., Dajles, A., Koo, Y.D., Bacevac, S., Salisbury, J.L., Pereira, R.O., Glancy, B., Trushina, E., Abel, E.D.: A comprehensive approach to sample preparation for electron microscopy and the assessment of mitochondrial morphology in tissue and cultured cells. Adv. Biol. **7**(10), 2200202 (2023). https://doi.org/10.1002/adbi.202200202
29. Böhm, T., Felfer, P., Thiele, S.: A modular and automated serial section collection system for ultramicrotomy and subsequent imaging. Microsc. Microanal. **29**(1), 212–218 (2023). https://doi.org/10.1093/micmic/ozac007
30. Pavathuparambil Abdul Manaph, N., Ltaief, S.M., Nour-Eldine, W., Ponraj, J., Agcaoili, J., Mansour, S., Al-Shammari, A.R.: An optimized protocol for the preparation of blood immune cells for transmission electron microscopy. Micron **173**, 103517 (2023). https://doi.org/10.1016/j.micron.2023.103517
31. Monikandan, V.V., Joseph, M.A., Rajendrakumar, P.K.: Studies on artefacts induced in the specimen preparation routines of electron microscopy characterization. IOP Conf. Ser. Mater. Sci. Eng. **149**, 012016 (2016). https://doi.org/10.1088/1757-899X/149/1/012016
32. Graham, L., Orenstein, J.M.: Processing tissue and cells for transmission electron microscopy in diagnostic pathology and research. Nat. Protoc. **2**(10), 2439–2450 (2007). https://doi.org/10.1038/nprot.2007.304
33. De Carlo, S., Harris, J.R.: Negative staining and cryo-negative staining of macromolecules and viruses for TEM. Micron **42**(2), 117–131 (2011). https://doi.org/10.1016/j.micron.2010.06.003
34. Barreto-Vieira, D.F., Barth, O.M.: Negative and positive staining in transmission electron microscopy for virus diagnosis. In: Shah, M.M. (Ed.) Microbiology in Agriculture and Human Health. InTech (2015). https://doi.org/10.5772/60511
35. Moscheni, C., Malucelli, E., Castiglioni, S., Procopio, A., De Palma, C., Sorrentino, A., Sartori, P., Locatelli, L., Pereiro, E., Maier, J.A., Iotti, S.: 3D quantitative and ultrastructural analysis of mitochondria in a model of doxorubicin sensitive and resistant human colon carcinoma cells. Cancers **11**(9), 1254 (2019). https://doi.org/10.3390/cancers11091254

Chapter 6
Introduction to Cryo-TEM and Related Sample Preparation

Cryo-Electron Microscopy open a window into structure of life, allowing us to observe molecule as they function in their native environment
by ***Jacques Dubochet, Nobel Laurete in Chemistry 2017***

Abstract Cryo-TEM is a powerful and innovative imaging technique deals with preservation of sample structure at cryogenic conditions, during imaging. The basic principle, working with unique features related to respective techniques have been discussed in detail. Further, the importance and preference of cryo-TEM w.r.t. conventional TEM during specimen analysis also has been explained. Broadly w.r.t. specimen analysis under cryo-TEM, we have segregated respective samples into biological and soft specimen categories. Summary of key factors during cryo-TEM analysis viz. vitrification, slow or rapid freezing conditions, grid handling, artefacts generation, imaging precision w.r.t. innovative results and respective applications via emerging technologies has been presented.

Keywords Cryo-TEM · Sample preservation · Rapid freezing · Vitrification · Sample preparation

6.1 Introduction

TEM imaging of biological or soft material-based samples, will always be a challenging for researchers due to presence water in respective structure. In principle, stated specimens must be analysed under specialized electron microscopy techniques known as 'Cryo-TEM'. This technique is known as a high-end cutting-edge technique for visualization high resolution imaging of materials under cryogenic conditions. The novelty of Cryo-TEM is in viewing specimen closely in his native state with rapid or systematic freezing at ultra-low temperature as per requirement of sample. The important process known as 'vitrification' proceeds with formation of glasslike structure of water without ice formation maintaining specimen molecular structure. The unexplained mysteries about the structural biology of species like proteins, viruses,

R. Singh, *Transmission Electron Microscopy Sample Preparation*,
https://doi.org/10.1007/978-3-031-82967-3_6

nucleic acids and other biological macromolecules etc., will get explored insightly and reported through cryo-TEM very closely to their native state. With the help of cryo-TEM principle and working, researchers enable in observation of different dynamic processes like protein folding, variable mutation behaviour of virus or can understand and visualize about the different dynamic biological mechanisms. Similarly, any material belongs to non-biological category, like nanoparticles, polymer, lipids-based vesicles etc., will also get imaged in respective natural state. The whole approach under Cryo-TEM sample preparation and analysis, will help researchers and scientist to understand relationship between respective materials structure and functional properties, which can contribute in development and advancement of novel materials. With the novel outcomes of respective material analysis in their native state through cryo-TEM, will direct solution-oriented approach w.r.t. different existing problems of society and environment.

With the exploration of material properties under nearly native environment with optimized sample preparation in Cryo-TEM, we are very sure about the novel innovation and scientific understanding of structural biology and material design in coming future.

6.2 Basics of Cryo-TEM

Cryo-TEM is advanced imaging techniques deals in explicating two dimensional (2D) and three dimensional (3D) biological and molecular structure of especially different living species at high resolution. During processing of respective specimens, sample will be cooled below – 150 °C temperature in order to transform structural water into vitreous ice form. Stated vitrification process brings negligible interference of vitreous water in EM imaging during cryo-TEM analysis. In addition, the imaging of sample for multiple 2D images [1] at different tilting angles can transform respective specimen images into 3D model with suitable computational algorithm [2].

6.2.1 Features of Cryo-TEM

In addition to working and operation of conventional TEM, here we have discussed about the working and operation of cryo-TEM, through which users and readers credited with more clarity and understanding about the respective technique:

6.2.1.1 Unique Specimen Holder

Dedicatedly, Cryo-TEM deals in freezing the water-based specimen at low temperature ~ −150 °C with the help of specialized specimen holder in presence of liquid nitrogen or liquid ethane. The presence of cryogenic cooling system will help in maintaining the stability of specimen during interaction with electron beam. During operation of cryo-TEM, specimen loading environment onto respective holder prevents chances of frost deposition on specimen surface. In addition, hydrated state of specimen will be maintained with rapid cooling process bring formation of vitreous ice (amorphous ice), having no structural fingerprints during EM imaging [3]. This technique will prove to be best for having minimum specimen damage during sample processing in comparison to sample stabilization via conventional chemical fixation (fixation, dehydration etc.) process. Fig. 6.1a shows 200 kV field emission electron source-JEOL 2200FS image, (b) respective specimen transfer holder, and (c) demonstrate frozen grid positioning with cryo-transfer holder [3], respectively.

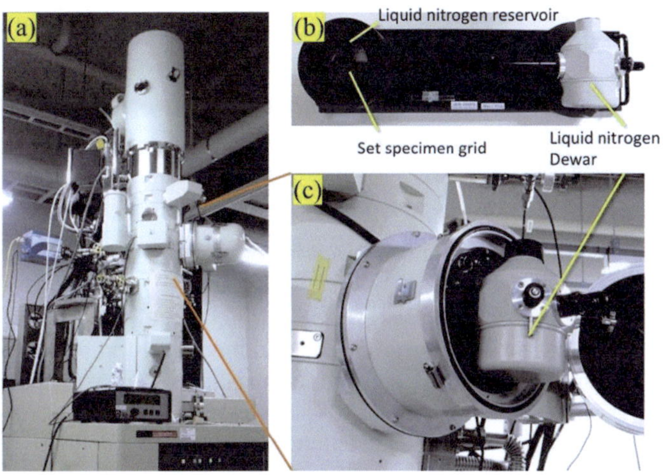

Fig. 6.1 **a** Cryo-TEM representative image (200 kV field emission electron source-JEOL 2200FS), **b** cryo transfer Specimen transfer holder, **c** frozen grid positioned with cryo-transfer holder while inserting into TEM column (Adapted with permission from Murata et al. [3] under open access)

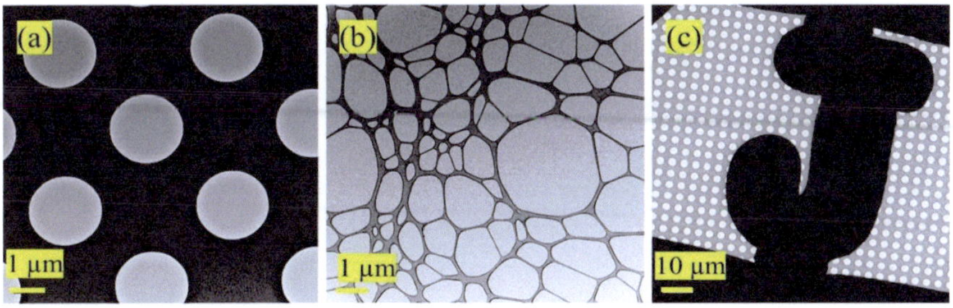

Fig. 6.2 TEM image of grid support film, **a** Holey carbon (Quantifoil) 2 µm hole separated by 2 µm, **b** Lacy carbon film (random network of carbon), **c** Finder grid (Adapted with permission from Thompson et al. [4] under open access)

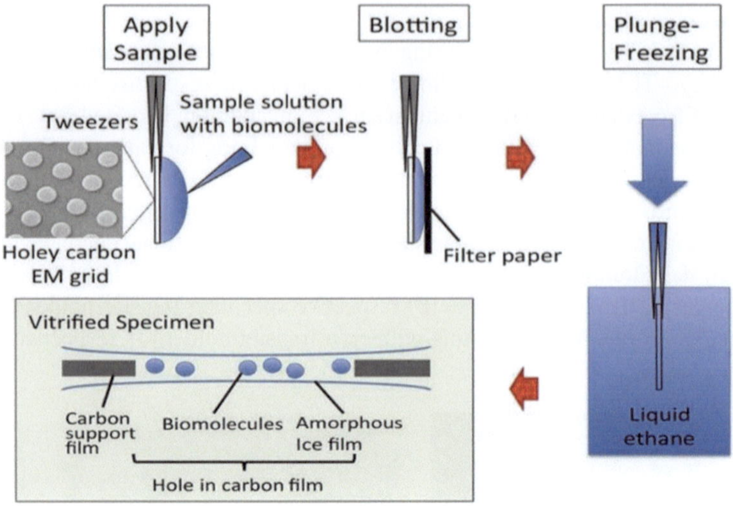

Fig. 6.3 Shows the handling of specimen loaded TEM grid for plunge freezing process (Adapted with permission from Murata et al. [3] under open access)

6.2.1.2 Cryo-TEM Grids Handling and Preparation

Cryo-TEM grids are specifically designed w.r.t. different grid preparation technique via different freezing processes and vitrification mechanism in presence of liquid ethane or nitrogen. Optimally designed grids having different type of support surfaces [4], will act as strong base for respective specimen during freezing process [3, 5]. This will be very much helpful in maintaining specimen integrity during in-process as well in EM imaging stage.

6.2.1.3 Anti Contamination Device (ACD)

The movement and induction of volatile phase called ‘frost’ inside column, exist due to high energy electron beam interaction specimen. This will create interference during EM imaging process. The presence of ACD system near to specimen holder, will keep specimen and electron beam-specimen region bring volatile component free path during imaging cycle. ACD system work on active gas flow mechanism for maintaining high precision precise environment at cryogenic condition. Figure 6.4, schematically demonstrated the working of ACD w.r.t. TEM operation.

6.2.1.4 Automated Specimen Transfer System

Chances of minimum errors and deviation from natural state of specimen visualization under TEM, will be enhanced in case of cryo-TEM analysis with the help

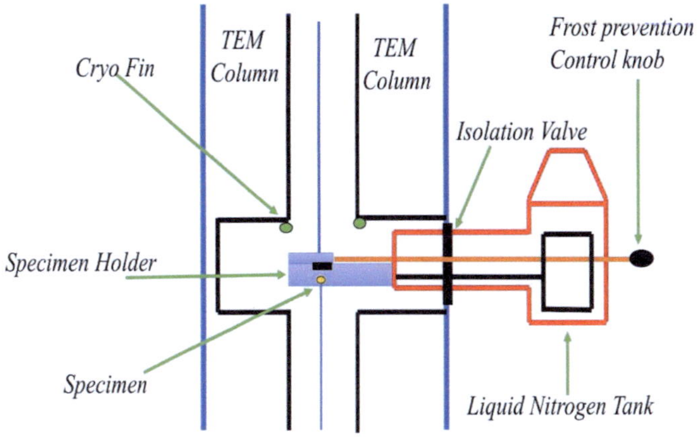

Fig. 6.4 Schematic representation of ACD position w.r.t. TEM column design

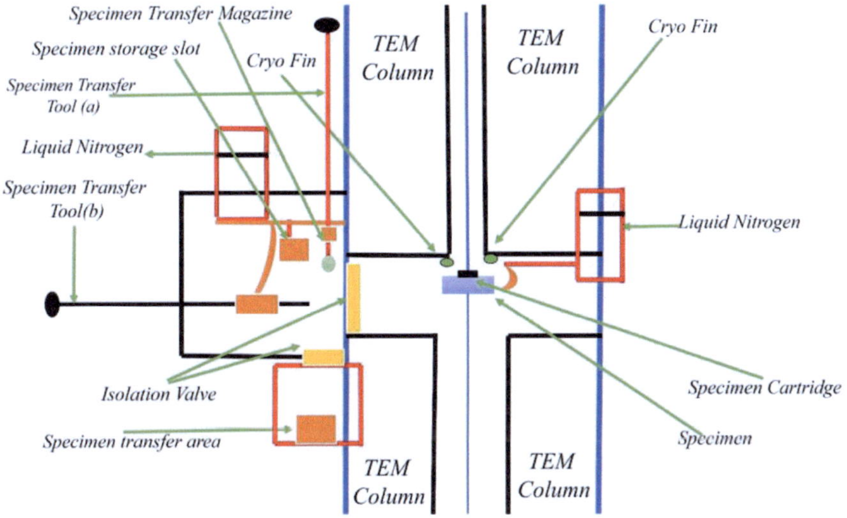

Fig. 6.5 Schematic representation view of automatic specimen transfer system during Cryo-TEM operation

of automated system for specimen transfer into electron microscope column. This device will be very much helpful in maintaining the specimen integrity and actual behaviour during its loading and unloading process. Figure 6.5, diagramically shows automatic specimen transfer system involved in transferring the TEM grid inside cryo-TEM column during its respective operation.

6.2.1.5 Low Dose Imaging Mode

The conditions of maintaining the integrity of specimen as well parallel high-resolution imaging, will be challenging for an electron microscopist. In addition to optimized sample preparation at standard conditions, delicate specimen can be analysed through low dose imaging mode under Cryo-TEM. Setting of low beam current, small spot size (small beam diameter), shorter specimen exposure time, use of appropriate energy filters and phase plate etc., parameters are very useful in generating sufficient contrast and high-resolution imaging w.r.t. specimen under study [6, 7].

6.2.1.6 Other Sample Preparation Techniques

In addition to availability of core technique i.e. Cryo-TEM, during processing of delicate specimen analysis, respective laboratory must be equipped with specialized sample preparation techniques like plunge freezing device, cryo-preservation, freeze fracture system, cryo-ultramicrotome etc. All stated techniques will be used for conditioning of hydrated specimen before inserting inside Cryo-TEM instrument. In addition, before proceeding for sample preparation and analysis in Cryo-TEM laboratory, lab manager must have to ensure and monitor routinely about controlled temperature, humidity, dusting, hygiene, safety etc. Ideally, a standard operating procedure (SOP) for entering, exist and operation related to respective laboratory must be practiced and followed.

Specialized and dedicated sample preparation tools and techniques w.r.t. cryo-TEM working and operation, facilitate the ideal imaging condition of biological or soft specimen having minimum artifacts and maximum functional information. The integration of cryogenic technologies with basic TEM instrumentation revolutionized the specimen study at nanoscale for insightful information.

6.3 Importance of Cryo-TEM in Comparison to Conventional TEM

Nature and properties of specimen will direct the selection and use of respective TEM for desired analysis. Biological or soft samples can be processed and analysed under Cryo-TEM instrument, in addition to their initial investigation under conventional TEM [8]. There are following basic and advanced factors related to cryo-TEM which make it demanding in comparison to conventional TEM.

6.3.1 Preservation of Native Structure

The presence of low temperature environment (cryogenic condition) will protect the biological or soft specimen from any stress and alteration w.r.t. respective basic structure. Conventional chemical fixation and dehydration-based techniques have possibility of shrinking and damaging the specimen natural state [9]. The ultimately the integrity of specimen will be maintained and preserved through standardized sample preparation protocols as per nature of sample.

6.3.2 Visualization of Dynamic Processes at High Resolution

Most of dynamic processes related to physiological working in biological species will be diminished through improper stabilization procedure. Under optimized cryogenic conditions w.r.t cryo-TEM analysis, researchers can capture/imaged/monitor different biological dynamic processes like protein folding, membrane dynamics and molecular interactions etc., nearly in their native states. Rarely reported molecular movement and transformation of delicate specimen from life or material sciences, will be reported with the help of cryo-TEM analysis [3, 10].

6.3.3 Advancement in Structural Biology

Cryo-TEM will have potential in visualization of specimens in hydrated state provides fundamental insights w.r.t. biomolecular natural state imaging with evaluation of innovative and efficient drug delivery system. Regenerated three-dimensional (3D) biomolecular structure of species like protein, viruses, nucleic acids or biological macromolecules etc., will be determined under 3D tomography mode of cryo-TEM (Cryo-ET). Under 3D Cryo-ET mode, specimen will be imaged for multiple images at different angles via specimen tilting features [11, 12]. Further, through suitable computational programming software's/models, 3D structural image of respective specimen will be generated to understand the wider functional aspect of respective material under study.

6.3.4 Nanomaterial Analysis

Conventional TEM will work normally on air drying of specimen loaded TEM grid before observing under suitable EM machine. Normally, direct air-drying methods is the basic cause of deviation in hydrated sample analysis under TEM analysis. The common challenges like shrinkage in original morphology, improper particle and respective distribution, aggregation and agglomeration etc., will be observed during imaging. Cryo-TEM will follow the maximum natural conditions specimen drying at low temperature without disturbing its natural molecular or chemical structure setup. With the observation and understanding of material physical, chemical or structural properties, one can develop novel synthesis method and can design innovate material-based technologies [13].

6.3.5 Multidisciplinary Applications

Cryo-TEM have diverse range of applicability in physics, chemistry, botany, zoology, pharmaceutical, environment science, medical science, material science etc. As in current scenario of research, synthesized material may have multidimensional features and applications, which may get implemented and validated via hybrid material development under Cryo-TEM [13].

The importance of Cryo-TEM is not about to underestimate the role of conventional TEM in research, but is in choosing an appropriate technique i.e. Cryo-TEM for appropriate sample analysis of biological samples under stable conditions. We are very sure that every sample will give novel results under electron microscopy analysis, unless it will be processed under optimized sample preparation procedure and analysed under appropriate instrumentation technique as per nature and type of specimen.

NOTE: Native state of living specimen will be visualized through respective vitrified state, via preservation of structural integrity of specimen facilitates insightful ultrastructural molecular imaging.

6.4 Category of Samples Analysis Under Cryo-TEM

Cryo-TEM is a versatile technique widely utilized in analysis of variety of samples which need careful preservation of their hydrated state. There are following category of specimen and related information which can be analysed under Cryo-TEM.

6.4.1 Biological Specimen

There are following type of biological species and related components, which can be analysed under Cryo-TEM.

6.4.1.1 Cell to Organelle

Biological species like tissue, cell or any other related component will be analysed under Cryo-TEM at maximum hydrated state for ultrastructural detail, membrane dynamics or intracellular interaction behaviour. Related species components like blood plasma, extracellular matrix, mucus etc., can be examined very delicately under Cryo-TEM [11].

6.4.1.2 Viruses

Well known and horrible COVID-19 virus make everyone aware about their adverse impact on human life on earth. On same line, research scientist with help of cryo-TEM can identify and explore about viruses' morphology and their assembly pathways w.r.t. different host environment, virology etc. With the help of analysis of viruses' species in their natural state under Cryo-TEM technique, will be very much helpful in respective vaccine development [14].

6.4.1.3 Protein and Macromolecule

Any living species on the earth have protein as the one of major component in physiological working mechanism. In order to understand the morphological aspect of individual or complex proteins and macromolecule assemblies for structural and functional aspect, can be elaborated and analysed under Cryo-TEM insightly [15].

6.4.2 Soft Materials

Species other than biological category, which have very delicate structure due to water-based network categorized as soft material. Stated specimens' analysis under Cryo-TEM will be very useful and informative due to respective imaging in nearly natural state. Related categories have been elaborated as mentioned below:

6.4.2.1 Lipid Bilayer and Membranes

Conventional TEM will lead to shrinkage and distortion of lipids bilayer, vesicles etc., during their imaging cycle. Low temperature environment under Cryo-TEM for different samples like lipid, fats, cholesterol based nanoparticles (NPs), vesicles etc., will lead to precise analysis of respective bilayers, membrane dynamics as well their interaction with different drugs or NPs [16].

6.4.2.2 Colloids

Colloidal nanoparticles are stable normally under respective dispersion form whereas solvent air-drying step led to aggregation or inhomogeneous distribution behaviour of respective active components. Cryo-TEM under controlled conditions bring stabilized and uniform imaging and evaluation of respective specimen behaviour with minimum drying and homogeneity challenges [17].

6.4.2.3 Gel and Hydrogel

Due to wide range of application of gel and hydrogel materials in tissue engineering, contact lenses, bone cement for orthopaedics, wound dressings etc., suggest respective material analysis under cryo-TEM for reliable and reproducible behaviour [18].

6.4.2.4 Nanomaterials

In addition to analysis of different nanomaterials analysis under normal TEM or HRTEM, respective materials can also be analysed under cryo-TEM for more insight. Materials like gold, silver colloidal suspension, semiconductor (TiO_2, ZnO etc.) or insulator (glasses etc.), will be analysed and imaged for investigating growth mechanism, aggregation behaviour under Cryo-TEM instrument more precisely [19].

6.4.2.5 Complex Environment Samples

Analysis of samples which directly extracted from natural source of material, will also be analysed under Cryo-TEM for accurate investigation. Specimen like contaminated water, adulterated milk, refined oil, catalyst, geological rocks analysis and respective minerals investigation etc., can be analysed for studying the different mechanisms in respective specimens [20].

6.4.2.6 Drug Delivery System

Novel fabrication and analysis of active pharmaceutical ingredient (API) with their stability study, drug delivery carriers' formulations (liposomes etc.) etc., will be performed very precisely in handling limitations as well for revised formulations for upcoming demands. Further, with the modification of different API's via active protein molecules bonding for novel efficient drug or biomolecule designs as biopharmaceutical compounds, which further can be imaged in realistic domain via extraordinary capabilities of Cryo-TEM [21].

From above mentioned samples categories analysis under cryo-TEM, researchers become able to imaged and credited certain basic and advanced scientific information of fragile and delicate specimen behaviour. The proper knowledge of specimen nature and properties, researchers can utilize maximum potentialities of instrumentation in simple to advance research accomplishments.

6.5 Crucial Phenomenon Related to Cryo-TEM

6.5.1 Vitrification

Vitrification is process which solidifies the liquid component of specimen into amorphous form via rapid cooling process. During cryofixation mechanism, it would not allow sample liquid component to crystallized and form non-vitreous ice crystal. Normally, most of physiological mechanism of any living species will propagates in fraction of seconds time will be freezes through vitrification step, will facilitate natural state imaging of specimen [22, 23]. Stated procedure facilitates the immobilization of different biological components constituents in current technique via cryofixation.

6.5.1.1 Challenge with Application of Vitrification

The rate of cooling is very crucial step during vitrification process. Slow as well fast rate of cooling may bring formation of ice crystallization. For example, slow rate of cooling brings hexagonal ice crystal at ambient pressure condition whereas fast cooling bring formation of cube ice crystal with specimen, in presence of nucleation centre. Liquid water will be supercooled to about – 25 °C with 9 μM tiny droplet diameter to – 46 and – 92 °C at 2048 MPa [5]. During cooling above stated temperature range, will facilitates the uniformly distribution of nucleation centre which good for proper freezing of specimen [5]. Under similar study, Thompson et al. [4] under Fig. 6.6 clearly shows the behaviour of specimen water freezing in (a) empty vitreous, (b–c) shows presence of ice crystal, whereas Fig. 6.6d depicts the probable ethane contamination during vitrification process.

Due to variation in interior cellular composition of different biological species like proteins, sugar, cations or anions etc., will shows variable freezing behaviour mechanism. The availability of variable concentration of salts or solutes in the interior and exterior cellular system, promote rupture or damage of respective cell walls and other biological functionaries. In order to restrict the ice formation process, inside and outside cellular system, specimen must be vitrified uniformly. Tokuyasu method is also known for use of cryoprotected chemically fixed specimen for rapid cooling (vitrification) in liquid nitrogen [24].

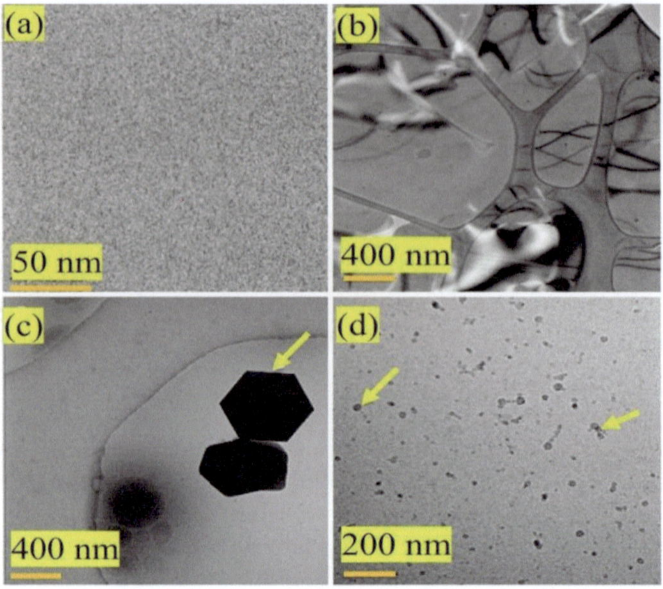

Fig. 6.6 Shows Vitreous and non-vitreous ice, **a** empty vitreous, **b** hexagonal ice, **c** large ice crystal, **d** probable ethane contamination (Adapted with permission from Thompson et al. [4] under open access)

6.5.1.2 Plunge Freezing

Cryo-immobilization of any cellular system, suspension etc., will be achieved with immersion of specimen thin liquid film into cryogen viz. ethane or propane, cooled in presence of liquid nitrogen [25]. Specimen layer must be as thin as possible, so as to ensure the rapid and uniform freezing of specimen during plunging process. As the process of cooling rate is at the rate of ~ 10^8 K/s, the overall sample vitrification process will depend on the cooling conditions of cryogen with nature of specimen under study. Preference for mixture of cryogens like ethane and propane etc., will be suggested in place of individual use. Specifically, ethane will exist in solid state at 77 K whereas combination of ethane and propane will be liquid state in similar temperature range. Due to stabilized and liquid environment of appropriate cryogen medium during vitrification having least damage on delicate support film on copper grid [26]. Figure 6.7a–f demonstrated the cryo-TEM images of eukaryotic cells, prokaryotic cells, isolated organelles, synthetic liposomes, viruses, macromolecular complexes specimen prior to their optimized sample preparation [4] respectively.

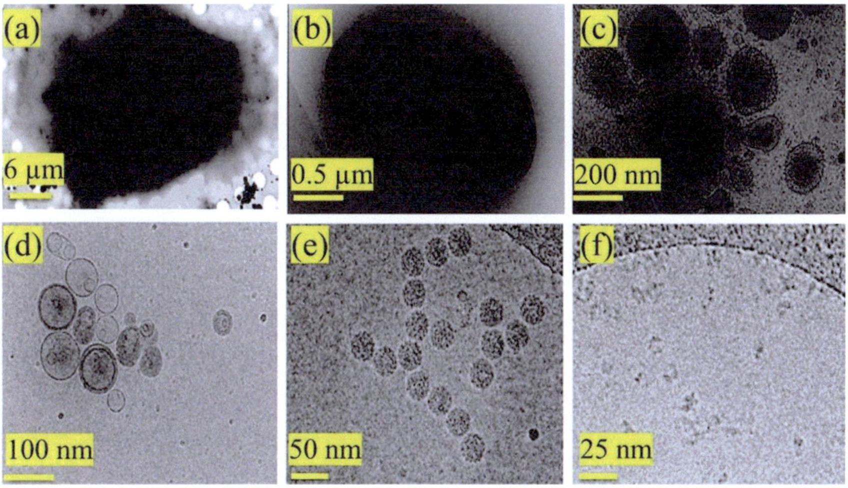

Fig. 6.7 Shows the cryo-TEM image of **a** Eukaryotic cells, **b** Prokaryotic cells, **c** Isolated organelles, **d** synthetic liposomes, **e** viruses, **f** macromolecular complexes (Adapted with permission from Thompson et al. [4] under open access)

6.5.1.3 High Pressure Freezing (HPF)

Thicker specimen like nuclear section of eukaryotic cell or tissue sections etc., which cannot be freeze under plunge freezing mode, will be processed via HPF. Basically, water expand its volume under appropriate conditions during crystallization. In continuation, as per well-known Le chatelier's principle, enhancement in ice volume will be hindered by external medium pressure which suppresses the both i.e. ice nucleation and respective growth behaviour. Means at high pressure condition i.e. 2048 bar, the specimen get lowering in both melting and freezing temperature to − 22 and − 92 °C respectively [27]. In addition, biological specimen having thickness upto 200 µm, will be vitrified at 2048 bar pressure at − 196 °C temperature in milliseconds with liquid nitrogen jet. Furthermore, with the higher pressure cryoprotectant medium environment, one can vitrify the specimen of thickness even high thick specimen (~ 600 µm) range [28].

The effect of high pressure frozen versus chemically fixed rat brain tissue specimen has been demonstrated under Fig. 6.8a–d [28]. Figure 6.8a, c demonstrate the high pressure frozen, freeze substituted with 2% osmium tetroxide specimen images has been presented whereas Fig. 6.8b, d depicts same specimen processing via chemical fixation with glutaraldehyde and osmium tetroxide. Figure 6.8a, c clearly shows high contrast images showing synaptic vesicles, fusion of vesicles, and uniform mass distribution etc. features, which are less clearly visible in chemically processed specimen under Fig. 6.8b, d [28].

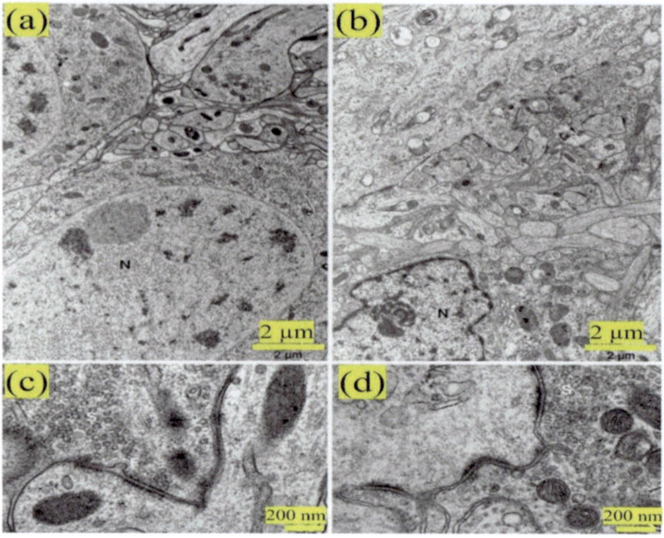

Fig. 6.8 **a**, **c** Demonstrate the high pressure frozen, freeze substituted with 2% Osmium tetroxide specimen whereas **b**, **d** depicts same specimen processing via chemical fixation with glutaraldehyde and osmium tetroxide respectively (Reprinted with permission from Studer et al. [28] under open access)

HPF directed stabilized specimen with electron transparent (~ 40–100 nm thickness) w.r.t. TEM analysis, will be precisely processed by cryo-ultramicrotome. Challenge of collapse of intercellular air-filled spaces specimen during HPF treatment for specimen like lungs tissue or plant leaves etc., will be protected via saturating the respective space with solvent not miscible with water. One similar study showing importance of HPF guided sample preparation has been presented in Fig. 6.9a–d [29]. Figure 6.9a shows ultrastructure image of ivy leaf with (b) respective cell organelle through high pressure frozen and freeze substituted process. Further, Fig. 6.9c shows of cellular as well related neuropil imaging of organotypic brain tissue culture of hippocampus of mouse. Similarly, under Fig. 6.9d depicted langerhans blood cell imaging having healthy cells adsorbed on sapphire disc whereas top position cell shows DNA localized based in nucleus with empty vesicles in respective cytoplasm. Whole observation of state imaging has been preserved through high pressure frozen and freeze substituted process [29].

6.5.1.4 Self-pressurized Rapid Freezing (SPRF)

SPRF will proceed in plunging of specimen under defined tube of copper or aluminium material in presence of suitable cryogen [30]. Under this technique, water will expand inside tube having pressure under definite volume (isochoric freezing). Presence of tube wall will support growing ice crystal concentrate cryoprotectant for

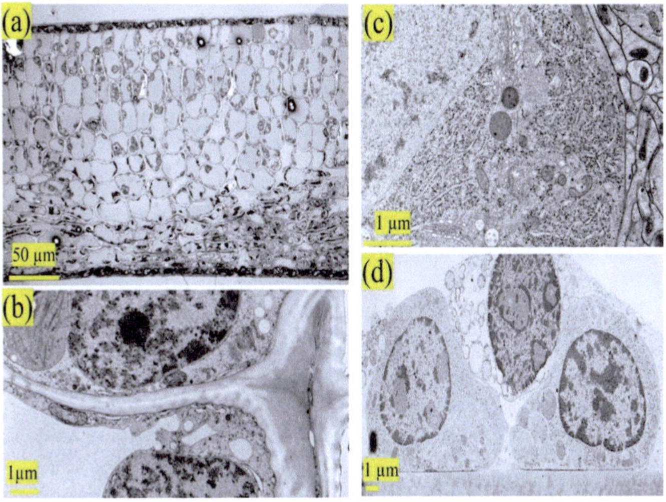

Fig. 6.9 Shows high pressure frozen and freeze substituted process-based demonstration, **a** ultra-structure image of ivy leaf with **b** respective cell organelle, **c** cellular as well related neuropil imaging of organotypic brain tissue culture of hippocampus of mouse, **d** langerhans blood cell imaging having healthy cells adsorbed on sapphire disc whereas top position cell shows DNA localized based in nucleus with emplty vesicles in respective cytoplasm (Reprinted with permission from Vanhecke et al. [29])

vitrification process. Further, faster cooling system will be felicitated via higher heat diffusion coefficient of crystal ice [30].

It is reported in the literature that vitrification rate for both HPF and SPRF mode is comparable. In addition, in case of eukaryotic cell vitrification via SPRF for (30–60) s, lead to loss in native state of respective species under study [31]. Either the cellular non-reactive coating inside the copper wall tube or use of aluminium tube would be the best alternatives while working with SPRF technique.

6.6 Freezing Techniques w.r.t. Cryo-TEM Analysis

The preservation of specimens prior to vitrification process need to preserved below devitrification temperature i.e. − 136 °C. As per limited penetration ability of TEM w.r.t. specimen thickness ~ 1 µm, specimen like bacteria, virus, subcellular cells etc., will be imaged directly under cryo-TEM. Whereas thick specimen needs proper vitrification process, optimized under ultrathin sectioning with cryo-ultramicrotome below devitrification point, will be imaged under cryo-TEM termed as CEMOVIS. In addition, focussed ion beam (FIB) technique will also be utilized during precise thinning of specimen.

6.6.1 Cemovis

This is technique which deal with imaging of biological or delicate specimen under Cro-TEM through vitrification, ultrathin sectioning under cryo-ultramicrotome steps. The only challenge in current technique is maintaining the integrity of specimen just below its devitrification temperature. Proper vitrified specimen will be optimally fix, dehydrate and stained as requirement of sample, bring atomic structure preservation and quality imaging [32, 33]. Use of appropriate amount of chemicals like dextran (20%) in HPF or SPRF process, will bring minimum possibility of ice formation during vitrification cycle. In addition, the vitreous form of water based stabilized specimen ultrathin sectioning may lead to deformation during cutting process. The resin embedded specimen will be sliced through water boat surface of diamond knife surface whereas with CEMOVIS mode have non-availability of any liquid surface for specimen slice floating. Due to which issues of chattering, compression etc., will be faced during thin slices of vitreous specimen. Condition like humidity of cryo-ultramicrotome chamber below 1%, use of un-damaged knife cutting edge, optimized cutting speed, cryo-cutting tool free from frost contamination etc., will lead to ultrathin section having minimum artefacts. Handling and transfer of vitreous specimen section from diamond knife edge to TEM grid will be felicitated by very important tool called micromanipulator. Due to much delicacy and sensitivity in stated process w.r.t. specimen vitrification, thin section handling from knife surface to grid etc., poses it as a tedious assignment for researchers [5].

6.6.2 FIB of Vitreous Specimen

The ultimate goal of whole vitrification and ultrathin sectioning of specimen will for stable electron transparent sections for Cryo-TEM analysis. Under FIB technique, vitreous specimen will be bombarded with gallium ion beam for ablation via sputtering principle. The conditions like 10pA current at 30 kV accelerating voltage of ion beam during thinning of specimen surface, will avoid the chances of devitrification [34]. In addition, cryo-FIB technique will also be preferred in biological or soft specimen to get more concise and valid results of specimen. In addition to CEMOVIS and HPF technique for delicate specimen EM preparations, FIB and Cryo-FIB techniques, will also valuable support and new insight in specimen physiological and metabolic working visualization [35].

6.6.3 Freeze Substitution (FS)

FS technique meant for preparing sample via room temperature ultramicrotomy prior to vitrification process. FS process will follow fixation and dehydration process of specimen preparation with keeping specimen below devitrification temperature. During vitrification process, transition from ice crystal formation to hexagonal crystal will be followed ~ −80 °C. The structural preservation of specimen will be supported by rearrangement of water molecules without any specimen structural segregation [36]. Figure 6.10a–k shows multiple artefacts (crystallization of ice) dominated images during specimen rapid freezing processing in cryo-TEM [37]. Figure 6.10 shows multiple artefacts (a) hexagonal ice crystal during rapid freezing, (b) presence of cubic ice crystal through warming of vitreous ice, (c) formation of large ice crystal (frost mechanism) during atmospheric exposure. In continuation Fig. 6.10(d) demonstrated contamination in column, (e) under-focus TEM image, with (f) high contrast image (at 1 μm under-focus). Simultaneously, Fig. 6.10g, h depicts radiation damage effect to high resolution specimen feature at 10 and 90 e/Å^2 beam parameter, (i)bobble gas formation of ice whereas (j) shows specimen movement during imaging lead to blurriness, (k) modern direct detection system recue useful information respectively [37].

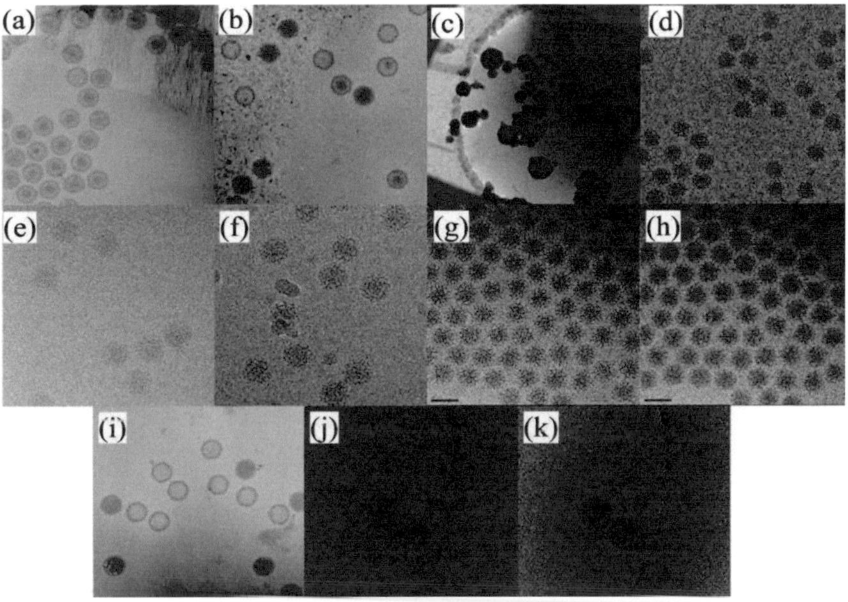

Fig. 6.10 Shows multiple artefacts. **a** Hexagonal ice crystal with rapid freezing, **b** cubic ice crystal during warming of vitreous ice, **c** formation of large ice crystal (frost) during atmospheric exposure, **d** subtle mottled contamination due to contamination in column, **e** under-focus (1 μm underfocus) TEM image, **f** greater contrast image (1 μm underfocus), **g**, **h** Radiation damage effect to high resolution specimen feature at 10 and 90 e/Å^2, **i** bobble gas form of ice, **j** specimen movement during imaging lead to blurriness, **k** modern direct detection system recue useful information (Adapted with permission from Bhella et al. [37] under open access)

From above all discussion about the cryogenic sample preparation and analysis under cryo-TEM, we can achieve insight about the actual state of existence of cellular system, physiological behaviour of different specimen under EM analysis.

6.7 Optimized Cryo-TEM Imaging

In coming paragraph, an attempt has been made to demonstrate the minimum artefacts-based specimen analysis under cryo-TEM. Ultimate goal of current subsection is to make researchers aware about factors affecting quality sample preparation, handling of delicate specimen and cryo-TEM image processing with precise interpretation of respective data.

In addition to controlled and finely tuned rapid freezing parameters according to method like plunge freezing, high pressure plunge freezing etc., there are following major and minor factors which will affect directly and indirectly vitrification process.

6.7.1 Preservation of Specimen State

Before proceeding for vitrification stage of specimen, most of time need to stabilized through optimized fixation or dehydration procedure. In case of delicate suspension specimen state, it must have minimum aggregation before proceeding for low temperature stabilization process [22].

6.7.2 Grid Preparation

Properly standardized grids having suitable support film of carbon, lacy carbon, holey carbon or graphene etc., will be used during respective vitrification process. Stable and non-reactive support film based stable TEM grid will be main factor in stabilizing the specimen during rapid freezing as well in during cryo-EM imaging. In case of suspension-based specimen preparation, prior glow discharge treated grids must be used to ensure maximum deposition of particles on grid support surface. In addition, controlled sample volume dispensing tool on TEM grid led to uniform vitrification and minimum artefacts formation [3, 4].

6.7.3 Controlled Blotting Procedure

Prior to dispensing of appropriate volume of solution on suitable TEM grid, formation of uniform layer of specimen on grid surface is highly expected. Manual use of suitable filter paper shape or blotting instrument etc., will be used to obtain a uniform, even surface of specimen deposition on grid surface. Blotting time and pressure during removal of excess of solution will be decided and optimized as per desired and nature of specimen during the process [3].

6.7.4 Controlled Temperature and Humidity

Equal importance for freezing chamber as well laboratory environment during sample preparation under cryo-TEM w.r.t. controlled temperature and humidity control, will be mandatorily required. Very well controlled and standardized temperature conditions, will lead to have minimum chances of ice formation, thermal drift during vitrification process. Temperature mapping conditions must be utilized during imaging to ensure the temperature variation range during imaging. Use of controlled desiccators and desiccants must be used during the whole procedure to ensure low humidity to avoid devitrification conditions of specimen [38].

6.7.5 Storage and Transfer of TEM Grid

There are maximum chances in devitrification of specimen on grid during exposure to open air while transportation or during their preservation. User must have to preserve vitrified specimen in cryo-TEM holder or cryogenic boxes during transportation and preservation time till imaging under cryo-TEM. Handling of vitrified specimen grids will require very expertise and delicate care to ensure minimum mechanical damage to specimen [3].

6.7.6 Use of Imaging Filters

Cryo-TEM technique face challenge of low signal to noise ratio, poor contrast, beam induced damage etc., which can be improved through use of suitable imaging filters during imaging cycle [39]. There are following type of imaging filters:

6.7.7 Energy Filters

Cryo-TEM equipped with energy filters have ability to block inelastic scattered electron based on energy loss after beam interaction with specimen during imaging process. Reduction in inelastic electron signal during imaging will contribute in improved image contrast whereas quality elastic scattered beam lead to enhance the respective image resolution [40].

6.7.8 *Phase Plate*

Issue of low contrast and distortion during delicate specimen imaging will be optimized and improved with the use of suitable phase plate. It will work on the principle of generating in shift the phase of electrons (like 90° phase shift) w.r.t unscattered electrons. It will improve the quality and visibility of specimen detail with minimum distortion during cryo-TEM imaging [41].

6.8 Application of Energy Filters/Phase Plate in Cryo-TEM

6.8.1 *Contrast Enhancement*

The low contrast images during Cryo-TEM analysis, will be improvised to high contrast with the use of energy filter or phase plate via selectively filtering the desired energy or phase of electrons during imaging. The use of stated accessories will bring visualization of very minute information of delicate or biological specimens [40, 41].

6.8.2 *Reduced Beam Damage*

The challenge of cryo-TEM high energy electron beam adverse impact on integrity of specimen will be protected via use of energy filters/phase plate. Use of energy filters/phase plate will block the specific high energy electrons before exposure on specimen surface. This will protect specimen with radiation damage having minimum impact of beam induced specimen imaging [40, 41].

6.8.3 *Improved Signal to Noise Ratio (SNR)*

During routine imaging of specimen, operator handling cryo-TEM will face low SNR due to interference phase present in specimen commonly due to impurities, debris etc. The use of suitable energy filters/phase plate etc., during TEM imaging will remove/block stray signal of electron beam (inelastic electron) from main signal. This will enhance the SNR with highlighting very fine detail of specimen having even low contrast problem [40, 41].

The use of energy filters/phase plates will help in explaining the physiological functioning of biological or soft specimen very insightfully through EM imaging. The selection and use of appropriate energy filter type and phase shift with their compatibility with respective EM instrument. Proper calibration of whole setup with main EM instrument will further improve and enhance the overall imaging and information domain of specimen study.

6.8.4 Specimen 3D Construction

The three-dimensional (3D) reconstruction of specimen visualization will be executed by single particle reconstruction (SPR) and cryo-electron tomography (Cryo-ET) modes of cryo-TEM operation [11, 12]. Broadly, homogenous specimen like viruses, vault particles or DNA origami frames etc., will be analysed via single particle construction with averaging projection process. Whereas collection of multiple images of inhomogeneous structures for specimen like lipids or polymer nanomaterials (polymorphous nature) based formulations will be analysed via tilting of the specimen [19]. Figure 6.11a shows the JEOL CryoARM 300 instrument having robotic system in sample loading and unloading, whereas Fig. 6.11b shows reconstruction image of complex lumazine synthase having 2.2 Å resolution [37].

SPR mode of operation under Cryo-TEM have higher resolution due to large number of images averaging feature in comparison to Cryo-ET analysis [11]. Limited information aspect of 2D images has been resolved via 3D construction of specimen under SPR and cryo-ET mode of operation. SPR have equipped with reconstruction of images with insights for wedge or cone aspect of high-resolution image of specimen whereas Cryo-ET have limited resolution in one direction. Study of specimen

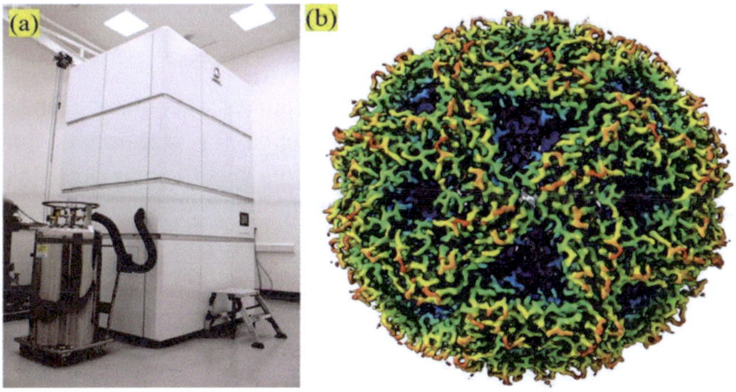

Fig. 6.11 **a** Shows the JEOL CryoARM 300 instrument, **b** shows reconstruction image of complex lumazine synthase having 2.2 Å resolution respectively (Adapted with permission from Bhella et al. [37] under open access)

through current mode of study will be really helpful in developing next generation nanoparticles or nanodrug or novel nanomaterial having predefined functionality and possible activity [42, 43].

6.9 Application of Cryo-TEM

As the imaging of any sensitive specimen is difficult due to their delicate structure, cryo-TEM technique has achieved the high-quality visualization via high resolution imaging. This will be really helpful in predicting and explaining many operational mechanisms of different cellular functions, metabolism system etc., very closely. There are following areas under which cryo-TEM capabilities can be utilized.

6.9.1 Dynamic Structural Behaviour

Any novel drug delivery mechanism or cellular functional behaviour, will be observed and explained with the help of cryo-TEM imaging very accurately. The optimized sample preparation via vitrification process will enables researchers in visualization of phenomenon like protein conformation, molecular interactions or cellular functions etc. Figure 6.12a shows cryo-TEM images of dynamic assembly pathways of polymer (Poly (ethylene oxide-*b*-poly (octadecyl methacrylate) (PEO-*b*-PODMA)), (b–d) shows respective specimen dispersion at fix amount of water, whereas (e–g) shows images with increasing temperature and (h–j) shows behaviour with decreasing temperature respectively [13].

6.9.2 High Resolution Imaging

In addition to observation of dynamic behaviour of specimen, respective high-resolution (HR) imaging was always a challenge for researchers during TEM imaging. Due to optimized stabilization of delicate specimen at suitable conditions bring specimen imaging possible at high resolution regime bring explanation of insightful atomic and molecular level phenomenon [19].

6.9.3 Multimodal Application

Combining the cryo-TEM mode of operation with advance imaging modalities like cryo-tomography, high resolution fluorescence microscopy etc., will enhance the

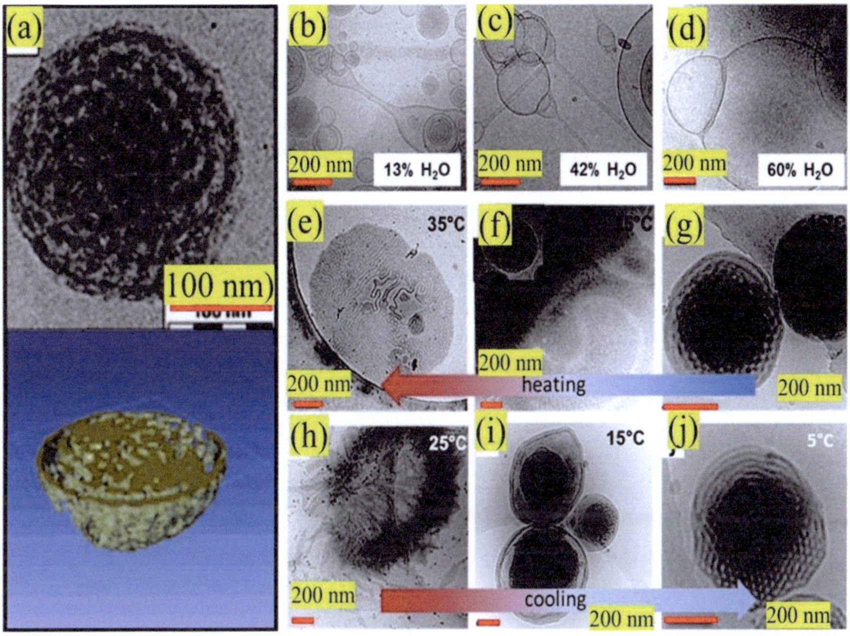

Fig. 6.12 **a** Shows cryo-TEM images of dynamic assembly pathways of polymer (Poly (ethylene oxide-*b*-poly (octadecyl methacrylate) (PEO-*b*-PODMA)), figure **b–d** shows respective specimen dispersion at fix amount of water, figure **e–g** shows images with increasing temperature, figure **h–j** shows behaviour with decreasing temperature respectively (Adapted with permission from Patterson et al. [13] under open access)

scope of interpretation and application of respective materials in present for future updations [11, 19].

6.9.4 Emerging Area of Medicine and Biotechnology

The use of cryo-TEM technique in drug delivery mechanisms, different viruses growth and mutations, insight behind various diseases spreading mechanism with development of targeted therapies etc., has unlimited chances in understanding respective areas very precisely and closely [21].

6.9.5 Single Particle Analysis w.r.t. Cryo-ET

Through cryo-TEM analysis of biological or soft specimen, one can analyse single particle and tomography analysis for 3D structure of respective materials. Different image reconstruction logarithms and computational methods while analysing large data sets, will be very much helpful in explaining, exploring the complex biological physiological behaviour [11, 12]. For example, electron micrograph of frozen hydrated section of human skin (desmosomes) has been shown at Fig. 6.13a with averaged sub-tomogram of desmosomes section representation (left) and respective density mapp (right) (b) whereas (c) shows molecular model of two cadherin tetramers, and (d) molecular cadherin model fitted with density mapp respectively [28].

From all above stated applications, we can claim a full proof database for unexplored world of scientific facts related to biological metabolism, different diseases behaviour, nanomaterials growth mechanisms, in form of realistic imaging database through Cryo-TEM and its related modes of operation.

NOTE: Cryo-TEM analysis revolutionize the research areas belongs to medical research, drug delivery through exploration of insightful functional aspect in their native state, supporting towards diseases remediation and novel drug development.

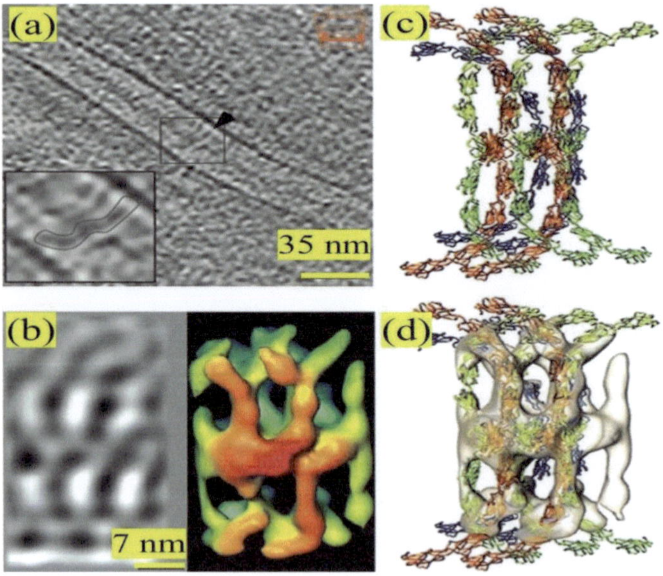

Fig. 6.13 **a** Electron micrograph of frozen hydrated section of human skin depicting desmosomes, **b** averaged sub-tomogram of desmosomes section (left) and respective density mapp (right), **c** molecular model of two cadherin tetramers, **d** molecular cadherin model fitted with density mapp (Adapted with permission from Studer et al. [28] under open access)

6.10 Protocol w.r.t. Specimen Analysis Under Cryo-TEM

Specimen analysis under cryo-TEM, will be observed with a validated and standardized protocol. In current paragraph, a protocol has been presented for two broad categories of specimen w.r.t. Cryo-TEM analysis (1) biological specimen (animal and plant tissue etc.), (2) Suspended specimen (bacteriophage, bacteria, viruses, nanoparticles suspension, lipid nanoparticles, emulsions etc.).

6.10.1 Analysis of Biological Specimen

There are following general steps which can be followed while preparing for biological sample under cryo-TEM analysis:

Step 1: Fixation:

(a) **Sample Extraction**: Take appropriate size like ~ (1–3) mm of specimen (animal or plant tissue).
(b) **Cryo-Fixation**: Use the suitable cryofixation technique like plunge freezing, high pressure freezing, self-pressurized rapid freezing, will be directly applied for washed fresh specimen.

Step 2: Embedding

Optimally fixed biological specimen will be embedded with freshly prepared resin on silicone capsules or embedding plate. Detail procedure will be at Chap. 5, Sect. 5.5.3.

Step 3: Cryo Sectioning

Ideally cryo-ultramicrotome or normal ultramicrotome will be utilized in ultrathin sectioning of specimens in range from 50 to 100 nm as nature of specimen.

Step 4: Staining

Post staining procedure of specimen will heavy metals like uranyl acetate or lead citrate etc., will be performed on above specimen supported on TEM grid. Related detail of staining procedure has been summarized at Chap. 5, Sect. 5.4.5.

Step 5: Cryo-TEM Imaging

Cryo-TEM instrument at optimum accelerating voltage (80–300 kV) as per observed contrast of specimen, will be utilized in order to capture quality imaging.

Step 6: Interpretation of Results

Most importantly, cryo-TEM respective data interpretation will need deep knowledge and understanding of biological specimen working mechanism with ability to distinguish between artefacts from actual organelles behaviour.

6.10.2 Analysis of Suspension Based Specimen

There are following general steps need to follow while preparing for suspension sample under cryo-TEM analysis:

Step 1: Suspension Preparation

Well dispersed suspension of specimens needs to prepare in suitable solvent like buffer etc. Final suspension must be free from aggregates.

Step 2: TEM Grid Conditioning

In order to ensure maximum deposition of NPs on support film of TEM grid, respective grid will be exposed under glow discharge technique.

Step 3: Drop Casting

Apply (2–5) μl drop of suspension specimen on glow discharged TEM grid. Time to stay of specimen droplet on grid surface, will vary according to requirement of maximum spreading of NPs on support surface.

Step 4: Blotting

Remove excess of solution present on TEM grid after probable maximum deposition of desired material on grid surface. Removal of excess solution from grid surface will be take place with sharp edge-based filter paper pieces or blotting device. Over deposition or under deposition time of specimen on TEM grid will lead to issue of over thick or low concentration of specimen, respectively.

Step 5: Vitrification (Rapid Freezing)

The blotted TEM grid will be quickly proceeded for vitrification process via plunge freezing, HPF or more suitable technique.

Step 6: Cryo-TEM Imaging

Initially transfer the vitrified TEM grid into cryo-TEM holder with maintaining the respective environment during loading and imaging ~ −150 °C. Finally, capturing of specimen images under cryo-TEM will proceed via optimization of different factors like accelerating voltage, magnification, beam current etc.

Step 6: Interpretation of Results

Analyse and explain critically the respective data captured under cryo-TEM with expertise and experience in respective field.

In addition to stated protocol at Sects. 6.10.1 and 6.10.2, researchers/scientist may need to minor reschedule of sample preparation protocol w.r.t. cryo-TEM analysis, as per specimen nature and properties.

6.11 Conclusion

Impressive advancement and development in hardware and software w.r.t. TEM basic and advance operations, bring excellent improvement in data generation of hydrated sample through '*Cryo-TEM*' instrumentation. Challenges of hydrated specimen visualization w.r.t. conventional TEM, have been proposed with the use of Cryo-TEM at optimized low temperature conditions. The process of vitrification brings non-interfering amorphous water phase during imaging lead to quality specimen analysis with minimum artefacts generation.

Initially, we have explained about the basic features and working of cryo-TEM and supporting techniques. This includes information about cryo-TEM specimen holder, grid preparation procedure, specimen transfer mechanism and role of low dose imaging etc. The controlled sample preparation and precise analysis conditions under cryo-TEM operation, bring advancement in visualization of dynamic delicate structural analysis, advanced structural investigation via Cryo-ET or routine stabilized nanomaterial analysis. Wide variety of specimen under biological specimen category including different cellular systems, bacteria, viruses, proteins, macromolecules etc., can be analysed under Cryo-TEM. Parallely, suspension-based specimen includes lipid, emulsion, colloids, hydrogel, nanomaterials, drug delivery system etc., also has been analysed under respective mode EM analysis.

During Cryo-TEM imaging, sensitivity to high energy electron beam, beam induced artefacts on specimen surface, low imaging contrast or formation of ice crystal during vitrification etc., are the routine challenges, which need proper control and validation. Respective challenges has been controlled and minimized with level of expertise of operator and availability of advance techniques via controlling parameter of respective technique very precisely. Challenge of beam harsh behaviour due to specimen delicacy can also be handle with low dose imaging. Further, specimen drifting during imaging cycle, maintained via use of direct electron detector with frame averaging whereas low contrast imaging proceed with optimized phase contrast imaging through Cryo-TEM.

Further, in order to extract insightful information related to specimen through cryo-TEM imaging, we have elaborated about dos and don'ts during preservation of specimen, grid preparation and blotting, rapid freezing of specimen on grid, storage and handling of grid. Furthermore, the use of energy filters and phase filters during cryo-TEM operation have further improved the issues of low contrast, low signal to noise ratio and beam induced damage to specimen imaging. SPR and Cryo-ET mode of Cryo-TEM operation has further upgraded the in-depth explanation and interpretation high-resolution imaging of specimens.

Conclusively, cryo-TEM presented a novel and precise analysis procedure for hydrated specimen preparation and respective analysis. The imaging of biological physiological behaviour, diseases mechanism, realistic drug delivery system and nanomaterial growth and self-assembly trend etc., has been presented in more accurate and authentic way via Cryo-TEM analysis.

Declaration

Author declares that there is no personal or financial conflict of interest regarding publication of this chapter.

References

1. Williams, R.E.A., McComb, D.W., Subramaniam, S.: Cryo-electron microscopy instrumentation and techniques for life sciences and materials science. MRS Bull. **44**(12), 929–934 (2019). https://doi.org/10.1557/mrs.2019.286
2. Milne, J.L.S., Borgnia, M.J., Bartesaghi, A., Tran, E.E.H., Earl, L.A., Schauder, D.M., Lengyel, J., Pierson, J., Patwardhan, A., Subramaniam, S.: Cryo-electron microscopy—a primer for the non-microscopist. FEBS J. **280**(1), 28–45 (2013). https://doi.org/10.1111/febs.12078
3. Murata, K., Wolf, M.: Cryo-electron microscopy for structural analysis of dynamic biological macromolecules. Biochimica et Biophysica Acta (BBA) Gen. Subj. **1862**(2), 324–334 (2018). https://doi.org/10.1016/j.bbagen.2017.07.020
4. Thompson, R.F., Walker, M., Siebert, C.A., Ranson, N.A.: An introduction to sample preparation and imaging by cryo-electron microscopy for structural biology. **100**, 3–15. https://doi.org/10.1016/j.ymeth.2016.02.017
5. Mielańczyk, Ł., Matysiak, N., Klymenko, O., Wojnicz, R.: Transmission electron microscopy of biological samples. In: Maaz, K. (Ed.) The Transmission Electron Microscope - Theory and Applications. InTech (2015). https://doi.org/10.5772/60680
6. Fujiyoshi, Y.: Low dose techniques and cryo-electron microscopy. In: Schmidt-Krey, I., Cheng, Y. (Eds.) Electron Crystallography of Soluble and Membrane Proteins. Methods in Molecular Biology, vol. 955, pp. 103–118. Humana Press, Totowa (2013). https://doi.org/10.1007/978-1-62703-176-9_6
7. Spoth, K., Yu, Y., Nguyen, K., Chen, Z., Muller, D., Kourkoutis, L.: Dose-efficient cryo-STEM imaging of vitrified biological samples. Microsc. Microanal. **26**(S2), 1482–1483 (2020). https://doi.org/10.1017/S1431927620018279
8. Li, T., Nowell, C.J., Cipolla, D., Rades, T., Boyd, B.J.: Direct comparison of standard transmission electron microscopy and cryogenic-TEM in imaging nanocrystals inside liposomes. Mol. Pharm. **16**(4), 1775–1781 (2019). https://doi.org/10.1021/acs.molpharmaceut.8b01308
9. Mielanczyk, L., Matysiak, N., Michalski, M., Buldak, R., Wojnicz, R.: Closer to the native state. Critical evaluation of cryo-techniques for transmission electron microscopy: preparation of biological samples. Folia Histochem Cytobiol. **52**(1), 1–17 (2014). https://doi.org/10.5603/FHC.2014.0001
10. Bonilla, S.L., Kieft, J.S.: The promise of cryo-EM to explore rna structural dynamics. J. Mol. Biol. **434**(18), 167802 (2022). https://doi.org/10.1016/j.jmb.2022.167802
11. Nogales, E., Mahamid, J.: Bridging structural and cell biology with cryo-electron microscopy. Nature **628**(8006), 47–56 (2024). https://doi.org/10.1038/s41586-024-07198-2
12. Young, L.N., Villa, E.: Bringing structure to cell biology with cryo-electron tomography. Annu. Rev. Biophys. **52**(1), 573–595 (2023). https://doi.org/10.1146/annurev-biophys-111622-091327
13. Patterson, J.P., Xu, Y., Moradi, M.-A., Sommerdijk, N.A.J.M., Friedrich, H.: CryoTEM as an advanced analytical tool for materials chemists. Acc. Chem. Res. **50**(7), 1495–1501 (2017). https://doi.org/10.1021/acs.accounts.7b00107
14. Bodakuntla, S., Kuhn, C.C., Biertümpfel, C., Mizuno, N.: Cryo-electron microscopy in the fight against COVID-19—mechanism of virus entry. Front. Mol. Biosci. **10**, 1252529 (2023). https://doi.org/10.3389/fmolb.2023.1252529
15. Costa, T.R.D., Ignatiou, A., Orlova, E.V.: Structural analysis of protein complexes by cryo electron microscopy. In: Journet, L., Cascales, E. (Eds.) Bacterial Protein Secretion Systems.

Methods in Molecular Biology, vol. 1615, pp. 377–413. Springer, New York (2017). https://doi.org/10.1007/978-1-4939-7033-9_28.
16. Fox, Mulligan, S., Sung, J., Dowling, Q., Fung, H.W.M., Vedvick, T., Coler, R.: Cryogenic transmission electron microscopy of recombinant tuberculosis vaccine antigen with anionic liposomes reveals formation of flattened liposomes. IJN 1367 (2014). https://doi.org/10.2147/IJN.S56582
17. Frederik, P.M., Sommerdijk, N.: Spatial and temporal resolution in cryo-electron microscopy—a scope for nano-chemistry. Curr. Opin. Colloid Interface Sci. **10**(5–6), 245–249 (2005). https://doi.org/10.1016/j.cocis.2005.09.018
18. Da Silva, L.C.E., Borges, A.C., De Oliveira, M.G., De Farias, M.A.: Visualization of supramolecular structure of pluronic F127 micellar hydrogels using cryo-TEM. MethodsX **7**, 101084 (2020). https://doi.org/10.1016/j.mex.2020.101084
19. Stewart, P.L.: Cryo-electron microscopy and cryo-electron tomography of nanoparticles. WIREs Nanomed. Nanobiotechnol. **9**(2), e1417 (2017). https://doi.org/10.1002/wnan.1417
20. Hutchings, J., Zanetti, G.: Fine details in complex environments: the power of cryo-electron tomography. Biochem. Soc. Trans. **46**(4), 807–816 (2018). https://doi.org/10.1042/BST20170351
21. Filippov, S.K., Khusnutdinov, R., Murmiliuk, A., Inam, W., Zakharova, L.Ya., Zhang, H., Khutoryanskiy, V.V.: Dynamic light scattering and transmission electron microscopy in drug delivery: a roadmap for correct characterization of nanoparticles and interpretation of results. Mater. Horiz. **10**(12), 5354–5370 (2023). https://doi.org/10.1039/D3MH00717K
22. Weissenberger, G., Henderikx, R.J.M., Peters, P.J.: Understanding the invisible hands of sample preparation for cryo-EM. Nat. Methods **18**(5), 463–471 (2021). https://doi.org/10.1038/s41592-021-01130-6
23. Egelhaaf, S.U., Schurtenberger, P., Müller, M.: New controlled environment vitrification system for cryo-transmission electron microscopy: design and application to surfactant solutions. J. Microsc. **200**(2), 128–139 (2000). https://doi.org/10.1046/j.1365-2818.2000.00747.x
24. Loussert Fonta, C., Leis, A., Mathisen, C., Bouvier, D.S., Blanchard, W., Volterra, A., Lich, B., Humbel, B.M.: Analysis of acute brain slices by electron microscopy: a correlative light-electron microscopy workflow based on Tokuyasu cryo-sectioning. J. Struct. Biol. **189**(1), 53–61 (2015). https://doi.org/10.1016/j.jsb.2014.10.011
25. Tivol, W.F., Briegel, A., Jensen, G.J.: An improved cryogen for plunge freezing. Microsc. Microanal. **14**(5), 375–379 (2008). https://doi.org/10.1017/S1431927608080781
26. Carragher, B., Kisseberth, N., Kriegman, D., Milligan, R.A., Potter, C.S., Pulokas, J., Reilein, A.: Leginon: an automated system for acquisition of images from vitreous ice specimens. J. Struct. Biol. **132**(1), 33–45 (2000). https://doi.org/10.1006/jsbi.2000.4314
27. Kanno, H., Speedy, R., Angell, C.: Supercooling of water to −92 °C under pressure. **189**, 880–881. https://doi.org/10.1126/science.189.4206.880
28. Studer, D., Humbel, B.M., Chiquet, M.: Electron microscopy of high pressure frozen samples: bridging the gap between cellular ultrastructure and atomic resolution. Histochem. Cell Biol. **130**(5), 877–889 (2008). https://doi.org/10.1007/s00418-008-0500-1
29. Vanhecke, D., Graber, W., Studer, D.: Close-to-native ultrastructural preservation by high pressure freezing. Methods Cell Biol. **88** (2008). https://doi.org/10.1016/S0091-679X(08)00409-3
30. Rolle, K., Okotrub, K.A., Zaytseva, I.V., Babin, S.A., Surovtsev, N.V.: Self-pressurised rapid freezing at arbitrary cryoprotectant concentrations. J. Microsc. **292**(1), 27–36 (2023). https://doi.org/10.1111/jmi.13220
31. Han, H.-M., Huebinger, J., Grabenbauer, M.: Self-pressurized rapid freezing (SPRF) as a simple fixation method for cryo-electron microscopy of vitreous sections. J. Struct. Biol. **178**(2), 84–87 (2012). https://doi.org/10.1016/j.jsb.2012.04.001
32. Al-Amoudi, A., Norlen, L.P.O., Dubochet, J.: Cryo-electron microscopy of vitreous sections of native biological cells and tissues. J. Struct. Biol. **148**(1), 131–135 (2004). https://doi.org/10.1016/j.jsb.2004.03.010

33. Moriscot, C., Schoehn, G., Housset, D.: High pressure freezing and cryo-sectioning can be used for protein structure determination by electron diffraction. Ultramicroscopy **254**, 113834 (2023). https://doi.org/10.1016/j.ultramic.2023.113834
34. Marko, M., Hsieh, C., Moberlychan, W., Mannella, C.A., Frank, J.: Focused ion beam milling of vitreous water: prospects for an alternative to cryo-ultramicrotomy of frozen-hydrated biological samples. J. Microsc. **222**(1), 42–47 (2006). https://doi.org/10.1111/j.1365-2818.2006.01567.x
35. De Winter, D.A.M., Hsieh, C., Marko, M., Hayles, M.F.: Cryo-FIB preparation of whole cells and tissue for cryo-TEM: use of high-pressure frozen specimens in tubes and planchets. J. Microsc. **281**(2), 125–137 (2021). https://doi.org/10.1111/jmi.12943
36. Smith, A.K., Goff, H.D., Sun, B.D.: Freeze-substitution and low-temperature embedding of dairy products for transmission electron microscopy. J. Microsc. **213**(1), 63–69 (2004). https://doi.org/10.1111/j.1365-2818.2004.01264.x
37. Bhella, D.: Cryo-electron microscopy: an introduction to the technique, and considerations when working to establish a national facility. Biophys. Rev. **11**(4), 515–519 (2019). https://doi.org/10.1007/s12551-019-00571-w
38. Mills, D.J.: Setting up and operating a cryo-EM laboratory. Quart. Rev. Biophys. **54**, e2 (2021). https://doi.org/10.1017/S003358352000013X
39. Reimer, L. (Ed.) Energy-filtering transmission electron microscopy. Hawkes, P.W., Lotsch, H.K.V. (Eds.) Springer Series in Optical Sciences, vol. 71. Springer, Berlin, Heidelberg (1995). https://doi.org/10.1007/978-3-540-48995-5
40. Leijten, Z.J.W.A., Wirix, M.J.M., Strauss, M., Plitzko, J.M., De With, G., Friedrich, H.: Low-dose (S)TEM elemental analysis of water and oxygen uptake in beam sensitive materials. Ultramicroscopy **208**, 112855 (2020). https://doi.org/10.1016/j.ultramic.2019.112855
41. Obermair, M., Hettler, S., Hsieh, C., Dries, M., Marko, M., Gerthsen, D.: Analyzing contrast in cryo-transmission electron microscopy: comparison of electrostatic Zach phase plates and hole-free phase plates. Ultramicroscopy **218**, 113086 (2020). https://doi.org/10.1016/j.ultramic.2020.113086
42. Wu, M., Lander, G.C.: Present and emerging methodologies in cryo-EM single-particle analysis. Biophys. J. **119**(7), 1281–1289 (2020). https://doi.org/10.1016/j.bpj.2020.08.027
43. Bendory, T., Bartesaghi, A., Singer, A.: Single-particle cryo-electron microscopy: mathematical theory, computational challenges, and opportunities. IEEE Signal Process. Mag. **37**(2), 58–76 (2020). https://doi.org/10.1109/MSP.2019.2957822

Chapter 7
In-situ TEM: Principle, Working, Application and Challenges

By directly observing dynamic processes in real time, in-situ TEM open a window to nanoscale world, enabling discoveries that reshape our understanding of material science
*by **Dr. Frances M Ross.** Massachusetts Institute of Technology (MIT)*

Abstract Real time observation of materials dynamic properties at nanoscale under electron microscopy will be functionalize and revolutionize through operation and working of in-situ TEM. Starting from explanation with basics of in-situ TEM principle, working has been extended to correlation of different dynamic processes w.r.t. physical, chemical, thermal, optical etc., processes. Probable modification in specimen under in-situ TEM has been observed and analysed under external condition viz. temperature, pressure, moisture etc. Application of specimen analysis through specialized sample holder viz. sealed liquid or gas cell etc., have been also utilized in battery performance, catalysis investigation, junction analysis etc. Due to real time imaging of specimen in dynamic domains, respective major and minor challenges also have been resolved with best possible solutions. Finally, current chapter addresses versatile capabilities of in-situ TEM, which can be employed in development of battery material, catalysis, electrocatalysis and biological material for novel innovations.

Keywords In-situ TEM · Sealed liquid cell · Gas cell · Battery performance · Biological material

7.1 Introduction

Fast growing technological advancement shifted electron microscopy (EM) sector paradigm w.r.t. transmission electron microscopy (TEM) instrumentation, imaging of respective observations. The in-situ TEM analysis of specimens includes imaging of various dynamical physical, chemical, structural properties of nanoparticles facets,

R. Singh, *Transmission Electron Microscopy Sample Preparation*,
https://doi.org/10.1007/978-3-031-82967-3_7

heterojunctions, dislocations, intermetallic phases, core shell etc. Fast growing aberration corrected optics [1] and micro-electro-mechanical system (MEMS) technologies [2], enhances the depth of materials investigation through in-situ TEM operation. With the help of above technologies, in-situ TEM analysis referred in imaging and recording of structural evolution of materials under application of stress, heat, pressure, electricity, magnetic field or chemical reaction (oxidation/reduction) etc. conditions. In addition, with the use of different spectroscopic techniques such as electron energy loss spectroscopy (EELs) [3], x-ray absorption spectroscopy (XAS) [4], raman spectroscopy [5], mass spectroscopy [6] etc., one can monitor, analyze and quantify reaction products or byproducts very precisely during operando TEM. This will give a very precise idea about material intermediate dynamics behavior, which will be helpful in controlling and redesigning the reaction conditions and novel devices.

Interestingly controlled alteration of specimen environment w.r.t. its real behavior interaction to live conditions, will be produced inside the TEM column. Observed results will be correlated in the form of images, diffraction, spectroscopic data or optical, electrical, mechanical behavior through in-situ TEM operation. The microstructural inhomogeneities in specimen (metals, non-metals, catalyst, polymer etc.) before and after in-situ TEM analysis, bring understanding of different transient phase, nucleation sites and growth mechanism of nanocrystal, reaction kinetic behavior includes defects and dislocation movements, conductivity and melting behavior of material under study [7]. Further, the in-situ TEM experiments need to upgrade and functionalize with their spatial and spectral resolution with suitable peripheral equipment as per input stimuli environment like heating, cooling, light (photon), electrical biasing, liquid or gas environment etc. [8].

In current chapter, in-situ TEM technique has presented a versatile instrumentation technique in continuation of TEM basic capabilities, have improved and enhanced the understanding about material phase transformation, crystal growth, impurities phase, beam effect, under external liquid, gaseous, optical, electrical, thermal or mechanical or magnetic environment.

7.2 Basic of In-situ TEM

In-situ TEM technique deals with observation and analysis of specimen properties including various structural transformation and functional processes. In comparison to traditional TEM analysis, real time analysis of material under in-situ TEM, it will resolve various phenomenon like chemical reaction, stress, strain, phase transformation etc.

In recent time, the sample handling and processing under real time conditions under in-situ TEM became easy and user friendly. Further, with the development of micro-electrical–mechanical-system (MEMS) w.r.t. sample holder chip size, column design, pole piece area, electron beam propagation etc., facilitates respective imaging

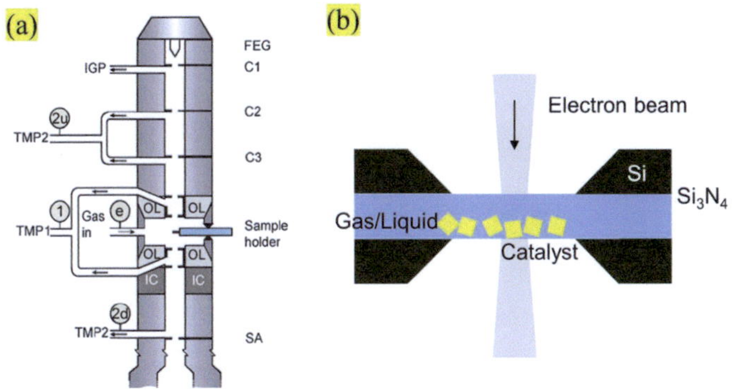

Fig. 7.1 **a** Shows the schematic representation of differential pumping system and **b** liquid cell assembly with specimen respectively (Adapted with permission from Jinschek et al. [9] and Qu et al. [10] under open access)

in realistic domain of specimen. Figure 7.1, has demonstrated the schematic representation of in-situ TEM having differential pumping system and gas/liquid cell assembly [9, 10].

In material science, in-situ TEM technique will be frequently utilized in study of colloids, metal, non-metals, semiconductor, ceramic, catalyst, corrosion, solar cell, polymer, semiconductor and many more. Whereas, in life sciences, in-situ TEM can be utilized in analysis and explanations of respective structural biology, protein transport, drug delivery, particle reconstruction etc. [7, 8, 10].

7.2.1 *Features of In-situ TEM*

There are following features of in-situ TEM technique w.r.t. working, specifications or results and analysis etc., will make it more demanding in comparison to basic TEM.

7.2.1.1 Real Time Observations

Real time analysis during in-situ TEM analysis, bring observation and analysis of dynamic process at nanoscale. Under the controlled environment of vacuum and exposure of high energy electron beam inside in-situ TEM, one can observe different changes and processes like growth, deformation, chemical reaction etc. Zhang et al. [11] has elobrtaed about the insitu gas flow arrangement inside the specimen chamber under Fig. 7.2a. Figure 7.2b–g has demonstrated anatase phase of TiO_2 phase transitions at 150 °C, with and without 1 Torr water (b) without presence of water, (c)

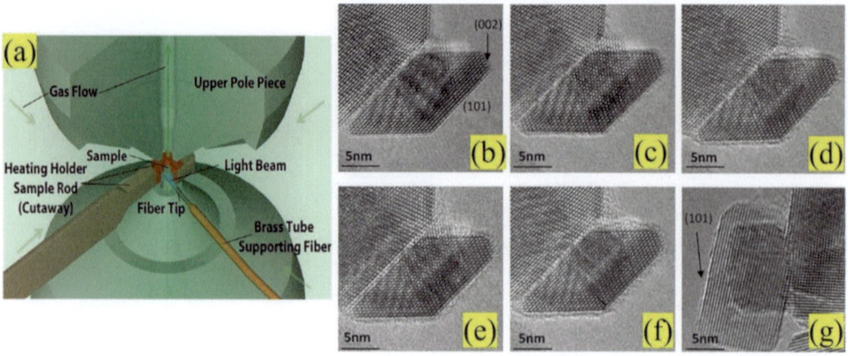

Fig. 7.2 **a** Elobrtaed about insitu gas flow arrangement in specimen chamber, **b–g** has demonstrated anatase phase of TiO_2 at 150 °C, with and without 1 Torr water **b** without presence of water, **c** 1 h water, **d** 7 h water, **e** 20 h water, **f** 40 h water, and **g** 40 h water gas with fresh area respectively (Each image was captured in 20 s exposure) (Adapted with permission from Zhang et al. [11] under open access)

1 h water, (d) 7 h water, (e) 20 h water, (f) 40 h water, and (g) 40 h water gas with fresh area respectively [11].

Specifically, researchers can also study the assembly behavior of NPs, atomic structure regime and growth kinetics etc., directly leads towards fabrication of novel material and respective efficient devices [7, 8, 10, 12].

7.2.1.2 High Spatial Resolution

In addition to in-situ TEM capturing and analyzing different dynamic processes, its feature to record and image finer detail of materials at nanoscale allow researchers to explore respective deep insights. At atomic level, one can track movement of individual atom during crystal growth, atomic rearrangement during phase transitions, evolution of different nanostructure at atomic scale. For example, under Fig. 7.3a, b studied anatase TiO_2 behavior under exposure of water and light. Specifically, image of anatase NPs under 40 h water gas at 150 °C temperature demonstrated at Fig. 7.3a whereas Fig. 7.3b observed after 12 light illumination shows high resolution (101) and (002) surfaces show behavior of roughening and amorphization [11].

In addition, spatial resolution features bring analysis about interfaces, grain boundaries, defects etc., features of material under study, which directly lead to describe and correlate different conduction, chemical reaction or mechanical aspects etc., in different research assignments [7, 8, 10, 12].

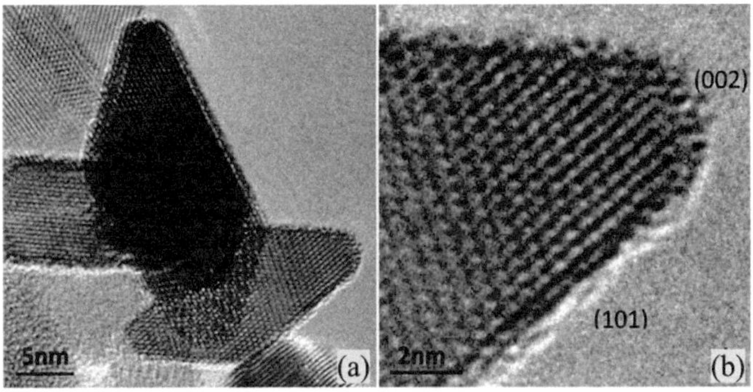

Fig. 7.3 **a** Anatase TiO_2 nanoparticles after 40 h in water gas at 150 °C, **b** after 12 light illuminations resolve the (101) and (002) phases of respective material (Adapted with permission from Zhang et al. [11] under open access)

7.2.1.3 Various Environmental Conditions

In-situ TEM designed in such a way that, it has possibility of different environmental conditions setup during live imaging like high temperature, high pressure, cooling, induction of gaseous etc. Different stated conditions combination during live imaging of specimen will brought many unseen and insightful behavior of material [7, 8, 10, 12].

7.2.1.4 Heat Generating Stage

Features of heating sample inside TEM column during imaging bring analysis for respective phase transformation, crystallization or respective thermal stability etc., behavior can be predicted. Stated heating mechanism of specimen will be further get utilized in catalysis, aerospace, or in nuclear reactor etc. areas respectively [7, 8, 10, 12].

For example, Falqui et al. [13] reported imaging of amorphous iron nanoparticles (NPs) under room temperature (RT) as well at extended temperature i.e. 500 °C through MEMS based sample holder. In comparison to amorphous feature (inset image of diffraction pattern) BF and DF image of Fe NP group as shown in Fig. 7.4a–c demonstrate similar amorphous nature of particle treated at 500 °C. In comparison to initial stage image at (a), image (c) shows layered accumulation around NPs surface like boundary, may be formed due to removal of residual component from specimen surface [13].

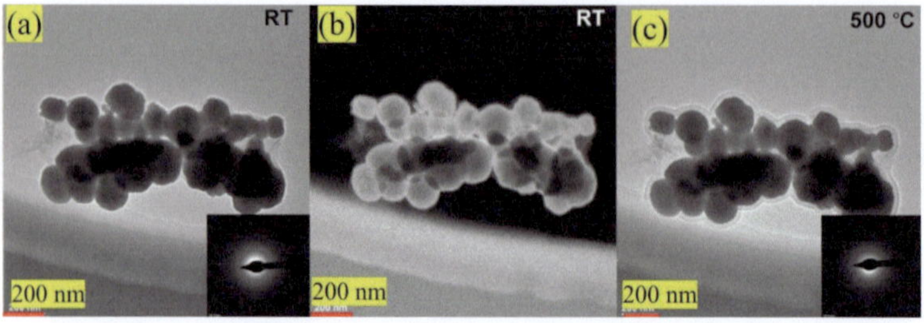

Fig. 7.4 Amorphous Fe NPs on heated MEMS holder **a** BF image of amorphous iron nanoparticles (NPs) under room temperature (RT), **b** DF image of amorphous iron nanoparticles (NPs), **c** BF image of amorphous iron nanoparticles (NPs) heated at 500 °C temperature, respectively (Adapted with permission from Falqui et al. [13] under open access)

7.2.1.5 Liquid Environment

Complex electrochemical reaction and insight behavior associated with devices like rechargeable batteries, fuel cell etc., will be analyzed with liquid cell sample holder of in-situ TEM. Under current mode, liquid based sample need not to freeze or dried as per requirement and further will be analyzed for different electrochemical reaction in real time at nanoscale [7, 8, 14].

7.2.1.6 Controlled Atmosphere

In one more unique mode of in-situ TEM operation, controlled atmosphere around specimen can be maintained and respective changes can be monitored and imaged w.r.t. nature of specimen. Effect of controlled supply of different gases like inert gases (nitrogen, argon etc.), reactive gases (oxygen or hydrogen etc.) or mixture of gases etc., will be studied during specimen-electron beam interaction during TEM operation. Different phenomenon like redox reaction, gas–solid reaction, gas–gas interaction etc., can be utilized/explained via oxidation/reduction of metal layers, reactivity behavior of catalyst surfaces etc. [7, 8, 15].

Ultimately with systematic variation in parameters like temperature, pressure or gas compositions inside in-situ TEM in real time imaging, facilitate researchers in discovering the insightful facts about the fundamental to advanced properties of materials for novel applications.

7.2.1.7 Versatility

Researchers can perform variety of experiments with in-situ TEM in real time at nanoscale. Due to versatile nature of in-situ TEM under controlled external conditions like heat, pressure, gases supply etc., following type of experiments can be conducted.

7.2.1.8 Nanomechanical Testing

In-situ TEM can be used to study the mechanical properties of material at nanoscale. Under application of variable mechanical loads in materials, researchers can analyze level of deformation, extent of fracture or plasticity etc., at nano-level. This type of information is very much useful during respective materials design and applications such as structural materials or micro electro mechanical system (MEMS) etc. [7, 16].

7.2.1.9 Nucleation, Growth and Assembly Kinetics

In-situ TEM enables researchers/scientists about nucleation, growth and respective assembly mechanism of nanomaterial in real time frame. Specifically, during interaction of electron beam with specimen, one can observe the nucleation of individual nanoparticles (NPs) with growth process for atomic layer deformation or atomic aggregation, which further may lead to growth into larger NPs via self-assembly mechanism. The precise and well-defined understanding of respective properties during in-situ TEM analysis, will play very crucial role in development of smart and novel materials in catalysis, electronics or biomedical applications etc., respectively [7, 8, 10, 12].

7.2.1.10 Dissolution and Phase Transformation

In addition to understand and explore the growth kinetics of materials under in-situ TEM study, respective material dissolution and phase transformation behavior also have important role. Under effect of external stimuli like temperature, heat, pressure, gases conditions etc., one can monitor and analyze respective material in-process dissolution and transformation w.r.t. phase, defect or restructuring etc. With the knowledge of above properties for material under investigation, researchers can explore materials for catalysis, nanodrug delivery or nanoelectronics etc., applications [7, 8, 17].

7.2.1.11 Chemical Reaction

Normally, it is not possible to observe any chemical reaction intermediates process in real time, but with updated in-situ TEM instrumentation will facilitate respective monitoring very closely. Observation and analysis of different processes like oxidation, reduction, or intermediate's reaction product etc. at nanoscale, will be helpful in designing novel sensors, catalyst and functional nanomaterials having active quality surfaces [7, 8, 18].

7.2.1.12 Electrical and Thermal Properties

In addition, in-situ TEM also have ability to analyze electrical and thermal properties of different nanomaterials and nanostructures. In-situ TEM suitably equipped with specialized holder having electrical bias features, will bring measurement of electrical conductivity behavior. Parallelly, with suitable heating holder analyze the thermal transport behavior like thermal transport behavior, thermal expansion etc., under real time analysis [13, 18].

Conclusively, in-situ TEM allows researchers to measure and analyze specimens' properties through mechanical, electrical, thermal etc. aspects at nanoscale in real time frame. Systematic investigation of functional properties of material under in-situ TEM will lead to development and design of next generation electronic and thermal efficient devices.

NOTE: In-situ TEM empowers researchers to bridge the gap between theory and reality of material with in-action image, not just by static images.

7.3 In-situ TEM Versus Conventional TEM

The limitation of traditional TEM has been optimized and updated in in-situ TEM through technological upgradations. There are following points which will differentiate between in-situ TEM from conventional TEM.

7.3.1 Static Versus Dynamic Imaging

Conventional TEM has ability to capture static images of specimen without any variation w.r.t. any variation in time, temperature or pressure etc. Whereas in-situ TEM has ability of analyzing real time features (phase transformation, chemical reaction, mechanical deformation etc.) of specimens having different dynamic behavior during electron beam interaction [7, 8, 12, 18].

7.3.2 Limited Versus Dynamic Environmental Conditions

There is no option in controlling environmental condition like pressure, heat, atmospheric etc., during sample analysis inside conventional TEM. Whereas in case of in-situ TEM analysis, it has capability of versatile option in creating artificial condition like pressure, temperature, gases supply etc., w.r.t. during electron beam-specimen interaction for respective dynamic imaging [7, 8].

7.3.3 Unique Sample Preparation

Under traditional TEM, most of time specimen will be exposed to harsh condition like high beam energy, high vacuum etc., lead to generation/development of artefacts during imaging. In case of in-situ TEM analysis, specimen will be exposed under native environment or relevant conditions to specific experiment, will validate for artefacts free insightful imaging. Respective specimen before mounting on specialized holder like MEMS, liquid cell etc., need to bring in specimen into electron transparent range with techniques like FIB or electropolishing etc. [7, 8].

In brief, both conventional and in-situ TEM has own importance regime with respect to nature of material under study and respective field of applications.

7.4 Specialized Sample Analysis Under In-situ TEM

In coming paragraphs, an effort has been made to investigate about different materials properties and respective applications through in-situ TEM analysis.

7.4.1 Sealed Gas Cell Mechanism

In conventional TEM, it works under high vacuum conditions ~ $\times 10^{-7}$ torr, which will not allow to analyze any physical and chemical transition or change of specimen specially under gaseous environment. Specifically, in order to explore and develop novel, efficient materials for catalysis, battery, chemical and biological dominated processes [15, 19], in-situ Environment TEM (ETEM) will analyze gas–solid interface under ambient pressure for insightful functional features of respective material in their real time frame. Specifically, real time monitoring and analysis properties for in-situ TEM of specimen under analysis, will be very much useful in development of nanomaterial-based technologies like energy conversion/storage/transportation/ environment remediation etc. areas [15, 19].

Gas cell design will maintain gas near sample by pressure limiting aperture through differential pumping scheme [20]. Sealed gas cell setup will expose precise specification w.r.t. electron transparent window with controlled supply of gas for few microns path length, without disturbing rest area of TEM column during respective operation. During controlled reaction conditions of imaging and related sample drift stabilization will be facilitated by low mass heating devices [21] or laser heating [22] techniques.

For example, Creemer et al. [15] studied transformation and stability behavior of Cu/ZnO material through window cell having two electron transparent faces with central hole of 1mm [2] covered by SiN_x membrane having amorphous nature (Fig. 7.5a).

The electron transparency requirement of window will be maintained via ultrathin specification through recession in central region of membrane as shown in Fig. 7.5a, c, d. MEMS based nanoreactor is mounted on custom made TEM holder with nanoreactor having leak tight features for gas flow as shown in Fig. 7.5b. Figure 7.5e–l shows growth and stability behavior of ZnO and CuO in presence H_2 atmosphere with heating upto 500 °C within 68.5 s. In comparison to image (e) having ZnO compact shape of 20–100 nm size, whereas under heating CuO get broken into small patches from 260, 330, 365, 410, 500 °C temperature shown in image (f–j). Image (k) shows sharp atomic fringes of both ZnO and CuO sample, which is heated at 500 °C and 1.2 bar pressure and with respective fourier transform pattern as shown under image (l) [15].

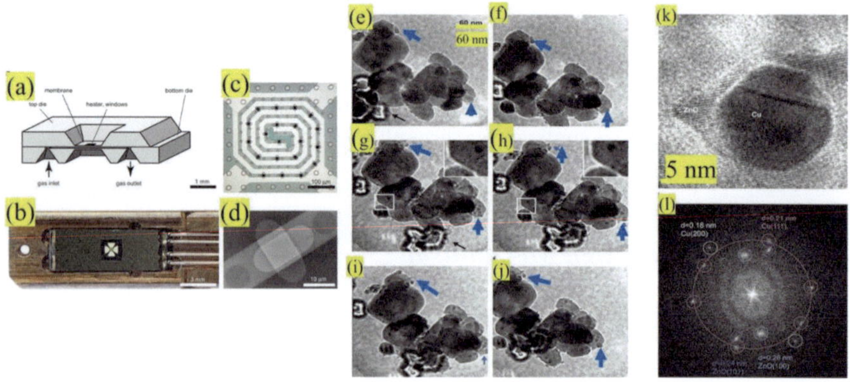

Fig. 7.5 **a** Cross-section view of MEMS based nanoreactor, **b** TEM holder mounted with nanoreactor connected with four connecting probe, **c** optical image of nanoreactor membrane having Pt heater (spiral), and (circles) SiO_2 spacer, **d** TEM image of 10 nm thick window; Images from (e-l) Shows growth of CuO on ZnO base and mobility under heating from room temperature to 500 °C at 1.2 bar H_2 with images frames recorded at (RT) **e**, **f** 260 °C, **g** 330 °C, **h** 365 °C, **i** 410 °C, **j** 500 °C with exposure time of 0.145 s time (right side), **k** shows Cu/ZnO high resolution image at 500 °C with 1.2 bar H_2 and **l** respective FFT pattern respectively (Adapted with permission from Creemer et al. [15])

Under sealed in-situ TEM environment, sealed gas cell holder will analyze biological specimen very gently and precisely. Due to maximum content of carbon in any biological or organic specimen, have maximum carbon dominated contamination. This contamination will be minimized by creating gas pressure of gases like H_2, N_2, He or Ar at pressure range of 100–200 torr during imaging just confined to specimen chamber. Bacterial specimen from respective culture will be directly applied in gas cell and investigated under ~ 97.5 torr pressure of saturated air with water vapor, which shows flagellated and non-spore-based morphology [23].

7.4.2 *Sealed Liquid Cell Mechanism*

In addition to gas cell assembly w.r.t in-situ TEM analysis, sealed liquid cell (SLC) assembly have promising applications in different electrochemical process [24] like electrodeposition [25], dendrite growth [26], nanoscale regime [27] etc. through electrode system [25] in liquid environment. Specifically, one of major application through SLC is investigation of lithium-ion battery (LIB). In comparison to ex-situ investigated distorted and deviated materials results from native environment [28], in-situ TEM electrochemical characterization bring insightful investigation of LIB study. For example, in addition to standard analysis of cathode/anode structural behavior, in-situ TEM is capable in analyzing solid-electrolyte interphase (SEI) through electrochemical oxidation–reduction cycles in presence of electrolyte setup [29]. Due to SEI sensitivity w.r.t. air, moisture etc. conditions, in-situ TEM controlled electrochemical setup investigation on dendritic growth of lithium metal will explore insights about batteries failure through short circuit [30].

In one more study, Niu et al. [14] investigated kirkendall effect dominated hollow bismuth oxide nanoparticles (NPs) by liquid cell equipped TEM. In presence of elevated temperature from 180 to 200 °C during reaction environment, in-situ TEM have ability to monitor the formation of hollow bismuth oxide NPs. Room temperature synthesized NPs shows slow oxidization process in absence of voids and diffusive ions which get diffused into respective inner shell homogeneously (Fig. 7.6b). Under controlled conditions of higher temperature i.e. 192 °C, bismuth oxide hollow NP will be formed through kirkendall effect with filling of voids (Fig. 7.6a). In current case, single particle based hollow bismuth oxide NPs fabrication and design alignment, has been guided for efficient mechanism via liquid cell equipped in-situ TEM [14].

Conclusively, liquid cell in-situ TEM have vast capabilities in exploration of structural and functional investigations of specimen under study. This is can be utilized in development of novel material design with their efficient performances in real time through monitoring of fast chemical reactions and transformations at nanoscale.

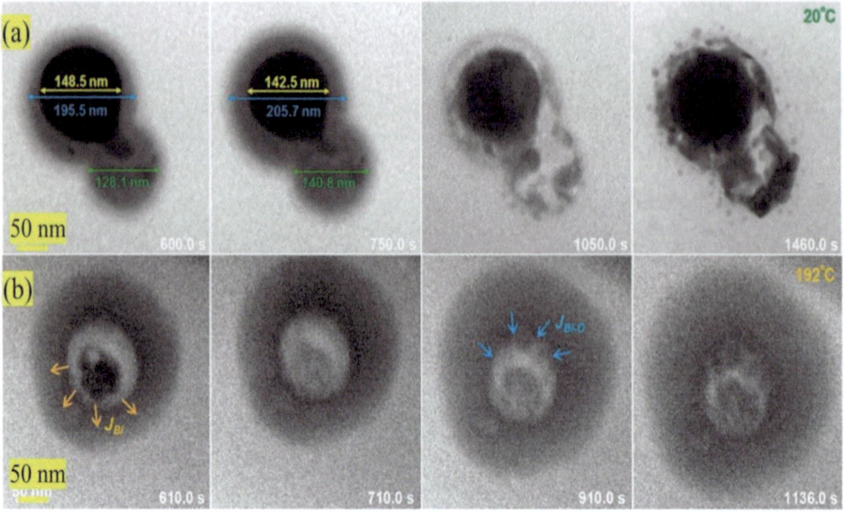

Fig. 7.6 **a** Kirkendall effect directed bismuth oxide NPs at RT, **b** Hollow NPs at 192 °C (Adapted with permission from Niu et al. [14] under open access)

7.4.3 Battery Performance

With rising demand of power, portable electricity, advanced storage setup, environment remediation etc., in-situ TEM [31, 32] fully capable in innovative development of material under study.

Development in battery research revolves around the electrode transformation which can be analyzed at atomic scale through in-situ TEM for electrode-electrode interface, solid-electrode interface (SEI) or structural modified electrode material etc., properties. In similar work, Qingyong et al [33] has analyzed the LiF modified positive charged titanium (Ti) cathode material behavior with in-situ TEM investigation via electrochemical liquid cell assembly as shown in Fig. 7.7a. LiF nucleation and growth kinetics was observed on Ti working electrode (WE) in SiN_x window (Fig. 7.7c) through electrochemical cyclic-voltammetry (CV) setup (Fig. 7.7b). Deposition of LiF on Ti working electrode has been schematically demonstrated in Fig. 7.7d. Further, Fig. 7.8a–p has elaborated about time series LiF deposition on Ti WE, corresponding to 3D image representation, current–voltage measurement, projected area of LiF nanosheet deposition in − 4 V to + 4 V. In addition, in-situ TEM image of LiF in liquid cell environment with selected area electron diffraction has been demonstrated in Fig. 7.7o, p [33] respectively. Through current study, in-situ TEM investigation of LiF deposition on Ti WE have been proven respective material morphing ability with self-healing features. This can be utilized for advancement in cathode material novel designs for efficient battery performances.

The performances and degradation of battery working mechanism will also be analyzed and improved via variable electrochemical reactions through lithiation,

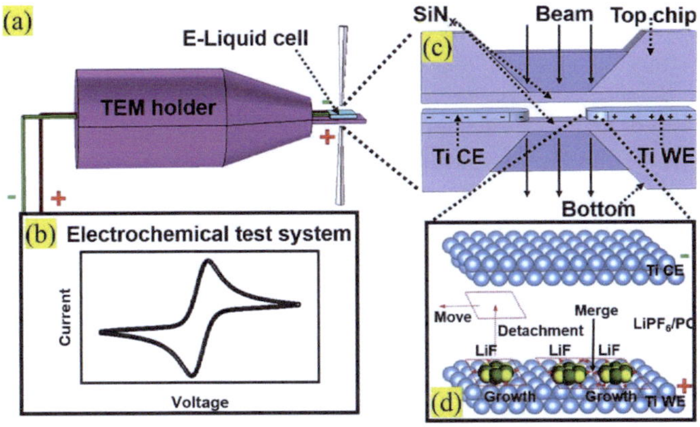

Fig. 7.7 **a** LiF modified positive charged titanium (Ti) cathode material with in-situ TEM investigation via electrochemical liquid cell assembly with electrochemical cyclic-voltammetry (CV) setup (**b**), with LiF nucleation and growth kinetics was captured on Ti working electrode (WE) in SiN_x window (**c**) (Adapted with permission from Zhang et al. [33])

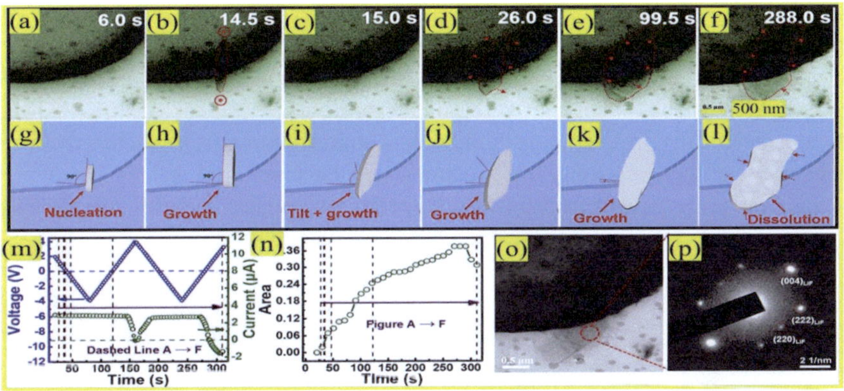

Fig. 7.8 **a–f** elaborated about time series LiF deposition on Ti WE, **g–l** corresponding 3D image representation, **m** current measurement with voltage load, **n** projected area of LiF nanosheet deposition in − 4 V to + 4 V, **o** in-situ TEM image of LiF in liquid cell and **p** selected area electron area diffraction image respectively (Adapted with permission from Zhang et al. [33])

de-lithiation, sodation or de-sodation etc. processes in real time imaging [34]. One more promising factor in battery performance is study of related interfacial dynamics w.r.t. electrode material, electrolyte or anode. In-situ TEM insightful investigation will analyze and monitor charge transport, charge transfer kinetics or interfacial stability etc. [35].

Particularly, lithium-ion battery working and efficiency will be affected by formation of dendrite and respective growth [26]. In-situ TEM capability of real time observation w.r.t. growth of dendrite at cathode or anode, will guide for minimum dendrite formation, safe working with long life span etc. features. Controlled synthesis methods like atomic layer deposition, chemical vapor deposition etc., bring homogenous and efficient nano-structuring w.r.t. cathode and anode material fabrications. In-situ TEM will play a very dynamic and crucial role in analysis of respective materials shape, size, thin film etc. features, for cycling stability, battery kinetics, storage and respective transport capacity etc., features.

With the help of above discussed features w.r.t. battery research w.r.t. failure and challenges, current field have vast possibilities and opportunities towards respective novel material innovation.

7.4.4 *Catalysis Investigation*

With the help of in-situ TEM, researchers/scientist can understand about the dynamic catalytic processes like transformation of catalyst structure, respective reaction activity during real time etc. In coming paragraphs, we have presented a simple and basic information based in-situ TEM guided investigation of different catalyst materials. Figure 7.9, has demonstrated the in-situ TEM role in analysis of heterogenous catalysis insightful processes at nanoscale [10].

In recent time, single atom dominated catalysis behavior will be studied at large extent which will be authenticated at atomic scale via capabilities of in-situ TEM technique. Specifically, investigation of individual atomic pathways, respective dynamic behavior, stability, reactivity etc., features will be monitored and analyzed very precisely. During catalyst investigation, respective material shape, size, morphology,

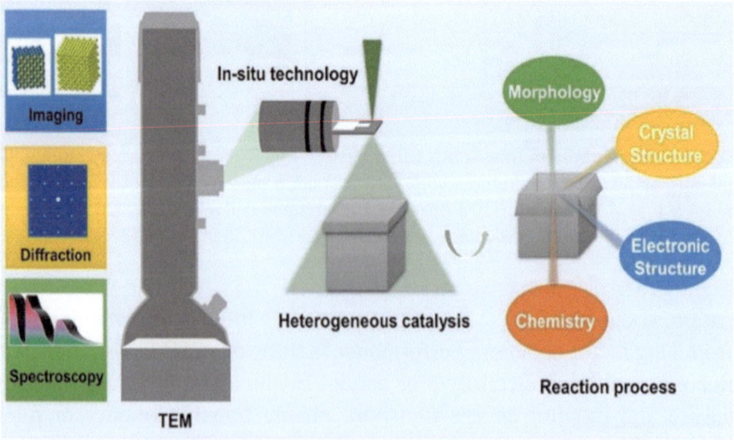

Fig. 7.9 Role of in-situ TEM in heterogenous catalysis (Adapted with permission from Qu et al. [10] under open access)

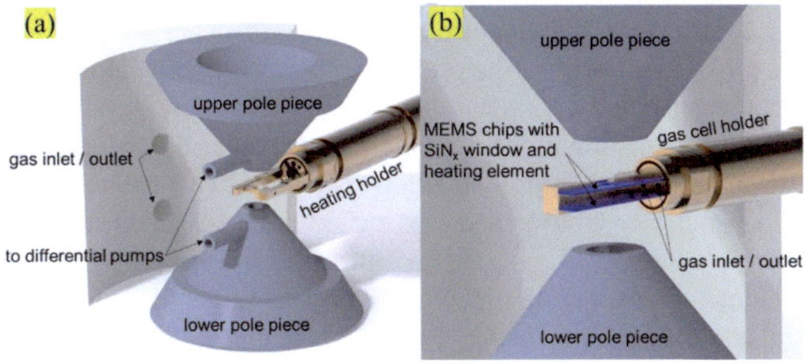

Fig. 7.10 **a** Environmental Transmission electron Microscope (ETEM), **b** windowed gas cell system (Adapted with permission from Ye et al. [37] under open access)

particles restructuring, surface reconstruction etc., will also be analyzed at nanoscale [36].

In order to get more clarity about inside view of environmental TEM working, Fig. 7.10a shows differentially pumped ETEM which alter the leak rate of ambient environment from ETEM specimen holder cell. Further, Fig. 7.10b depicts the positioning of nanoreactor based MEMS chip and gasket which will isolate the gaseous environment from rest of TEM column. Controlled high pressure conditions will be created around specimen inside column, will facilitate fast, precise and real time imaging with scanning electron transmission microscopy (STEM) imaging and spectroscopy [37].

Behavior of gas–solid phase on catalyst surface during catalysis mechanism, also have very dominating impact at nanoscale through gas adsorption, surface reaction, desorption, oxidation, reduction, hydrogenation or carbon dioxide conversion phenomenon via in-situ TEM investigation. Similarly, in-situ TEM have promising results in investigation through electrocatalysis at electrode–electrolyte interface [38]. Different structural evolution like oxygen reduction, generation of hydrogen, energies conversion and storage technologies, will be monitored critically with in-situ TEM for novel catalyst designs.

Conclusively, in-situ TEM will provide the insightful information about the catalyst working behavior w.r.t. electrolyte environment, interfacial structure, energy generations and storage etc. in-situ TEM dominated studies on catalysis will boost up different ongoing research projects on efficient catalysis through atomic utilization, surface modification and energies conversion strategies.

7.4.5 *Junctions Investigations*

The analysis and modification of junction or heterojunction of single phase or multiple phase-based material, will be facilitated in better way by in-situ TEM technique in comparison to other related EM techniques. With the monitoring of morphological, structural and electronic properties of materials w.r.t. junctions or heterojunction aspect, it will be helpful in development and fabrication of smart electronic, optoelectronic or photonic devices [39–41].

With proper visualization of interfacial interactions during materials analysis via in-situ TEM bring insight into conduction dynamics. The nature of defects like dislocation, vacancies or grain boundaries etc., at the interface of different material during their fabrication, will guide and control the for performance of respective material design, for specific applications. Qingyun et al. [41] investigated grain boundary relaxation behavior of CrMnFeCoNi, having high entropy-based alloy through in-situ TEM technique. Figure 7.11a shows one nanograin having size ~ 10 nm surrounded by two larger grain having size ~ 55 and 30 nm respectively. Further, Fig. 7.11b marked as code 'A' predicts low angle tilt boundary whereas right side grain marked 'B' shows twin boundary. Boundary dislocation at low angle grain boundary (LAGB) will be determined with the help of burger vectors. Under Fig. 7.11c shows three dislocation arrays with constant inter-dislocation distance of nine layers (111) at θ ~ 6°. Figure 7.11d–f shows dissociation and frank dislocation w.r.t. 'A' boundary during 3 min beam irradiation at 0′59″, 1′48″, 2′22″ elapse time [41].

During electronic and optical device integrations, respective interfaces (junction or heterojunction) between semiconductor (diodes, transistors etc.), optoelectronic devices (photodetector, solar cell etc.), electronic component (nanowire junction, quantum heterostructure etc.), will be analyzed at nanoscale under in-situ TEM. Under real time imaging of in-situ TEM researchers will find small morphological,

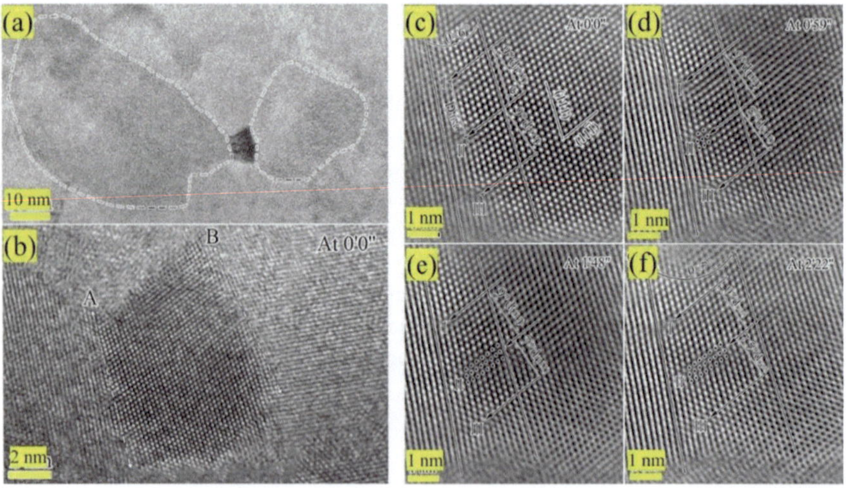

Fig. 7.11 **a** Bright field TEM image having 10 nm small grain surrounded with two adjacent large grain, **b** LAGB with low tilt angle boundary (A) and twin boundary (B), **c**–**f** HRTEM images of dislocation array w.r.t. boundary A during e-beam elapse time of **a** (0″), **b** 0′59″, **c** 1′48″, **d** 2′22″ respectively (Adapted with permission from Lin et al. [41])

structural based aligned or misaligned arrangements w.r.t. interfacial growth aspect. With fast growing technologies and rising demand of smart materials (2D material, quantum material, perovskite material etc.) in different sectors (electronical or optoelectronic devices), in-situ TEM will be very much helpful in respective device architectures, unlocking novel functionalities, helps in improving efficiencies and respective scalability factors [39–41].

With the proper investigation and analysis of junctions dominated study of materials through in-situ TEM technique, it will significantly contribute in development of respective material efficient improvements w.r.t. energy storage, catalysis, conduction, electronic features.

NOTE: Different modes of in-situ TEM ignite innovative materials studies by capturing dynamic phenomena, allowing researchers to tailor insights at the nanoscale.

7.5 Challenges During In-situ TEM Analysis

In real sense, performing real time analysis of preciseness specimen under in-situ TEM is biggest challenge in itself. It needs lot of expertise, patience and scientific vision. With the updated MEMS based specimen holder design, bring many challenges under control but still there are still something which need to improve through optimization.

7.5.1 Compatible Sample

During sample preparation for in-situ TEM analysis, specimen under analysis must be compatible with environment like heating, cooling, external gaseous or liquid environment, or electrochemical setup etc. [14, 15, 42]. In addition to compatibility of specimen w.r.t. in-situ TEM internal environment, optimize concentration and thickness, mounting of specimen on TEM grid via suitable sample holder (sealed gas cell or liquid cell etc.) etc., need to optimized for artefacts free imaging at nanoscale.

7.5.2 Environment Control

Control over working environmental during in-situ TEM analysis like pressure, temperature etc., will affect largely the respective specimen analysis. Before directly applying any condition like heating temperature like ~ 100–500 °C or variable pressure like ~ 100–200 torr etc., onto specimen need to optimize in systematic validation process w.r.t sample nature and type. Factors like heating rate, gas flow speed and pressure, uniformity of external condition (temperature or gas pressure etc.) around pole piece (around specimen) need to standardized properly [19].

7.5.3 Sample Stability

With reference to in-situ TEM specimen analysis, before inserting specimen inside TEM column respective sample must pre-stabilized as per nature of sample like emulsion, metal or biological etc. Precaution over factor like specimen mechanical drift, sample distortion or bean induced sample damage etc., factors need to take care before mounting specimen in respective holder in order to ensure accurate and reliable imaging and spectroscopic analysis.

7.5.4 In-situ TEM Operation Limitation

As in-situ TEM delicately work for achieving real time analysis of specimen under different condition of heating, cooling etc., during imaging process, many time user have to compromise with contrast, resolution factors. An optimum use of operational parameters like beam intensity, resolution, scan speed, exposure time, magnification etc., need to utilize efficiently for quality imaging with protecting specimen from over dose beam exposure etc.

7.5.5 Data Interpretation and Management

In-situ TEM results have ability in revealing many insightful processes of respective materials in real time imaging. Before analyzing the imaged data, one should have expertise in respective area with having sufficient knowledge and experience. Due to complexity of real time specimen imaging data or videos, respective interpretation and conclusion can be made with prior supporting experimental studies like normal TEM. HRTEM or theoretical modelling.

In addition to multiple challenges during operation of in-situ TEM, has vast potential in observation of dynamic process like phase transformation, atomic imaging, hidden processes etc. With optimally stabilize specimen will be imaged under real time frame under atmospheric or elevated temperature etc. conditions, guided new path towards development of novel and efficient materials and devices.

7.6 Application of In-situ TEM

In addition to earlier discussion about in-situ TEM guided studies, coming section have presented well defined areas which need more attention and research.

7.6.1 Lithiation Process

Anything which have material features i.e. shape, size, volume etc., will become more dominating and important when it grow in nano-range [43]. In order to develop and design new material, respective structural evolution of nanoparticles, nanowire, and different nanostructure during synthesis, fabrication and processing, in-situ TEM analysis will play very crucial and effective role [17].

Liu et al. [44] has demonstrated about ultrafast electrochemical lithiation process which is demonstrated at Fig. 7.12i, ii, iii and iv. Initially, Fig. 7.12(i)a, b shows schematic layout design of electrochemical device having silicon nanowires as anodes and $LiCoO_2$ film as cathode on Aluminum foil. Whereas Fig. 7.12b shows gap between anode and cathode. With respect to enhancement in electrical conductivity of silicon nanowire, doping effect of phosphorous (P) and carbon (C) has been studied, respectively. Figure 7.12(ii)a, b shows P doped Si nanowires having diameter 170 nm, (d) image after 3240 s of charging nanowire get bent with diameter expanded to 446 nm. In addition, lithiated nanowire structural identification has been further confirmed by diffraction oriented structural phases of bent nanowire as shown Fig. 7.12(ii)f. Like P doped Si nanowire, carbon doped Si nanowire at shows two charging and discharging cycles having fast charging, volume expansion and maximum lithiation process of c-$Li_{15}Si_4$ in first cycle, which is shown under Fig. 7.12(iii)a–p. During first charging cycle after 221 s, c-$Li_{15}Si_4$ nanowires get fully lithiated under Fig. 7.12(iii)b, m and respective diameter expanded to 303 nm (h). Further, Fig. 7.12(iii)a–i shows increase in axial charging rate of 213 nm/s with spiral and twisted lithiation of P doped Si nanowire lithiated to amorphous phase [44].

In summary, slow lithiation behavior of C and P doped Si nanowire led to amorphous Li_xSi alloy formation. Further, optimization process bring c-$Li_{15}Si_4$ crystalline phase of respective formulation has been investigated by in-situ TEM. Through, ultrahigh lithiation and ~ 300% volume expansion of Si nanowires shows stability of nanowires structure.

Conclusively, under external load condition like temperature, pressure etc., study of mechanical deformation behavior, phase transformation, nucleation, growth [45, 46] etc., of material under study, will be observed and analyzed very precisely through in-situ TEM for novel, advance scientific prediction.

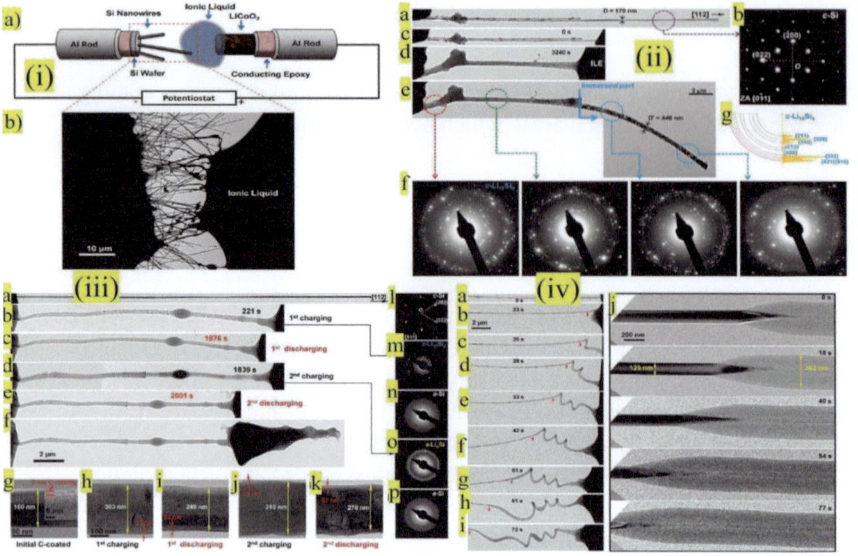

Fig. 7.12 **(i)** **a** Electrochemical device having silicon nanowires as anodes and $LiCoO_2$ film as cathode on Aluminum foil, **b** gap between anode and cathode, **(ii)** **a**, **b** P doped Si Nanowires having diameter 170 nm, **d** after 3240 s charging nanowire get bent and diameter expanded to 446 nm, **f** diffraction oriented structural phases of bent nanowire, **(iii)** **a**, **g**, **l** C doped Si pristine Nanowires having diameter 100 nm, **h** first charging cycle bring nanowire diameter to 303 nm, **d**, **j** radial and axial expansion of nanowire, **m**, **n**, **o**, **p** figure shows diffraction pattern of lithiation process, **(iv)** **a**–**i** shows increase in charging of P doped Si nanowire, **j** lithiated nanowires changes to amorphous phase (Adapted with permission from Liu et al. [44])

7.6.2 Catalysis

Due to well established capabilities of catalysis/photocatalysis/electrocatalysis science in material science for environmental remediation approach, in-situ TEM can play the crucial role. Monitoring of insight behind the chemical reactions, in-situ TEM have ability to monitor and analyze respective changes like shape, size, surface restructuring of catalysts etc., for efficient activity, selectivity and stability behavior can be studied. [24, 37]

In current paragraph, morphological evolution and degradation behavior of Pt-Fe photocatalyst has been studied via in-situ TEM during potential cycling [47]. Figure 7.13a, schematically demonstrate the liquid cell assembly having two silicon chips. Top view of silicon chip with inset showing modified working electrode with platinum NPs has been presented in Fig. 7.13b. Further, liquid cell effectiveness has been investigated with cyclic voltammogram (CV) measurement of Pt NPS deposited on electrochemical cell with 0.1 M H_2SO_4 as electrolyte with 100 mV/s scan rate as shown under Fig. 7.13c. Figure 7.13d–o shows TEM images of Pt-Fe catalyst during different electrochemical cycle with tracked particles respectively. Each micrograph get labelled on CV curve as shown in Fig. 7.13p, q [47].

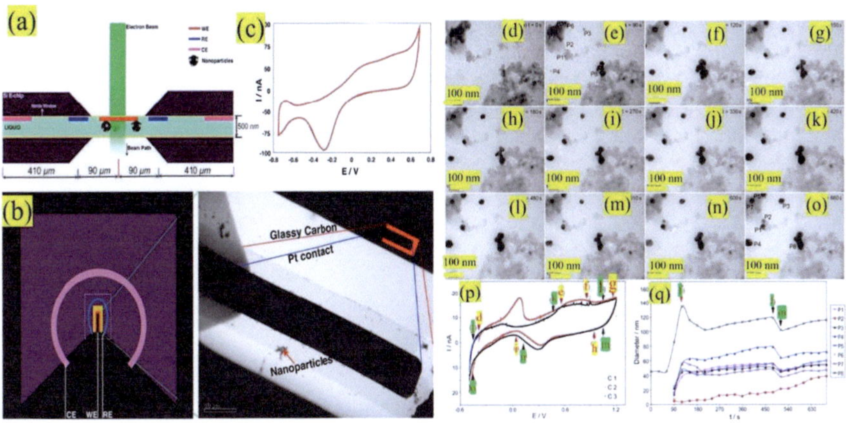

Fig. 7.13 **a** Liquid cell assembly having two silicon chips, **b** Top view of silicon chip with inset showing modified working electrode with platinum NPs on top of chip, **c** cyclic Voltammograms measurement using TEM liquid cell holder with 0.1 M H_2SO_4 as electrolyte with 100 mV/s scan rate; **images d–o** TEM images of Pt-Fe catalyst during different electrochemical cycle. **Image p** shows CV curves corresponding to different stages from **images d–o** and **q** shows corresponding particle size during cycling process (Adapted with permission from Zhu et al. [47] under open access)

Conclusively, in-situ TEM reported Pt-Fe catalyst growth behavior position and potential dependent and predicts insights about respective material structural evolution.

In addition, during chemical reaction, reaction kinetics can also be explained through observing absorption, desorption, surface reaction etc. behavior. With the understanding of catalyst growth dynamics and reaction mechanism through in-situ TEM, researchers can develop rational catalyst design for sustainable and efficient chemical process.

7.6.3 *Electrochemistry*

In-situ TEM will also be helpful in understanding and upgrading the battery research and electrodeposition mechanism through real time monitoring of materials and interfaces through electrochemical processes at nanoscale [24, 25]. Battery material's structural and chemical changes during charging-discharging cycles lead many phases transformation, surface modification, solid-electrolyte interface formation [29] etc., will can microscopically monitored with in-situ TEM analysis. With the investigation in formation of undesired and desired phases during battery operation, researchers/scientists can optimize the respective performances, limiting factors, new

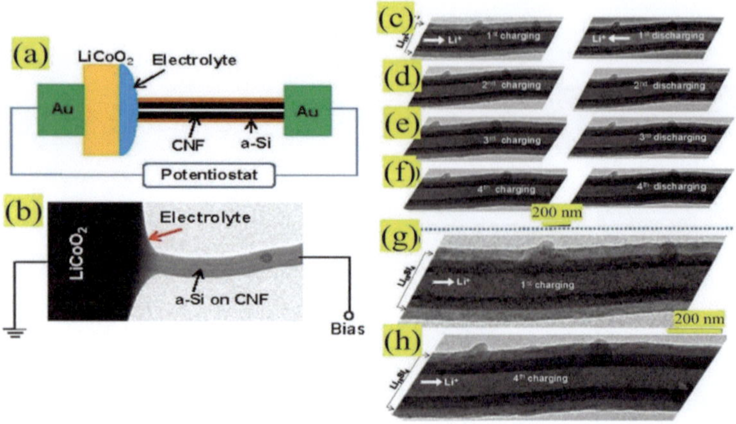

Fig. 7.14 **a** Experimental setup for nanobattery working with Si-CNF as anode, $LiCoO_2$ as cathode and ionic liquid as an electrolyte, **b** nanobattery working between cathode and anode via appropriate biasing during charging/discharging cycle, **c–f** left side column shows charging cycle whereas corresponding right side shows the respective discharging cycle, **g–h** first charging and fourth charging cycles inside in-situ TEM setup (Adapted with permission from Wang [45] under open access)

design strategies, battery failure reasons etc. In case of electrodeposition mechanism, in-situ TEM provide insight about formation of defects, grain boundaries, and microstructural defects mechanism [28].

In systematic work authors has shared structural evolution of silicon/carbon nanofiber (CNF) anode via in-situ TEM technique for charging/discharging process in battery working. Figure 7.14a shows an experimental setup for in-situ testing of battery working with Si-CNF as anode with $LiCoO_2$ as cathode and ionic liquid as an electrolyte. Further, Fig. 7.14b shows nanobattery working behavior between cathode and anode via appropriate biasing during charging/discharging cycle. Figure 7.14a–d left side column shows charging cycle whereas corresponding right-side have respective discharging cycle. During in-situ cycles study with in-situ TEM, minimum change in coating layers of respective Si-CNF has been observed. Further investigation about the modification of Si-CNF structure, fourth charging cycles shows little rough surface in comparison to first charging cycle Si-CNF [45].

7.6.4 *Biological Science*

In-situ TEM has very crucial role studying the various structural and dynamical properties of biological molecules [23]. For example, protein folding and protein aggregation dominated mechanism responsible in implication of diseases such as Alzheimer etc., will be monitored by in-situ TEM in real time domain. In addition, different cellular dynamics including cellular membrane, cell division, intracellular movement of vesicles and organelles, will also be analyzed for cellular function and dysfunction of health, through respective dynamic microscopy technique [48]. In addition, in-situ TEM have also wide capabilities in monitoring the molecular interaction between different cellular components like protein–protein interaction, protein-lipid interaction, protein-nucleic acid interaction etc. [19]. This will be really helpful in finding new undiscovered scientific remedies of existing diseases.

7.6.5 Investigation of Device Physics

Semiconductor devices are the backbone of modern electronics comprise from computer, smartphone or medical or solar panel devices etc. Operational mechanism of semiconductor devices includes diode, resistor, transistor or integrated circuit etc., for manipulation of charge carriers (electron or proton) need to analyzed in real time. With the analysis of in-situ TEM through appropriate sample preparation, manufacturing defects, electrical failure or material degradation behavior of different electronics devices will be analyzed and monitored.

In recent study, one dimensional nanostructure material analysis has been performed via in-situ TEM for tensile device fabrication [49]. Tensile device consists of three parts viz. electrostatic actuated chip, hollow base and varnished wire as shown in Fig. 7.15a. Sample holder device has hexagonal electrostatic chip having 706 pair of combs which provide tensile displacement of > 1 μm. Respective double tilt tensile layout and respective cross sectional specimen jaw has been demonstrated in Fig. 7.15a, b. Figure 7.15c–e shows y-axis tilting of image of sample holder capture from outside TEM whereas during x-tilting w.r.t. specimen jaw captured from inside the TEM (Fig. 7.15f–h). The feasibility of tensile system has been further investigated with Ag wire stretching having diameter 45 nm. Initially, Fig. 7.15i shows unstretched Ag wire whereas image (j) observe fracture in respective wire with actuating voltage. In addition, Fig. 7.15k, l have further confirmed the Ag nanowire crystal and high-resolution structure [49].

In addition, the miniaturized development of MEMS and nano-mechanical electro system (NEMS) become very important and demanding in recent times [50]. For example, in-situ TEM will help in investigating the accelerometer or gyroscopes for motion sensing, pressure sensor in medical devices, microfluidic system, resonator for frequency control etc.

In current section, we have presented best possible applications of in-situ TEM in fundamental or applied research and development belong to physical science, chemical science, life science, geological science. Figure 7.16, has demonstrated schematically about different application fields of in-situ TEM, modes of operations with probable challenges during its operation and analysis.

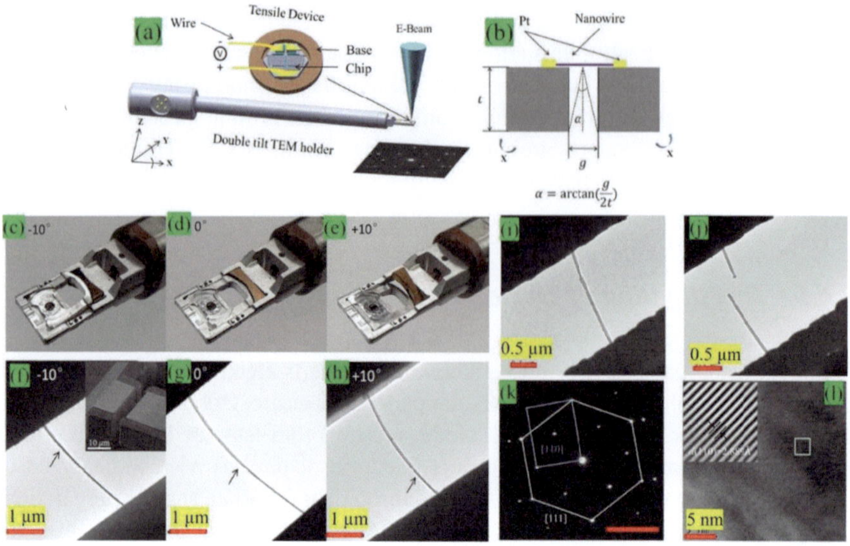

Fig. 7.15 **a** Shows double tilt tensile layout, **b** respective cross sectional specimen jaw (**c–e**). Picture of y-axis tilting of sample holder outside the TEM, **c** − 10°, **d** 0°, **e** + 10° holder capture from outside TEM, **f–h** during x-tilting w.r.t. specimen jaw captured from inside the TEM **i** TEM image of Ag nanowire before tensile testing, **j** image of Ag wire after facture, **k** SAED image of optimized X and Y tilting position of nanowire, **l** high resolution image of respective specimen (Adapted with permission from Yang et al. [49])

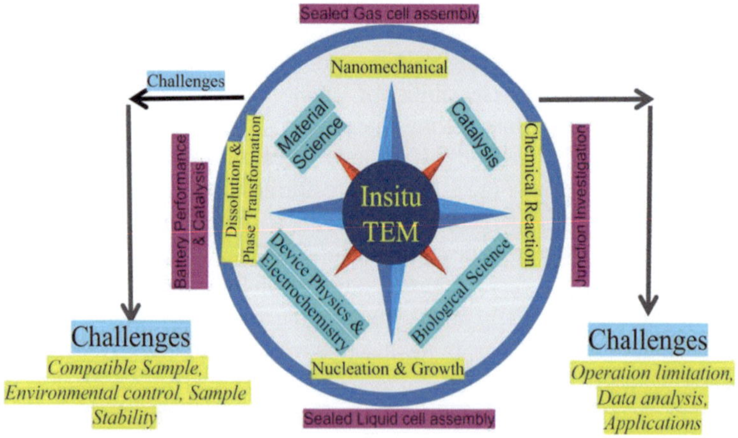

Fig. 7.16 Schematic representation of application areas of in-situ TEM, respective modes of operation and probable challenges faced during its operation and analysis

NOTE: Study of dynamic behavior of material via in-situ TEM w.r.t. real world conditions, guiding in fabrications of advanced material with efficient technologies.

7.7 Protocol for In-situ TEM Analysis

In order to perform quality sample analysis under in-situ TEM need a proper standardized protocol w.r.t. nature of specimen. Still with wide variety and nature of specimen belong to biological, life science or geological science, we have presented here a generalized sample preparation and analysis protocol under in-situ TEM.

Step 1: Sample size and Thickening

Selection of appropriate specimen size from micrometer to nanometer having electron transparent thickness via suitable thinning techniques like focus ion beam (FIB), electropolishing or ultramicrotomy etc.

Step 2: Mounting of Specimen

Electron transparent specimen will be mounted on suitable sample holder like MEMS etc. through proper handling and expertise.

Step 3: Instrument Setup

Respective mode of in-situ TEM operation as per nature of sample need to calibrate and aligned. Activate respective mode of operation like heating, cooling, mechanical testing or atmospheric conditioning etc., till stabilization of respective environment inside the instrument. In addition, there is need to optimize in-situ TEM operational parameters like beam intensity, magnification or aperture size etc.

Step 4: Experiment Design and Imaging

Design the imaging and other experiment process as per requirement of study like heating, cooling etc. Perform real time analysis of specimen at regular interval of time in order to capture desired behavior or changes w.r.t. study requirement.

Step 5: Validation and Reproducibility

In order to claim and report insightful analysis of specimen under in-situ TEM, validated and reproducible data must be needed. Standardized analysis of specimen under in-situ TEM will guide researchers globally for advance research.

Step 6: Interpretation of data

Before explaining and analyzing respective data under in-situ TEM, one should have sufficient knowledge about material's physical, chemical, electrical, optical properties or biological metabolism or catabolism etc. properties. In addition, certain theoretical models must be proposed related to real time analysis of specimen-beam interaction and probable outcomes, so that one can understand and analyze respective data to more precise and accurate manner.

With respect to above mentioned steps to perform in-situ TEM analysis, we have presented a generalized approach from sample selection to instrument conditioning to imaging and the interpretation of respective data. Although, sample analysis under in-situ TEM will vary from sample-to-sample nature, instrument conditions or expertise behind machine etc.

7.8 Conclusion

In current chapter, an attempt has been presented about in-situ TEM fundamentals, principle, working, and future scope. Here stepwise, we have explained, discussed and proposed about the present potential with future possibilities related to in-situ TEM working and respective analysis. Initially, we have discussed about the basic of in-situ TEM followed by active features/working conditions like real time observation, high resolution imaging, exposure of environmental conditions etc. Due to insightful imaging capabilities of in-situ TEM brought it as much more informative and useful through dynamic imaging. Controlled environmental condition inside TEM column, precise sample preparation and wide range of applications in different research and industrial areas, stand in-situ TEM as a dominating role in fundamental and device development research. The real time imaging of specimen under in-situ TEM will easier and more applied with the development of conditions like sealed gas cell and liquid cell assemblies, through respective holder design like MEMS/NEMS etc. Specially, technological advancement and rising demand in battery research sector for its efficient working, will explore in better way by in-situ TEM guided electrochemical analysis. In addition, research area like atomic structuring and restructuring, catalysis dynamics, cellular metabolism or catabolism behavior, junction/heterojunction investigation etc., will be monitored in real time during variable modes of in-situ TEM operation. It will be very helpful in finding each and every growth dynamic, impurities phase during in-process cycles of material processing at nanoscale.

In addition to capabilities of in-situ TEM, it has many challenges which need to optimized as per nature of sample and instrument operation. It includes issue of sample compatibility inside TEM column, equilibrating of environmental conditions inside column, limited manipulation freedom during real time imaging and respective data interpretation for novel results or insightful data. The rising demand of in-situ TEM expand its applicability in areas like material science (nucleation, growth, phase transformation etc.), catalysis (surface restructuring, reaction kinetics etc.), electrochemistry (batteries failure, efficiency enhancement, innovative design fabrication etc.), biological sciences (insight about cellular interactions, metabolism behavior, protein folding etc.). It has been also capabilities in catering the investigation of drug delivery system (uniform drugs uptake, targeted drug release, fabrication of nanodrug etc.), analyzing the operational or failure aspect of electronic system nano-level defects or respective device failures observations in real time domain.

Ultimately, the goal of explaining and discussing about in-situ TEM story right from basic features to advance applications, is to make readers aware about the depth and potential of respective technique. Specifically, objective is to make students/researchers/scientists aware about the insightful scientific explanations and logics behind the state of existence of any material. This approach will very much helpful in understanding and explaining the studied material for finding exact solution or explanation towards path breaking research. This regime of information/data/images/videos related to material under in-situ TEM study, will equip respective material extraordinary database which can be utilized in novel innovations for efficient device/system developments.

Declaration

Author declares that there is no personal or financial conflict of interest regarding publication of this chapter.

References

1. Urban, K.W.: Studying atomic structures by aberration-corrected transmission electron microscopy. Science **321**(5888), 506–510 (2008). https://doi.org/10.1126/science.1152800
2. Allard, L.F., Overbury, S.H., Bigelow, W.C., Katz, M.B., Nackashi, D.P., Damiano, J.: Novel MEMS-based gas-cell/heating specimen holder provides advanced imaging capabilities for in situ reaction studies. Microsc. Microanal. **18**(4), 656–666 (2012). https://doi.org/10.1017/S1431927612001249
3. Miller, B.K., Barker, T.M., Crozier, P.A.: Novel sample preparation for operando TEM of catalysts. Ultramicroscopy **156**, 18–22 (2015). https://doi.org/10.1016/j.ultramic.2015.05.003
4. Li, Y., Zakharov, D., Zhao, S., Tappero, R., Jung, U., Elsen, A.P.H., Baumann, Nuzzo, R.G., Stach, E.A., Frenkel, A.I.: Complex structural dynamics of nanocatalysts revealed in operando conditions by correlated imaging and spectroscopy probes. Nat. Commun. **6**(1), 7583 (2015). https://doi.org/10.1038/ncomms8583
5. Bañares, M.A., Wachs, I.E.: Molecular structures of supported metal oxide catalysts under different environments. J. Raman Spectrosc. **33**(5), 359–380 (2002). https://doi.org/10.1002/jrs.866
6. Vendelbo, S.B., Elkjær, C.F., Falsig, H., Puspitasari, I., Dona, P., Mele, L., Morana, B., Nelissen, B.J., Van Rijn, R., Creemer, J.F., Kooyman, P.J., Helveg, S.: Visualization of oscillatory behaviour of Pt nanoparticles catalysing CO oxidation. Nat. Mater. **13**(9), 884–890 (2014). https://doi.org/10.1038/nmat4033
7. Hawkes, P.W., Spence, J.C.H. (Eds.): Springer Handbook of Microscopy. Springer International Publishing, Cham (2019). https://doi.org/10.1007/978-3-030-00069-1
8. Tang, D.-M.: In Situ Transmission Electron Microscopy Studies of Carbon Nanotube Nucleation Mechanism and Carbon Nanotube-Clamped Metal Atomic Chains. Springer Theses. Springer, Berlin, Heidelberg (2013). https://doi.org/10.1007/978-3-642-37259-9
9. Jinschek, J.R., Helveg, S.: Image resolution and sensitivity in an environmental transmission electron microscope. Micron **43**(11), 1156–1168 (2012). https://doi.org/10.1016/j.micron.2012.01.006

10. Qu, J., Sui, M., Li, R.: Recent advances in in-situ transmission electron microscopy techniques for heterogeneous catalysis. iScience **26**(7), 107072. https://doi.org/10.1016/j.isci.2023.107072
11. Zhang, L., Miller, B.K., Crozier, P.A.: Atomic level in situ observation of surface amorphization in anatase nanocrystals during light irradiation in water vapor. Nano Lett. **13**(2), 679–684 (2013). https://doi.org/10.1021/nl304333h
12. Taheri, M.L., Stach, E.A., Arslan, I., Crozier, P.A., Kabius, B.C., LaGrange, T., Minor, A.M., Takeda, S., Tanase, M., Wagner, J.B., Sharma, R.: Current status and future directions for in situ transmission electron microscopy. Ultramicroscopy **170**, 86–95 (2016). https://doi.org/10.1016/j.ultramic.2016.08.007
13. Falqui, A., Loche, D., Casu, A.: In situ TEM crystallization of amorphous iron particles. Crystals **10**(1), 41 (2020). https://doi.org/10.3390/cryst10010041
14. Niu, K.-Y., Park, J., Zheng, H., Alivisatos, A.P.: Revealing bismuth oxide hollow nanoparticle formation by the Kirkendall effect. Nano Lett. **13**(11), 5715–5719 (2013). https://doi.org/10.1021/nl4035362
15. Creemer, J.F., Helveg, S., Hoveling, G.H., Ullmann, S., Molenbroek, A.M., Sarro, P.M., Zandbergen, H.W.: Atomic-scale electron microscopy at ambient pressure. Ultramicroscopy **108**(9), 993–998 (2008). https://doi.org/10.1016/j.ultramic.2008.04.014
16. Kiener, D., Minor, A.M.: Source truncation and exhaustion: insights from quantitative in situ TEM tensile testing. Nano Lett. **11**(9), 3816–3820 (2011). https://doi.org/10.1021/nl201890s
17. Chou, Y.-C., Tang, W., Chiou, C.-J., Chen, K., Minor, A.M., Tu, K.N.: Effect of elastic strain fluctuation on atomic layer growth of epitaxial silicide in Si nanowires by point contact reactions. Nano Lett. **15**(6), 4121–4128 (2015). https://doi.org/10.1021/acs.nanolett.5b01234
18. Arita, M., Hamada, K., Takahashi, Y., Sueoka, K., Shibayama, T.: In situ transmission electron microscopy for electronics. In: Maaz, K. (Ed.) The Transmission Electron Microscope Theory and Applications. InTech, 2015. https://doi.org/10.5772/60651
19. Wu, F., Yao, N.: In situ transmission electron microscopy studies in gas/liquid environment. Microsc. Anal. (2016). https://doi.org/10.5772/62551
20. Sharma, R.: Design and applications of environmental cell transmission electron microscope for in situ observations of gas-solid reactions. Microsc. Microanal. **7**(6), 494–506 (2001). https://doi.org/10.1007/S10005-001-0015-1
21. Shreyas, R., Khalid Mikhiel, H., Blythe, C.: Hydride Formation in Cladding Materials Studied via In-Situ Environmental Heating Transmission Electron Microscopy. United States (2012)
22. Mehraeen, S., McKeown, J.T., Deshmukh, P.V., Evans, J.E., Abellan, P., Xu, P., Reed, B.W., Taheri, M.L., Fischione, P.E., Browning, N.D.: A (S)TEM gas cell holder with localized laser heating for in situ experiments. Microsc. Microanal. **19**(2), 470–478 (2013). https://doi.org/10.1017/S1431927612014419
23. Daulton, T.L., Little, B.J., Lowe, K., Jones-Meehan, J.: In situ environmental cell-transmission electron microscopy study of microbial reduction of chromium (VI) using electron energy loss spectroscopy. Microsc. Microanal. **7**(6), 470–485 (2001). https://doi.org/10.1007/S10005-001-0021-3
24. Liu, X.H., Zhang, L.Q., Zhong, L., Liu, Y., Zheng, H., Wang, J.W., Cho, J.-H., Dayeh, S.A., Picraux, S.T., Sullivan, J.P., Mao, S.X., Ye, Z.Z., Huang, J.Y.: Ultrafast electrochemical lithiation of individual Si nanowire anodes. Nano Lett. **11**(6), 2251–2258 (2011). https://doi.org/10.1021/nl200412p
25. Williamson, M.J., Tromp, R.M., Vereecken, P.M., Hull, R., Ross, F.M.: Dynamic microscopy of nanoscale cluster growth at the solid-liquid interface. Nature Mater **2**(8), 532–536 (2003). https://doi.org/10.1038/nmat944
26. White, E.R., Singer, S.B., Augustyn, V., Hubbard, W.A., Mecklenburg, M., Dunn, B., Regan, B.C.: In situ transmission electron microscopy of lead dendrites and lead ions in aqueous solution. ACS Nano **6**(7), 6308–6317 (2012). https://doi.org/10.1021/nn3017469
27. Min Yuk, J., Park, J., Ercius, P., Alivistos, A.P.: High-resolution EM of colloidal nanocrystal growth using graphene liquid cells. Science **336**(Issue 6077). https://doi.org/10.1126/science.12176

28. Holtz, M.E., Yu, Y., Gunceler, D., Gao, J., Sundararaman, R., Schwarz, K.A., Arias, T.A., Abruña, H.D., Muller, D.A.: Nanoscale imaging of lithium ion distribution during in situ operation of battery electrode and electrolyte. Nano Lett. **14**(3), 1453–1459 (2014). https://doi.org/10.1021/nl404577c
29. Aurbach, D., Markovsky, B., Levi, M.D., Levi, E., Schechter, A., Moshkovich, M., Cohen, Y.: New insights into the interactions between electrode materials and electrolyte solutions for advanced nonaqueous batteries. J. Power. Sources **81–82**, 95–111 (1999). https://doi.org/10.1016/S0378-7753(99)00187-1
30. Zeng, Z., Liang, W.-I., Liao, H.-G., Xin, H.L., Chu, Y.-H., Zheng, H.: Visualization of electrode-electrolyte interfaces in $LiPF_6$ /EC/DEC electrolyte for lithium ion batteries via in situ TEM. Nano Lett. **14**(4), 1745–1750 (2014). https://doi.org/10.1021/nl403922u
31. Lv, H., Zhu, X., Mei, J., Xia, Y., Wang, B.: Recent progress of in-situ characterization of LiNi1−x−yCoxMnyO2 cathodes for lithium metal batteries: a mini review. Nano Res. **17**(3), 1384–1401 (2024). https://doi.org/10.1007/s12274-023-5986-2
32. Zeng, Z., Zhang, X., Bustillo, K., Niu, K., Gammer, C., Xu, J., Zheng, H.: In situ study of lithiation and delithiation of MoS_2 nanosheets using electrochemical liquid cell transmission electron microscopy. Nano Lett. **15**(8), 5214–5220 (2015). https://doi.org/10.1021/acs.nanolett.5b02483
33. Zhang, Q., Ma, J., Mei, L., Liu, J., Li, Z., Li, J., Zeng, Z.: In situ TEM visualization of LiF nanosheet formation on the cathode-electrolyte interphase (CEI) in liquid-electrolyte lithium-ion batteries. Matter **5**(4), 1235–1250 (2022). https://doi.org/10.1016/j.matt.2022.01.015
34. Zou, R., Cui, Z., Liu, Q., Guan, G., Zhang, W., He, G., Yang, J., Hu, J.: In situ transmission electron microscopy study of individual nanostructures during lithiation and delithiation processes. J. Mater. Chem. A **5**(38), 20072–20094 (2017). https://doi.org/10.1039/C7TA05768G
35. Wang, Z., Santhanagopalan, D., Zhang, W., Wang, F., Xin, H.L., He, K., Li, J., Dudney, N., Meng, Y.S.: In situ STEM-EELS observation of nanoscale interfacial phenomena in all-solid-state batteries. Nano Lett. **16**(6), 3760–3767 (2016). https://doi.org/10.1021/acs.nanolett.6b01119
36. Tao, F. (Feng), Crozier, P.A.: Atomic-scale observations of catalyst structures under reaction conditions and during catalysis. Chem. Rev. **116**(6), 3487–3539 (2016). https://doi.org/10.1021/cr5002657
37. Ye, F., Xu, M., Dai, S., Tieu, P., Ren, X., Pan, X.: In situ TEM studies of catalysts using windowed gas cells. Catalysts **10**(7), 779 (2020). https://doi.org/10.3390/catal10070779
38. Jinschek, J.R.: Advances in the environmental transmission electron microscope (ETEM) for nanoscale in situ studies of gas-solid interactions. Chem. Commun. **50**(21), 2696–2706 (2014). https://doi.org/10.1039/C3CC49092K
39. Harada, K., Matsuda, T., Kasai, H., Kamimura, O., Tonomura, A.: Observation of dynamic interaction of vortices with ion irradiated defects by lorentz microscopy. Ultramicroscopy **67**(1–4), 133–141 (1997). https://doi.org/10.1016/S0304-3991(96)00100-3
40. Merkle, K.L., Thompson, L.J., Phillipp, F.: Collective effects in grain boundary migration. Phys. Rev. Lett. **88**(22), 225501 (2002). https://doi.org/10.1103/PhysRevLett.88.225501
41. Lin, Q., An, X., Liu, H., Tang, Q., Dai, P., Liao, X.: In-situ high-resolution transmission electron microscopy investigation of grain boundary dislocation activities in a nanocrystalline CrMnFeCoNi high-entropy alloy. J. Alloy. Compd. **709**, 802–807 (2017). https://doi.org/10.1016/j.jallcom.2017.03.194
42. Yang, R., Mei, L., Fan, Y., Zhang, Q., Liao, H.-G., Yang, J., Li, J., Zeng, Z.: Fabrication of liquid cell for in situ transmission electron microscopy of electrochemical processes. Nat. Protoc. (2022). https://doi.org/10.1038/s41596-022-00762-y
43. Banhart, F.: The transformation of graphitic onions to diamond under electron irradiation. J. Appl. Phys. **81**(8), 3440–3445 (1997). https://doi.org/10.1063/1.365040
44. Liu, X.H., Zhang, L.Q., Zhong, L., Huang, J.Y.: Ultrafast electrochemical lithiation of individual Si nanowire anode **11**, 2251–2258. https://doi.org/10.1021/nl200412p
45. Wang, C.-M., Li, X., Wang, Z., Xu, W., Liu, J., Gao, F., Kovarik, L., Zhang, J.-G., Howe, J., Burton, D.J., Liu, Z., Xiao, X., Thevuthasan, S., Baer, D.R.: In situ TEM investigation of

congruent phase transition and structural evolution of nanostructured silicon/carbon anode for lithium ion batteries. Nano Lett. **12**(3), 1624–1632 (2012). https://doi.org/10.1021/nl204559u

46. Liu, Y., Zheng, H., Liu, X.H., Huang, S., Zhu, T., Wang, J., Kushima, A., Hudak, N.S., Huang, X., Zhang, S., Mao, S.X., Qian, X., Li, J., Huang, J.Y.: Lithiation-induced embrittlement of multiwalled carbon nanotubes. ACS Nano **5**(9), 7245–7253 (2011). https://doi.org/10.1021/nn202071y
47. Zhu, G.-Z., Prabhudev, S., Yang, J., Gabardo, C.M., Botton, G.A., Soleymani, L.: In situ liquid cell TEM study of morphological evolution and degradation of Pt–Fe nanocatalysts during potential cycling. J. Phys. Chem. C **118**(38), 22111–22119 (2014). https://doi.org/10.1021/jp506857b
48. Han, Z., Porter, A.E.: In situ electron microscopy of complex biological and nanoscale systems: challenges and opportunities. Front. Nanotechnol. **2**, 606253 (2020). https://doi.org/10.3389/fnano.2020.606253
49. Yang, Y., Fu, Z., Zhang, X., Cui, Y., Xu, F., Li, T., Wang, Y.: In situ TEM mechanical characterization of one-dimensional nanostructures via a standard double-tilt holder compatible MEMS device. Ultramicroscopy **198**, 43–48 (2019). https://doi.org/10.1016/j.ultramic.2018.12.008
50. Kang, W., Merrill, M., Wheeler, J.M.: In situ thermomechanical testing methods for micro/nano-scale materials. Nanoscale **9**(8), 2666–2688 (2017). https://doi.org/10.1039/C6NR07330A

Chapter 8
Sample Preparation for Quantitative Analysis Under TEM

To extract meaningful quantitative data from electron microscopy, sample preparation must be precise and reproducible: This will ensure that measurements reflect the true properties of material
*by **Dr. Robert F Egreton,** Author of Physical Principles of Electron Microscopy*

Abstract One of important aspect of material analysis i.e. quantitative analysis using transmission electron microscopy (TEM), has been exhaustively discussed in current chapter. Briefly highlighting the importance of quantitative and respective probable mode analysis has been discussed. Individual explanation of electron diffraction (ED), energy dispersive x-ray spectroscopy (EDS), electron energy loss spectroscopy (EELS), scanning transmission electron microscopy (STEM) modes of operation w.r.t. principle, working, unique characteristics, application and probable challenges have been discussed in detail. Through current chapter, researchers/scientist become able to expand and explain imaging aspect of specimen analysis in thorough and insightful way, through optimized sample preparation techniques.

Keywords Electron diffraction · Energy dispersive spectroscopy · Electron energy loss spectroscopy · Scanning transmission electron microscopy

8.1 Introduction

Atomic or cellular level analysis of materials belong to material science or life science specimens, will be performed with precise and accurate way during TEM analysis. TEM will deal with investigation and analysis about the nucleation and growth kinetics, dislocation or defects, morphological driven properties. Main focus of current chapter is discussion about the different quantitative modes which will be possible under TEM analysis. Technique such as energy dispersive X-ray spectroscopy (EDS), electron energy loss spectroscopy (EELS), scanning transmission electron microscopy (STEM), tomography, holography, selected area electron

R. Singh, *Transmission Electron Microscopy Sample Preparation*,
https://doi.org/10.1007/978-3-031-82967-3_8

diffraction (SAED) etc., may be classified in respective category [1–5]. In addition to qualitative data (shape, size, texture etc.) of material during routine TEM imaging, above stated quantitative techniques (EDS, EELS, SAED etc.) use will make drastic difference in exploring insights about hidden properties of material under study. Collective observed image/graph/spectrum-based data of sample during TEM analysis, will lead to basic to advance analysis and interpretation of respective material analysis. Stated quantitative techniques will utilize in examining and explaining specimen behavior like elemental composition with respective distribution, unequal contrast, growth kinetics etc., as per sensitivity and spatial resolution of respective mode of TEM operation. For example, EDS and EELS techniques will report the compositional behavior of material whereas SAED mode will figure out about the quantitative aspect of crystal structure and phase identification. The cutting-edge technologies like STEM, tomography etc., has unprecedently enhance the quantitative domain of materials. Above all stated quantitative methodologies will setup the basic platform for in-depth investigation of material properties under TEM analysis.

Technological advancement in TEM basic instrumentation, data capturing system and respective data analysis software etc., have also excel the quantitative data aspect as well the respective in-depth interpretation. Historically, the journey of novel discoveries/innovations in different research areas, will initially locate and further authenticated/validated through imaging and quantitative modes of TEM operation. The features and capabilities of in-situ TEM, cryo-TEM, STEM or aberration corrected (C_S) TEM etc., bring new horizon for quantitative insight of respective materials w.r.t. phase quantification, impurity phase detection, defects identification etc. [1–5].

8.2 Importance of Quantitative Analysis

With vast capabilities and insights of TEM specimen analysis, respective quantitative exploration of material has wide potential in in-depth structural or functional investigations. In coming paragraph, we have summarized specimen investigation for possible quantitative analysis of material.

8.2.1 Elemental Composition and Distribution

In addition to morphological features of specimen-like shape, size, texture etc. under TEM imaging, site specific elemental analysis of respective material through EDS or EELS can be performed. This will further strengthen the detail of elemental makeup and respective distribution behavior. Respective study will locate the presence of impurity phase or active components positioning w.r.t. bulk material. Further, EELS techniques have also capability of analyzing respective chemical state of material under investigation [1–5].

8.2.2 Crystallographic Information

Selected area electron diffraction (SAED) will not predict directly about the crystal structure, but with minor calculation and measurements on TEM diffraction images, one can claim for specific information about crystal structure, orientation and defects behavior. This will be really helpful in designing the desired material having specialized structural alignments for specific applications [1–5].

8.2.3 Compositional Contrast

Under quantitative mode during TEM operation, STEM with dark field (DF) imaging mode, has ability to distinguish multicomponent/multiphase material from respective constituents through contrast differentiation. Through inelastic scattering, source electron beam gets diffracted through specimen at different angles in addition to elastic scattering. Inelastic scattered electrons will be captured via annular dark field (ADF) or high angle annular dark field (HAADF) detectors w.r.t. different scattering angles. It will generate sharp compositional contrast illustration explaining the purity and uniform distribution content of specimen [1–5].

8.2.4 Multidisciplinary Applications

Quantitative modes of TEM are not just limited to finding atomic or molecular predictions/calculations of material through quantitative modes of TEM operation, but will have potential to correlate and explain the reason of ineffective or highly efficient functional performances of materials under study. Dynamic behavior and respective data of quantitative techniques like EDS, EELS, diffraction etc., extend respective modes applicability in areas viz. applied sciences, geological science, cosmetic industry, paint industry, polymer industry, semiconductor industry. This will strengthen the existing material investigation for novel material to efficient device development [1–5].

Discussing the importance of quantitative modes under TEM, is not about the justification for the use of quantitative attachments like SAED, EDS, EELS etc., but it is about the strengthening of proposed experimental or theoretical research work hypothesis.

8.3 Quantitative Techniques Under TEM

As per demand and requirement of research hypothesis, researchers will purchase or upgrade their TEM instrumentation with quantitative attachment like SAED, EDS, EELS, STEM etc., to expand their research analysis domain. In coming section, we have discussed about principle, working, applications and challenges behind the techniques w.r.t. handling, sample preparation, interpretation of results etc.

8.3.1 Electron Diffraction Study

8.3.1.1 Meaning of Electron Diffraction (ED)

Electron diffraction simply means study of diffraction pattern observed when electron beam passes through electron transparent sample. ED will help in explaining and correlating about atomic or molecular structural data captured through TEM/HRTEM/Cryo-TEM/in-situ TEM etc., techniques [1, 6]. ED patterns will help in answering the question like:

(a) Is our material have amorphous or crystalline nature.
(b) If crystalline phase is present in specimen, what are the respective crystallographic parameter.
(c) Is material being monocrystalline or polycrystalline. What is grain morphology, grain size or grain orientation etc.
(d) Is there is more than one phase present in specimen.

8.3.1.2 Principle and Working of ED

On the basis of dual nature of electron i.e. wave as well particle nature, under interaction of electron beam with e-beam transparent specimen, respective wave nature become prominent. De Broglie well established relation have explained about the wavelength of electron as per Eq. (8.1) [1]:

$$\lambda = \frac{h}{p} = \frac{h}{\sqrt{2meV}} \tag{8.1}$$

where (h) is Planck's constant and (m) is mass of the electron, (e) is charge of electron and (V) is accelerating voltage.

Atomic size equivalent wavelength of electron beam (in Å) at higher accelerating voltage, will interact with atomic array of crystalline material, act like diffraction grating. Specific diffraction pattern will be observed in different specimens as per their crystal structure. Periodic potential of crystal lattice interaction with electron beam brings constructive and destructive interference behaviour. This will

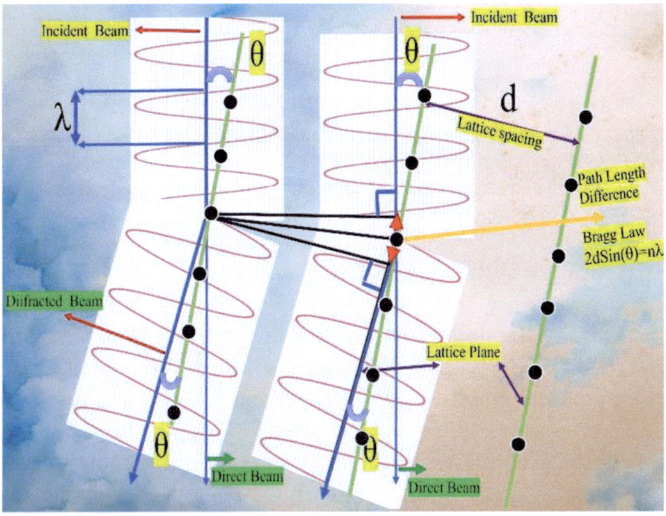

Fig. 8.1 Working of Braggs law

generate the respective diffraction pattern of specimen as per nature of specimen i.e. amorphous or crystalline.

In case of crystalline specimen, observation of diffraction pattern will be facilitated by Bragg's law as shown in Fig. 8.1, given in Eq. (8.2) [4]:

$$2d\sin(\theta) = n\lambda \tag{8.2}$$

where n is order of reflection, λ is wavelength, d is interplanar spacing, θ is bragg angle.

As the Bragg's angle during diffraction mechanism lies in low diffraction range of milli-radian (mrad), the respective specimen explanation will be correlated with reciprocal lattice domain of specimen for crystal structure exploration.

8.3.1.3 Types of Electron Diffraction

On the basis of availability of instrument specifications, respective diffraction analysis can be performed. Broadly, two type of diffraction behavior namely SAED and microdiffraction, primarily used for materials analysis [3, 5, 6]. Through incident electron beam, convergent electron beam is used to perform different type of diffraction studies viz. selected area diffraction, CBED, microdiffraction, large angle convergent diffraction etc. [7] Different beam convergence approach has been represented schematically under Fig. 8.2.

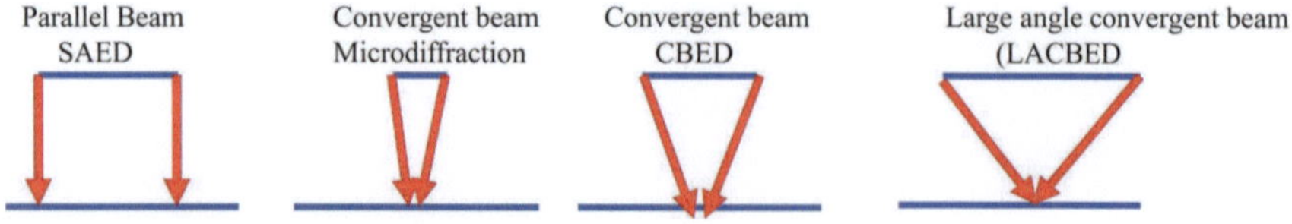

Fig. 8.2 Different beam convergence schematic representation has been depicted

Selected Area Electron Diffraction (SAED)

This is one of most basic diffraction mode, which will be used with different type of TEM, HRTEM, STEM, in-situ TEM etc. instrument. SAED is used to generate the diffraction patterns in wider area of specimen like 0.5 μm dimensions. With prior selection of appropriate area of specimen followed by use of suitable size of diffraction mechanical aperture, will produce respective diffraction patterns [3, 5, 6].

Steps to Perform SAED

There are following generalized step which may be followed to perform SAED analysis for appropriate specimen irrespective to model and design of TEM instrument:

(a) Locate the specific area of interest on TEM grid during normal TEM imaging.
(b) Objective aperture must be removed.
(c) Press SA button to put TEM into selected area diffraction mode. Set the specimen for optimum parameters i.e. magnification, center position of sample on fluorescent screen, focusing of sample with objective focus knob.
(d) Insert suitable size diffraction aperture followed by centering w.r.t. specimen position
(e) Focus the edge of diffraction aperture using DIFF Focus.
(f) Press DIFF button. Select an appropriate camera length ~ 20–40 cm.
(g) Adjust condenser lens (brightness knob) towards lowest intensity, in order to generate more coherent beam.
(h) Insert beam stopper in path of central beam
(i) Record the diffraction micrograph and save at desired place.

For example, in interesting work by Dai et al. [8] authors have studied the growth and phase identification of InSe for γ-InSe and γ-In_2Se_3 phases. γ-InSe single phase crystal structure having flakes morphology (Fig. 8.3a), has been confirmed for hexagonal structure (Fig. 8.3c) through six-fold symmetry via SAED measurement (Fig. 8.3b). Similar measurement has been performed for γ-In_2Se_3.

Similarly, Shen et al. [9] authors have studied for lithiation/de-lithiation behaviour of ball milled Si and porous Si after different charge–discharge cycles. Clear structure evolution and phase transition has been observed for ball milled Si and porous Si in Li-Si cell with voltage window 0.01–2 V at current density of 400 mA/g has been observed. Inset image of Fig. 8.4a, e shows crystalline nature via SAED study for both ball milled Si and Porous Si whereas during different charge-discharging cycles

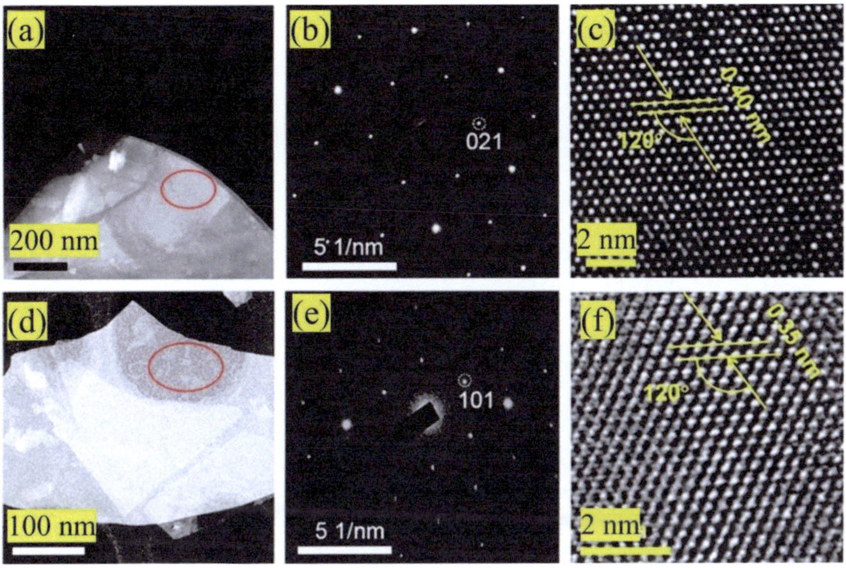

Fig. 8.3 **a** TEM images of γ-InSe, **b** SAED pattern, **c** HRTEM Images of marked area; whereas **d–e** images show TEM images of γ-In_2Se_3, **b** SAED pattern, **c** HRTEM Images of marked area respectively (Adapted with permission from Dai [8] under open access)

for respective specimens shows formation of amorphous phase has been confirmed which is depicted in inset of Fig. 8.4b–c, f–h. In order to further authenticate the porous silica nanostructure behaviour with LiSi cell, both solid Si nanowire and porous Si nanowire has been studied and detail in depicted in Fig. 8.4i–p. With reference to Si nanowire image before lithiation process at Fig. 8.4i shows diameter of 120 nm with polycrystalline pattern through SAED analysis under Fig. 8.4o. Just with lithiation process of Silicon nanowire (Fig. 8.4m–n), coating of Li on the surface of Si nanowire has been observed clearly as shown in Fig. 8.4l–n. Further, transformed phase of Si nanowire after lithiation i.e. c-$Li_{15}Si_4$, has shown modified SAED pattern for Fig. 8.4p [9].

Normally, recorded diffraction micrograph pattern will be depend on nature of crystal growth orientation of specimen. If specimen is amorphous in nature, destructive interference of diffracted beam gives diffuse concentric ring pattern whereas single crystalline pattern shows bright spots arranged in regular pattern. Similarly, polycrystalline specimen shows concentric ring with spot pattern during diffraction study.

Micro-diffraction (Nano-Diffraction)

As the name 'micro-diffraction' predicts, is going to deal with diffraction of specimen in micro range i.e. ~ 10–500 nm in diameter. In comparison to SAED study where

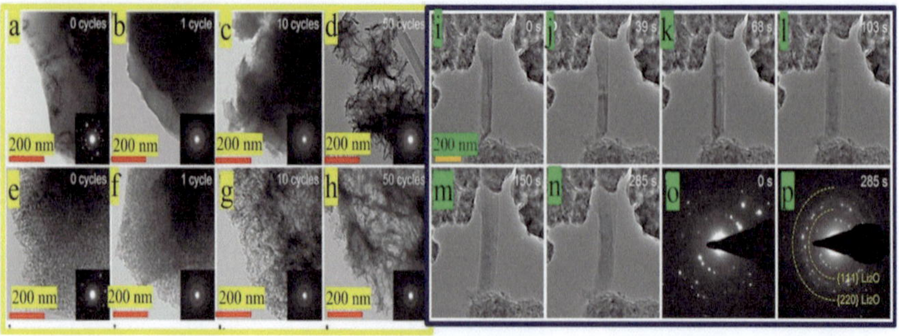

Fig. 8.4 Ex-Situ TEM characterization of ball milled Si and porous Si after different charging-discharging cycles with **a–d** shows respective SAED pattern, **a** Ball milled Si before lithiation, **b–d** after 1, 10 and 50 cycle; **e** TEM Images of porous Silicon before lithiation, **f–h** shows lithiation cycles for 1, 10, 50 cycles with **e–h** shows respective SAED pattern; In-situ TEM Si nanowire lithiation process **a** before lithiation, **j–n** time dependent lithiation of Si nanowire, **o–p** SAED pattern of respective specimen for before and after lithiation respectively (Adapted with permission from Shen et al. [9] under open access)

diffraction aperture will outline the area of diffraction whereas in microdiffraction mode respective aperture get utilizes in converging the electron beam for generating diffraction pattern. As per suitability in TEM instrument, nano-diffraction behavior of specimen can be explored having specimen area in ~ 1 nm diameter range. For example, convergent beam electron diffraction (CBED) will use convergent electron beam to get specimen diffraction pattern exploring crystal structure symmetry and defect analysis.

Kattan et al. [10], studied about the identification and analysis of Cu_2ZnSnS4 (CZTS) crystal structure through SAED and CBED in addition to XRD and HRTEM study. The presence of small and larger size nanoparticles distribution of CZTS material has been observed under Fig. 8.5a, d. Figure 8.5b through SAED study shows polycrystalline nature of CZTS with 112, 200, 211, 224, 332 kesterite plane reflections. Specifically (211) reflections, will confirm for presence of larger tetragonal unit cell for kesterite and stannite materials. Further, (112) diffraction planes have been further authenticated with HRTEM image d-spacing value of 3.1 Å as shown in Fig. 8.5c. CBED analysis of large size NPs for CZTS confirms the weak superlattice reflections w.r.t. tetragonal units in presence of hexagonal disc close to central disc in [010] phase (Fig. 8.5e).

In order to make more clarity about diffraction regime of CZTS, the SAED and CBED patterns has been taken for individual particles at different crystal zone axis Fig. 8.5g–i. Different pattern for low indexed crystal plane has been extracted with the help of Kikuchi band in current diffraction study. (001) zone axis view unit cell along tetragonal structure having four-fold symmetry whereas (010) zone axis has two-fold symmetry. In addition, different superlattice reflections i.e. (002), (101), (110) of respective tetragonal unit cell has been also demonstrated in Fig. 8.5g.

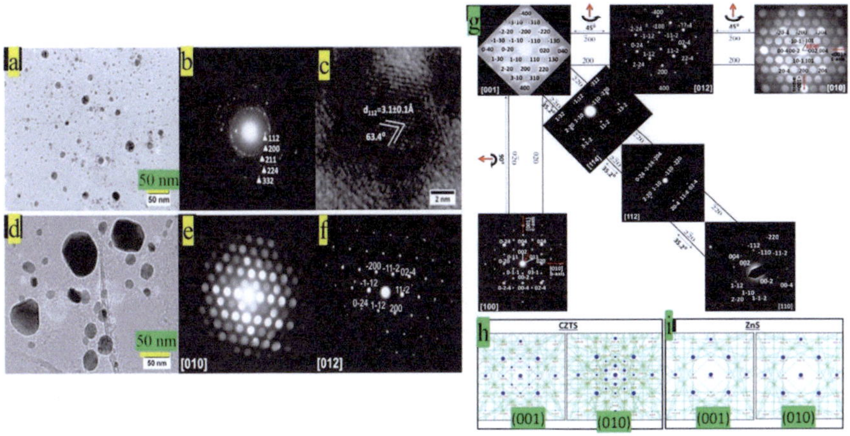

Fig. 8.5 **a**, **d** TEM image of as gowned CZTS small and large size NPs, **b** SAED of smaller population NPs, **c** high resolution image w.r.t. 112 planes, **e–f** shows CBED and SAED of larger nanostructure; **g** CBED and SAED pattern identification for CZTS specimen through Kikuchi band whereas simulation study for **h** [001], **i** [010] zone axis of CZTS and ZnS respectively (Adapted with permission from Kattan et al. [10] under open access)

In addition, simulation studies for diffraction pattern also have been performed for kesterite CZTS and ZnS w.r.t. (001) and (010) zone axis [10], as shown in Fig. 8.5h–i.

There are following step which may be followed to perform micro-diffraction analysis for appropriate specimen irrespective to model and design of TEM instrument.

Steps to Perform Microdiffraction

(a) Locate the area of interest on TEM grid during normal TEM imaging at 20,000–30,000x.
(b) Set specimen height (z) in eucentric position so that during specimen tilt, specimen shift will not take place.
(c) Insert diffraction aperture followed by sharp focusing of aperture edge with DIFF focus knob.
(d) Take diffraction aperture out and bring TEM to normal imaging mode.
(e) Insert suitable size C2 aperture, followed by focusing through objective lens control.
(f) Focus the specimen again by specimen height control (z height).
(g) Press DIFF button and observe the respective diffraction pattern.
(h) Adjust condenser lens (brightness knob) towards lowest intensity, in order to generate more coherent beam.
(i) Insert beam stopper in path of central beam
(j) Record the diffraction micrograph.

With above steps, suitably transparent specimen become able to disclose the insightful crystal structure, symmetry and defects behaviour very closely.

8.3.1.4 Application of Diffraction Studies in TEM

Normally, electron diffraction mode under TEM will be utilized for exploring that whether the material under analysis is amorphous or crystalline in nature [1]. Specifically, diffraction mode will be utilized in identification of materials crystalline or amorphous or mix state phase, during the in-process as well at the final stage of respective materials synthesis. Growth kinetics with dynamics behavior of material will also be investigated through quantification of different lattice parameters as per material crystal structure [11]. Further, the orientation aspect of different grains w.r.t. respective bulk or polycrystalline material, can also be predicted and analyzed very precisely at optimum specimen thickness with single or double axis tilt TEM specimen holder. Furthermore, in depth diffraction studies leads to defect analysis of crystalline material includes identification of different dislocations, twin boundaries etc., analysis at nanoscale [8].

8.3.1.5 Challenges Behind Electron Diffraction Analysis

There are following factors during pre and post quality diffraction imaging w.r.t. variable properties of specimen as well of TEM instrument.

Quality Sample Preparation

Optimum specimen thickness in range of ~ <100 nm, through appropriate synthesis method with minimum artifacts suitable for diffraction analysis. Process oriented defects like mechanical stress, chemical oxidation etc., incorporation into specimen structure, must be minimized in order to achieve precise diffraction imaging [3, 4].

Beam Induced Damage

Over or under beam exposure during TEM analysis on specimen surface will bring damaged or ill-analyzed specimen behavior. Specially, sensitive specimen under over beam exposure leads to damaging or modifying actual the material properties, leads to misleading diffraction results [3, 4].

Aligned TEM Instrument

As per capabilities of TEM instrument, calibrated TEM parameters w.r.t. diffraction study (camera length etc.), low intensity beam, improper beam alignment, vacuum stability, diffraction aperture centric position w.r.t. specimen position etc., are the factors which must be upkeep during respective diffraction analysis [3, 4].

Multiphase Identification with Respective Orientation

Insight understanding w.r.t. multiphase crystal structures and respective grain orientation of different material under diffraction study under TEM, will always be demanding and essential to predict about respective material quality. Due to overlapping of different phases in polycrystalline material will create difficulty in individual phase identification in respective composite samples. Optimum and uniform thickness of specimen with sufficient beam energy and beam size (in nano-range) at appropriate size diffraction aperture, will help in identifying multiphase and respective material orientation more precisely [3, 4].

Through above stated details related to diffraction study of material via SAED or microdiffraction mode in TEM technique, researchers can explore respective material structural or functional aspect in more insightful manner. Researchers can identify respective material crystalline or amorphous nature, defects domain, single or multiphase identification with respective grain orientation, or texture analysis etc.

NOTE: Diffraction Data is Essential in TEM for Identifying the Crystal Structure and Orientation of Material at Atomic Level.

8.3.2 Energy Dispersive X-Ray Spectroscopy (EDS or EDX)

Energy dispersive x-ray spectroscopy (EDS or EDX) is one of powerful analytical technique to be used in conjunction with TEM for elemental composition and quantification of material under study [12].

8.3.2.1 Principle and Working of EDS

EDS will work on the principle that high energy beam bombarded on material surface causes emission of x-ray energy having characteristic fingerprint w.r.t. element present. Specifically, high energy beam will eject or remove electron from specimen surface which is further filled by higher energy level electron during relaxation. Energy released during relaxation process is unique for each element in material which will be further used in identification and proportion assessment of respective element. Figure 8.6a demonstrated the generation of x-ray during interaction of specimen surface with high energy electron beam and (b) shows the generalized interaction behavior of electron beam with specimen surface.

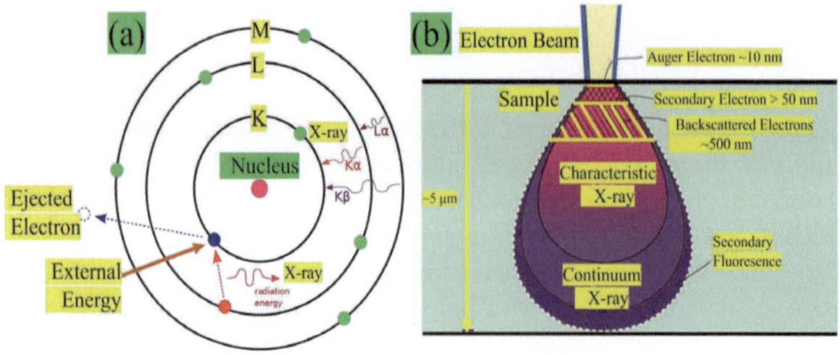

Fig. 8.6 **a** Demonstrated the generation of x-ray during interaction of specimen surface with high energy electron beam, **b** the generalized interaction behavior of specimen with incident electron beam

Steps to Perform EDS Analysis

There are following generalized steps which can be followed in order to perform EDS analysis through TEM:

(a) Prepare the ultrathin specimen have electron transparent thickness.
(b) Mount respective specimen on suitable TEM grid.
(c) Before loading specimen holder inside TEM, TEM must be optimally aligned and calibrate for imaging.
(d) Calibrate the EDS detector for accurate quantification.
(e) Locate the area of interest in TEM imaging mode for EDS in bright field or dark field mode as per instrument capability and specimen nature.
(f) Set the imaging conditions like accelerating voltage, spot size, beam current, condenser aperture size etc., as per sample requirement.
(g) Collect the EDS spectrum through suitable detector to accumulate the x-ray count for clear signal w.r.t. optimum values of dead time and x-ray count etc.
(h) Save the acquired spectrum.

Recorded spectrum through EDS analysis will be used in qualitative and quantitative analysis of material under study. As per nature of sample, scientist/operator have freedom to manipulate the beam current, condenser aperture, orientation of specimen, acquisition time etc., to get sufficient x-ray count for nearly accurate and precise quantification.

8.3.2.2 Advance Correction Algorithms for Elements Quantification

Modern EDS systems have capabilities in precise elemental quantification of material through x-ray intensity w.r.t. count in comparison to standard data. There are following approaches which can be utilized for accurate elemental quantification of material.

ZAF Correction

ZAF correction is one of crucial step in precise quantification of elemental concentration. Although, updated system will automatically apply the respective correction in final calculation results. Firstly, Z-correction (Z) deal with corrections in quantification of specimen through respective atomic number of elements. Current correction will consider the differences in ionization behavior and backscattering of electrons with variation in different atomic number. Secondly, absorption correction (A), which will be prominent and important due to presence of variable element atomic number and respective specimen thickness during x-ray absorption mechanism. This correction is significant in low x-ray energy and thicker samples analysis. Thirdly, fluorescence (F) correction which will be prominent in case of high energy generating-ray which have ability to excite the characteristic x-ray of lighter element also during individual detection. Collective ZAF correction, will generate a precise and accurate quantitative analysis of specimen in EDS through TEM imaging [1, 13].

CLIFF LORIMER Method

This is an important method, also known as k-factor method is widely used for quantification in EDS analysis via TEM. Specifically, use of Cliff-Lorimer approach is effective and useful over thin specimens where matrix-based effect like absorption and fluorescence are minimum. This method will study the proportionality between intensity of characteristic x-ray peak and corresponding concentration of respective element in specimen [14, 15]. Fundamentally, Cliff-Lorimer approach will work as per Eq. (8.3) as given below:

$$\frac{C_A}{C_B} = K_{AB}\frac{I_A}{I_B} \tag{8.3}$$

where C_A and C_B are the concentration of element A and B, I_A and I_B are the characteristic x-ray intensity of respective element. K_{AB} correspond to sensitivity factor known as k-factor for x-ray generation and detection efficiencies of element A and B.

During application of Cliff-Lorimer approach, initial collection of desired EDS spectrum followed by peak identification of respective element in specimen. Precise peak intensity of respective elements will achieve with integrating corresponding peak via ignoring related background area [16]. Finally, known k-factor will be applied for element pair of interest w.r.t. Eq. (8.3). In addition, respective k-factor can also be determined from related software database or from literature respectively.

8.3.2.3 Modes of EDS Analysis

EDS analysis in TEM can be performed in different modes as per requirement of data and objective of research hypothesis will be with respect to specimen nature. Modes of EDS analysis will be discussed as below.

Point Analysis

Localized compositional analysis of specimen in TEM will be performed with point mode analysis of EDS. Presence of defects, impurity phase or identification of different phases in specimen, will be authenticated and analyzed in current mode of quantification [1, 3]. In addition, challenges of beam damage to specimen surface, limited spatial resolution due to constrained interaction volume, interference in quantification for low atomic number through absorption and fluorescence factors etc., need to optimized during respective specimen precise analysis.

Line Scan Analysis

Quantification of specimen under line scan mode will be performed along the linearly from one point to other across the sample. Under this mode, interface identification w.r.t. multiple phases, composition variation along the specific direction or boundary of composite material etc., can be performed [1, 3].

Area-Mapping Analysis

With identification of particular area during TEM imaging, area mapping credits data about 2-dimensional mapped area w.r.t. composition of sample. Area map mode will give idea about the compositional dispersion, impurities or multiple phase detection according to specimen behavior [1, 3].

Above discussed modes of EDS analysis in TEM, will be utilized as per requirements of research objective and nature of specimen. Many times, we have to use most of mode under EDS, in order to get insightful data which matching with pre-proposed theoretical hypothesis.

8.3.2.4 Applications of EDS

In order to get structural, compositional and functional clarity about the sample, EDS analysis in TEM proven as an indispensable tool for material science, life science, nanotechnology, semiconductor sector. In coming paragraph, we have explained about versatile applications of EDS.

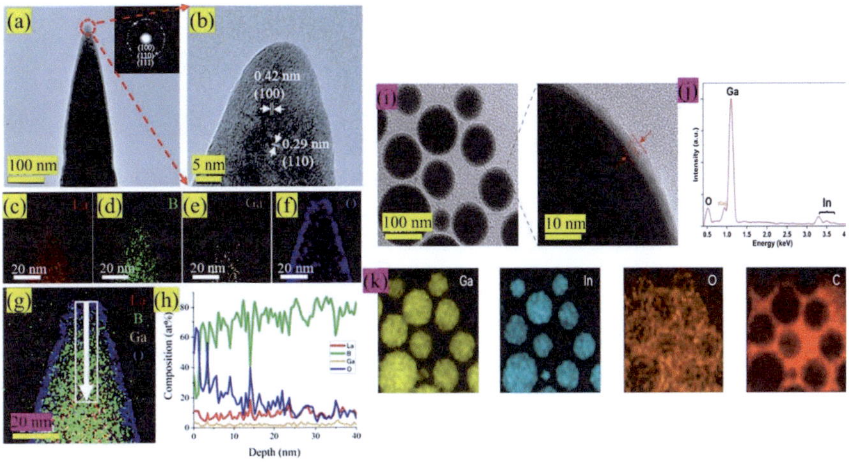

Fig. 8.7 **a** Shows nanoneedle LaB_6 tip image with respective SAED pattern, **b** HRTEM image shows excellent lattice fringes free from vibration, **c–g** shows respective elemental mapping profiling for **c** La, **d** B, **e** Ga, **f** O, **g** La + B + Ga + O, **h** shows depth elements profiling along arrow in **g** (Adapted with permission from Tang et al. [17] under open access); **i** shows TEM image of EGaIn ND, **j** respective EDS spectrum, **k** EDS mapping of Ga, In, O and C elements for EGaIn ND respectively (Adapted with permission from Xu et al. [18] under open access)

Material Sciences

EDS analysis in TEM, will help researchers in analysis and characterization of sample in phase identification, compositional and defects analysis, unwanted phase detection etc. In addition, to establish correlation between microstructural features with respective chemical composition of sample, EDS area scan or area map analysis will be very useful.

In one interesting work, Tang et al. [17] analyzed purity and quality of nanoneedle of LaB_6 for field emission. In addition to HRTEM and SAED oriented analysis of LaB_6 nanoneedle (Fig. 8.7a, b), the chemical composition of respective material has been verified with EDS-mapping mode under TEM. Figure 8.7c–f shows presence of lanthanum (La) and boron (B) as the main component of needle whereas Gallium (Ga) incorporated due to FIB milling and oxygen element attributed due to exposure with exposure of open air. More interestingly, line profiling of specimen under Fig. 8.7g, h shows uniform distribution of La whereas B increases from surface to interior side. This will be the ideal condition for lowering the work function condition in respective material [17].

In similar work, Xu et al. [18] has reported the analysis of surfactant coated liquid eutectic Gallium indium nanodroplet (EGaIn ND). Novel stability features of metal droplets have become most demanding in drug delivery, conductive inks, printed circuit etc. research areas. Under Fig. 8.7i, j shows uniform particle size of EGaIn ND i.e. 100 nm after 240 min shaking. Specifically, EDS mapping shows confined and uniform distribution of Ga and In element w.r.t. shape of ND whereas oxygen

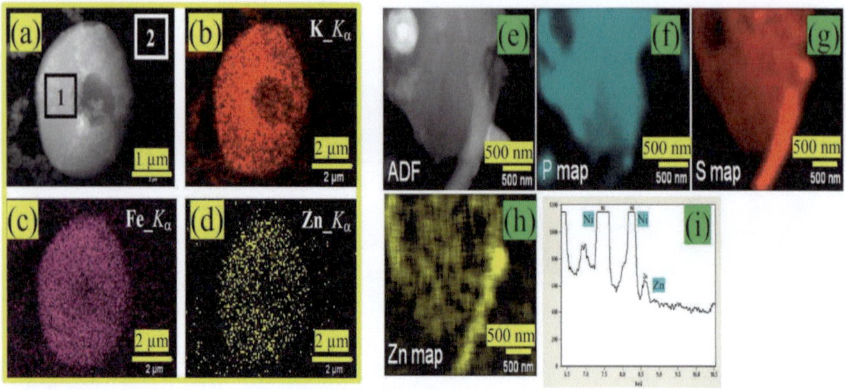

Fig. 8.8 **a** STEM-ADF (dark field imaging) of RBC cell, **b** dual EDS spectra mapping **of** respective cell for **b** K, **c** Fe, **d** Zn with rectangle 1 marking for collection of elemental distribution whereas rectangle 2 shows area used for background collection; **e** shows sperm cell Z-contrast annular dark STEM image, **f–h** X-ray mapping for P, S and Zn element, **i** EDS spectra of respective cell (Adapted with permission from Wu et al. [19])

and carbon distributed in scattered manner due to presence of polymer and oxide layer [18], as shown in Fig. 8.7k.

Biological Science

Identification of cellular system or organelles of biological specimen can be performed with EDS analysis. Tissue engineering and tissue implantation materials interaction with different biomaterial, will be analyzed very closely with respective modes viz. point, area, line scan or mapping. In addition, detection of specialized trace elements in biomaterial will also be monitored while EDS analysis.

Wu et al. [19] reported high performance elemental and mapping analysis of biological specimens. The morphological and spatial distribution of chemical species in red blood cell (RBC) has been demonstrated in Fig. 8.8a–d. Intact morphology of RBC Cell has been observed in Fig. 8.8a under STEM-dark field imaging mode whereas uniform elemental composition of K, Fe and Zn in respective cellular system has been observed as shown in Fig. 8.8b–d. Authors has also investigated sperm cell analysis under X-ray map mode. The confirmation of phosphorous rich DNA with dense packing of sulfur containing protamines in sperm head has been confirmed in Fig. 8.8f–h with STEM-ADF imaging. In addition, EDS spectra of respective cell also has been performed confirmed [19] which is depicted at Fig. 8.8i.

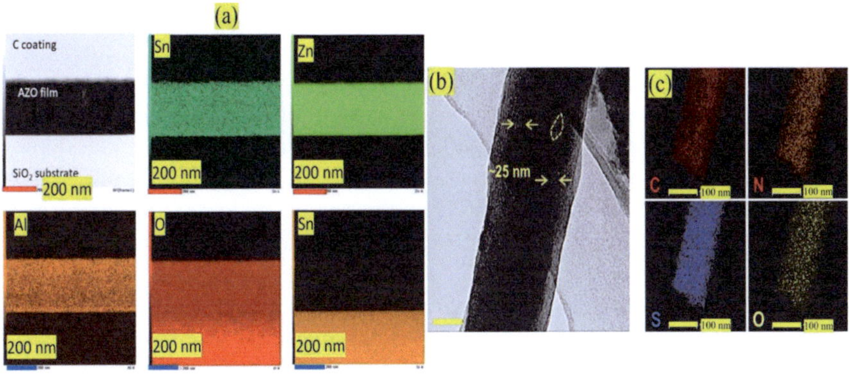

Fig. 8.9 **a** EDS mapping of AZO + SnO_2 2% on silica thin film (AZO_2S) for Sn, Zn, Al, O and Si (Adapted with permission from Latronico et al. [20] under open access), **b**, **c** TEM and EDS-mapping of S/N-KCNFs nanofiber respectively (Adapted with permission from Xiong et al. [21] under open access)

Nanotechnology

Due to rising dominance of nanotechnology technologies in different sectors like power sector, energy sector, cosmetics, pharmaceutical, textiles industries etc., respective materials nanostructures and composition analysis become very important. This will help scientist/researchers to tailor specialized properties of materials for specific applications. Thin film and coating industry will also get benefited with EDS technique in TEM analysis, for quality assessment and development of advanced, economical and durable material.

Latronico et al. [20] reported SnO_2 doped Al-ZnO (AZO) thin film fabrication on Silica and Al_2O_3 substrate investigated materials for respective thermoelectric power capabilities. Out of multiple specimens, AZO + 2%SnO_2 thin film specimen grown on silica substrate, shows power factor values of 211.8 $\mu W/mk^2$ and 8.56 W/mK at 300 and 573 K temperature respectively. TEM-EDS modes has been utilized to study the uniformity of elemental distribution in AZO_2S. Figure 8.9a shows uniform distributions of Al, Zn, O with Sn elements in respective specimen. The uniform distribution of Sn on the AZO thin film without any aggregation, proposed respective metal uniform substitution or interstitial entry [20] has been confirmed. In one more similar work, Xiong et al. [21] reported porous kink carbon nanofiber thin film having high potassium ion storage ability. Sulfur and nitrogen co-doped kinked carbon nanofiber (S/N-KCNFs) has shown high performance rate of 270 mAh/g at current density 2000 mA/g with retention capacity rate of 93.3% after 2000 cycles. With the help of TEM imaging under Fig. 8.9b, mesoporous nature (~ 25 nm in diameter) of carbon nanofiber has been confirmed. Importantly, the uniform incorporation of nitrogen (N) and carbon (c) into respective nanofiber has been observed with TEM-EDS mapping mode [21] as shown in Fig. 8.9c.

Semiconductor Industry

Most of electronic sector devices will be dominate by semiconductor technologies. With rising demand of electronic devices w.r.t. efficiency, respective updated technologies will bring fast modifications through structural tuning like doping, heterojunction formation etc. Elemental composition during failure of semiconductor system, detection of composition contrast in layered semiconductor system etc., can be analyzed under TEM-EDS system for efficient, reliable and economical technologies [22].

EDS analysis in TEM technique will be extended to geological science, environment science, metallurgy, archeological science, catalyst research etc. The ultimate goal of specimen analysis under EDS is for understanding of compositional investigations of materials for efficient futuristic technologies.

8.3.2.5 Challenges Under EDS Analysis

In addition to wide capabilities of EDS analysis under TEM, there are certain challenges which must need to discuss [1, 3]. Here are some prominent challenges which are presented below.

Spatial Resolution

Ability of TEM electron beam to scan the specimen surface in localized manner is always challenging. Specifically, small beam diameter with high beam current, minimal beam spreading with thinner specimen surface (~ 50 nm) will lead difficult in maintaining spatial resolution of respective analysis. In addition to optimized detector specification with its relative position w.r.t. around the specimen etc., will contribute towards feature of improved spatial resolution [1, 3].

Quantification Challenge

Its look very simple to us as we credit with quantified spectrum in quick time during EDS analysis. Being electron microscopist, we must have to understand factors behind actual quantification process. Effect of absorption and fluorescence, inaccurate detector efficiency, overlapping between different elements peak positions, matrix effect etc. w.r.t. instrumental and operational factors, will restrict improper quantification of material under study. Stated challenges will be optimized and minimized with uniform thin specimen (~ 100 nm), ultrathin detector window or windowless detector, peak deconvolution algorithms etc., for peak overlapping, matrix corrected algorithms with standard database having minimum errors etc. [1, 3].

Low Signal to Noise Ratio (SNR)

EDS coupled with TEM has issue of low SNR with many samples poses as a significant challenge during precise elemental quantification. Optimum beam intensity with protection of specimen from beam damage with longer acquisition time and sufficient thickness, will bring high x-ray signal intensity from specimen surface. In addition, proper grounding and shielding from electromagnetic interference for TEM-EDS system with respective detector advance resolution and efficiency, will be required. Use of appropriate size of condenser and objective aperture without affecting beam current, optimum accelerating voltage, stabilized specimen from organic contaminant etc., factors bring minimum noise, maximum signal during elemental detection and quantification [1, 3].

Detection Limitation

Role of efficient generation of x-rays is equally important as their efficient detection. Low energy x-ray (1 keV) generating from light element ($Z < 5$) will have lowest detection efficiency. Poor energy resolution and high-count rate, high dead time etc., factors will deteriorate the respective specimen efficient quantification. Respective elements precise and lowest range quantification will be improved with lowest background noise and highest detector efficiency and proper calibration [1, 3].

Sample Preparation

The approach used in thinning of specimen will be depend on nature of sample. Broadly, sample can be belonged to metal, alloy, polymer sheet or biological sample or nano/bulk powder form. According to nature and properties of sample, respective specimen will be prepared for respective elemental quantification. For example, any metal or hard alloy will proceed with grinding, polishing, dimpling followed by FIB thinning and ion milling for precise thinning. Whereas. biological specimen will follow fixation, dehydration, embedding, infiltration and ultramicrotomy steps in respective specimen preparation. In case of nanoparticle respective analysis which is in powder or liquid form, will proceed with appropriate dispersion in suitable solvent, followed by drop casting on TEM grid for elemental detection [1, 3].

From above discussion, researchers get credited insight about different pre and post specimen information related to TEM-EDS analysis. Through above systematic discussion, researchers/scientists will get aware about probable areas of mistakes and chances of error during EDS analysis, which can be minimized, towards efficient and precise quantitative analysis.

NOTE: EDS Technique in TEM Identifies and Maps Elemental Composition at Nanoscale.

8.3.3 *Electron Energy Loss Spectroscopy (EELS)*

EELS is the one of powerful analytical technique, can used in analysis and detection of materials w.r.t. their electronic and chemical composition.

8.3.3.1 Principle and Working of EELS

EELS measure the energy loss of few electrons during transmission of electron through specimen under inelastic scattering. Loss of transmitted electron will be captured through specialized electron spectrometer elaborating about specimen excitation mechanism including electronics transition, plasmon or phonon behavior.

Fundamentally, EELS system design will varied w.r.t. position of spectrometer, energy filtering system and field emission source with strong electromagnetic lenses system [23], whose detail is under Fig. 8.10a–c.

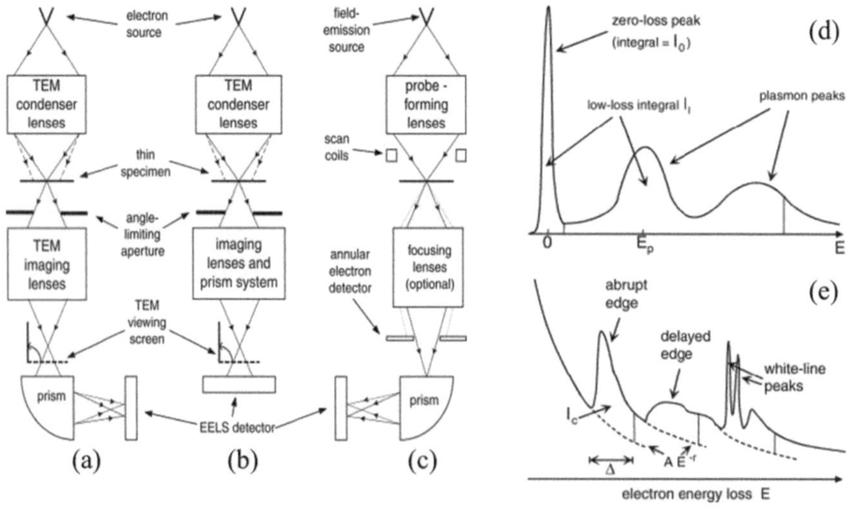

Fig. 8.10 TEM–EELs system **a** conventional TEM with magnetic prism spectrometer beneath the viewing chamber, **b** in column imaging filter, **c** STEM system; Schematic energy loss spectrum in **d** Low loss region, **e** core loss region, showing ionization edges with associated background edges (dashed curves) (Adapted with permission from Egerton et al. [23])

Further, Fig. 8.11a, b demonstrated the microscope configuration in STEM mode with illustration of low loss and core loss region EELS during inelastic scattering. Further, STEM-HAADF mode has captured atomic resolution image of GaN-Ge specimen interface with core loss spectrum of N_K edge of N_2 under Fig. 8.11c, d [24].

EELS spectrum normally consists of intensity versus energy loss behavior of specimen. Spectrum consist of zero loss peak having no loss in energy during transmission through sample. Further, low loss region peak claim collective excitation i.e. plasmon and inter-band transition having energy < 50 eV. Whereas core loss region of EELS spectrum corresponds to ionization edges to specific elements inner shell with energy > 50 eV, providing element specific information [24].

Zero Loss Peak (ZLP)

Zero loss is initial information of ELLS spectrum showing minimum loss electron energy (0 eV) through inelastic scattering during specimen compositional analysis.

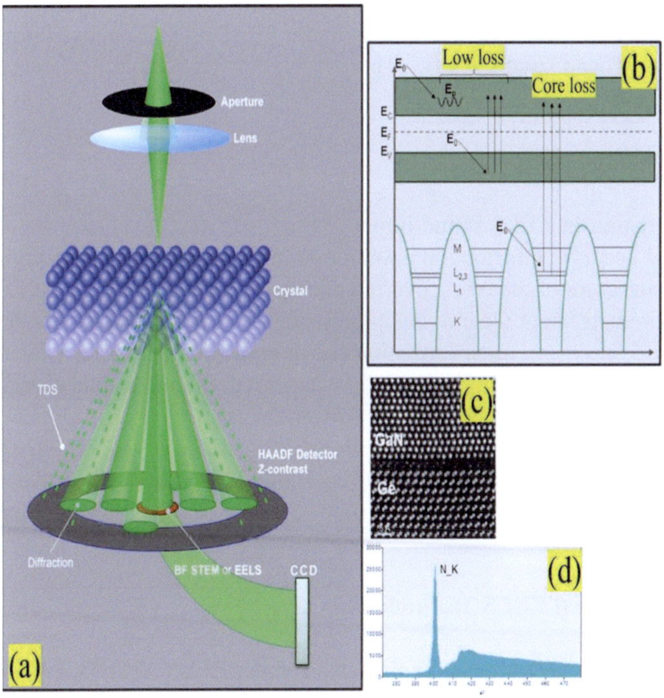

Fig. 8.11 Schematic representation of the principle in STEM-EELS. **a** Microscope configuration in STEM mode, **b** illustration of low loss and core loss region EELS during inelastic scattering, **c** atomic resolution image of GaN-Ge interface, **d** core loss spectrum showing N_K edge of N_2 (Adapted with permission from Zhang et al. [24] under open access)

The intensity of zero loss peak will serve as a reference point for calibration process under EELS analysis. Any respective shift in zero loss peak will alert user about probability of deviation in calibration or drift in EELS elemental quantification. In addition to drifting in positioning of ZLP, respective peak symmetry and narrowness predicts about energy resolution and stability of electron source or detection mechanism. Whereas broad ZLP characteristics directs defected electron source or misaligned spectrometer. Respective mechanism has been demonstrated under Fig. 8.10d, e [23, 24].

Low Loss Region (LLR)

Low loss region in EELS will provide valuable information about electronic and dielectric properties of material. This region starts from ZLP to onset of core loss edges of material in EELS spectrum, covering energy range from 0 to 50 eV. LLR region broadly comprised on plasmon excitation and inter-band transition originated energy loss peaks whose detail is comprised in Fig. 8.10d, e. During inelastic interaction of electron source beam with specimen free electron gas, lead to plasmon excitation predicting about density of electrons and nature of free electron. The transition between electronic bands of the material under EELS give respective information of electronic and band structure [23, 24].

Core Loss Region (CLR)

Core loss region in EELS is the important part of EELS analysis, which provide precise and accurate information about chemical state, elemental composition and electronic structure of material covering energy range > 50 eV. CLR of ELLS spectrum will predicts about the binding energy of core electrons at specific energy loss. Under EELS spectrum, the information above ionization edge is known as electron energy loss near edge structure (ELNES) whereas oscillation extend several hundred eV beyond the ionization edge termed as extended electron energy loss fine structure (EEELFS). Respective detail has been also demonstrated in Fig. 8.10d, e [23, 24].

Through, above presented information about EELS, one can prove the actual chemical state, compositional or electronic structure of respective material.

8.3.3.2 Advanced EELS Technologies

In addition to routine compositional analysis under EELS in TEM, certain advance in EELS techniques have improved and enhanced the detection and quantification capabilities of specimen. Detail is as mentioned below.

Dual EELS System

In comparison to single EELS analysis, dual EELS have capability of capturing two different spectra i.e. low loss region and core loss region, at different dispersion and at other related settings. Current system has capability of switching between two modes through single detector's unique capability with dual dispersion combinations [25].

Monochromated EELS

Use of monochromator in EELS will bring narrowing the beam size, before its interaction with specimen. Enhancement in high energy resolution will be achieved through filtering of electron beam with narrow energy spread of few milli electron volt (meV). Improved signal to noise ratio and better chemical sensitivity factors of EELS under current mode bring effective distinction between different energy loss quantification of respective elements with improvised chemical and bonding information [26].

Spectrum Imaging

Spectrum imaging of EELS with scanning transmission electron microscope (STEM), integrates EELS chemical sensitivity with STEM high spatial resolution ability. With the help of finely focused electron beam of ~ 1 nm diameter in STEM through high annular angle dark field imaging (HAADF) will analyze the respective interfaces or nanostructures. In same time domain, localized position of specimen will also be analyzed for complex elemental mapping, chemical state identification of material [27].

In related work, Arthur Losquin et al. [28] unveil information about the extinction and scattering phenomenon of gold nanoprism through EELS and cathodolumines-cences (CL) at nanoscale. Under Fig. 8.12a shows pictorial positioning of EELS and CL w.r.t. STEM system. With respect to Fig. 8.12b shows HAADF image of gold nano-prism of ~ 60 nm size lying on graphene sheet, whereas other two images correspond to EELS and CL mode of same area. Two dominant mode of gold nanoprism EELS data i.e. low energy dipolar and high energy non-dipolar mode have been also investigated. Dipolar mode has demonstrated charge density confined at tip whereas high energy mode shows charge density peaking of tips and edges of prism [28]. Above mentioned complete detail has been demonstrated under Fig. 8.12c–e.

Energy Filtered TEM (EFTEM)

EFTEM is one versatile mode of EELS operation in TEM, where specific electron energy loss region will be imaged for compositional and chemical sensitivity analysis. Under the application of specific energy window allowing specific energy loss

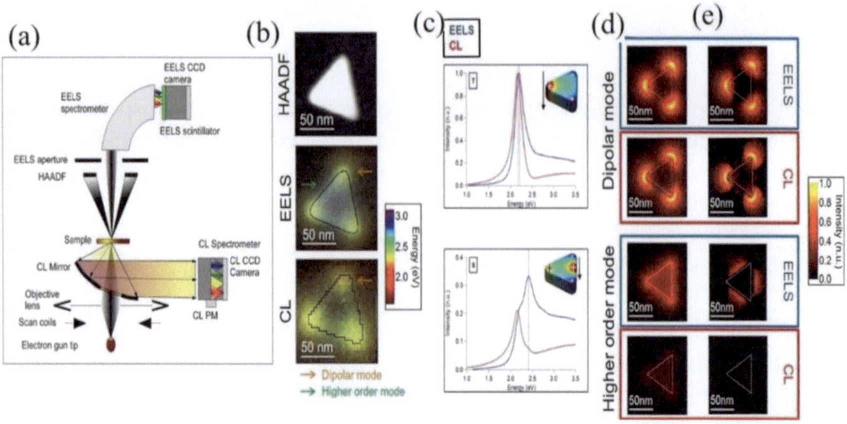

Fig. 8.12 **a** Scheme shows STEM equipped with EELS and CL, **b** (top) spatially resolved HAADF image, (middle) EELS image with acquisition of 16 s, (bottom) CL image with acquisition of 157 s, **c** simulated EELS (blue) and CL (red) spectra at tip (T) and side (S) of 60 nm long, 30 nm thick nanoprism with inset image showing induced by fast electron beam at tip and side surface, **d** simulated EEL and CL map filtered around energy of EEL and CL maxima, **e** simulated fitted amplitude map to dipolar (EELS and CL) and higher energy (EELS). The white lines under higher energy mode depicts shape of prism (Adapted with permission from Losquin et al. [28] under open access)

signal get utilized in respective image formation. Zero loss peak (ZLP) image will show high contrast, high resolution features through maximum elastic scattering of travelling electron. Whereas core loss region specific peaks will credit for elemental distribution imaging of specimen under EFTEM analysis [29]. In addition, quantitative comparison between ZLP image and core loss region gives idea about the specimen thickness.

In addition to above used technologies and techniques during elemental quantification and mapping through EELS mode in TEM, other modes like valence band specific EELS, aberration corrected EELS etc., also have more specific compositional analysis and precise elemental phase identification ability.

8.3.3.3 Application of EELS

Quality of sample w.r.t. compositional and chemical analysis, EELS study proven to be an important tool. It will have versatile capabilities in respective analysis of nanomaterials, semiconductors, energy materials, biological, soft materials, environmental science and quantum materials etc.

Nanomaterials Analysis

EELS specifically, analyze critically and provide very detailed information about elemental composition, chemical bonding, electronic structures of different nanomaterials. In addition, many complex nanostructures will also be interpreted and investigated for different phases for different structural or functional properties through mapping mode.

Semiconductor Analysis

Homogeneity and purity are critical factors in efficient working of semi-conductor technologies. TEM–EELS will help in investigation for doping and defects level of materials from laboratory scale to commercial scale. This will help in identification of semiconductor material failure explanations with possibilities of future upgradations in related efficient technologies.

Energy Materials

TEM–EELS will contribute in investigation of materials related energy transport at their nano as well bulk level. For example, battery and catalyst research have been working on analysis of electrode composition, charging-discharging cycles, battery failure, catalytic active sites localization, chemical interaction of catalyst with support surface etc., through different EELS technologies. Related detail has been already mentioned under this chapter, Sect. 8.3.3.

Dumaresq et al. [30] have optimized the side effect of high energy beam during TEM analysis for beam sensitive battery material (TiN, TiB_2, h-BN) through STEM-low voltage (10, 20, 30, 200 keV) regulated EELS analysis under Fig. 8.13a–e. During EELS analysis for TiN and TiB_2 (Fig. 8.13a, b, d), no major interference in peak shape and onset energy has been observed at 20, 30, 200 keV spectrum. Authors has further concluded about transition of core electron to unoccupied orbital not impacted by incident electron beam. Whereas Fig. 8.13c, e shows the considerable peak shape difference in boron k-edge and nitrogen k-edge of h-BN. In addition to anisotropic nature of h-BN, multiple orientation of respective nanosheet bring variable peak shape behavior [30].

Biological and Soft Materials

Investigation of biological specimen for their elemental distribution, structures, and respective functions will be performed very subjectively with TEM–EELS mode. For example, during bio-mineralization, release of specific mineral during respective process will be analyzed through respective EELS mapping mode.

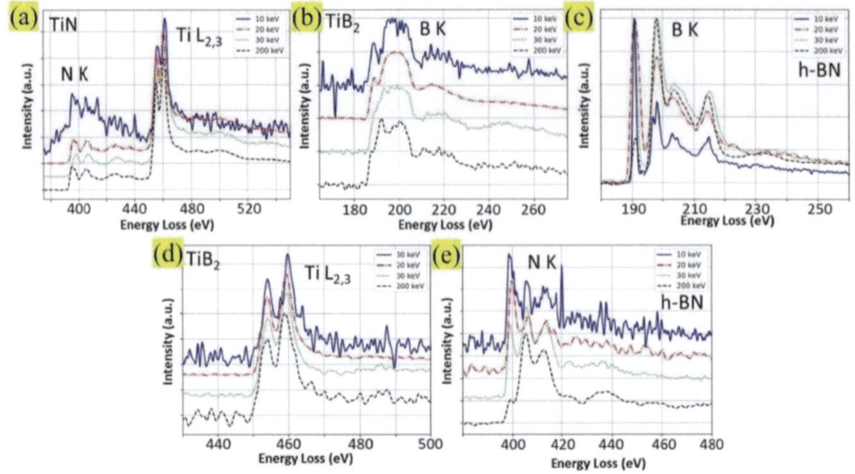

Fig. 8.13 Core loss EELS spectrum of **a** Ti $L_{2,3}$ and N K edge in TiN, **b** boron k edge of TiB_2, **c** boron k edge of h-BN, **d** titanium $L_{2,3}$ edge of TiB_2, **e** nitrogen k edge of h-BN at 10 keV (Blue), 20 keV (Red), 30 keV (green), 200 keV (black) (Adapted with permission from Dumaresq et al. [30])

EELS elemental analysis has been performed for mouse sperm cell ultrathin sections [19]. Dark field detector under STEM, collected mass-thickness dominated image highlighting cell head and middle piece clearly as shown in Fig. 8.14a. Through line scan EELS monitoring of respective cell shows presence of P, S, N elements respectively (Fig. 8.14b–d). Interestingly, high density of detected element has been found in head region of cell confirms high concentration of DNA and protamines predicting confirmation of cellular head region [19].

Similarly, soft materials like polymer, emulsions or gel specimen etc., can also be analyzed via EELS versatile capabilities for their composition, bonding, degradation mechanism etc., for operational and functional behavior.

Environmental Science

Presence and identification of different pollutants like heavy metal, organic dyes, cosmetics and pharmaceutical waste etc., from bulk to nano level in soil, air, water, will be analyzed through EELS mode. For example, formation of unbalanced aerosol in environment will be analyzed for probable reason of climate change [31].

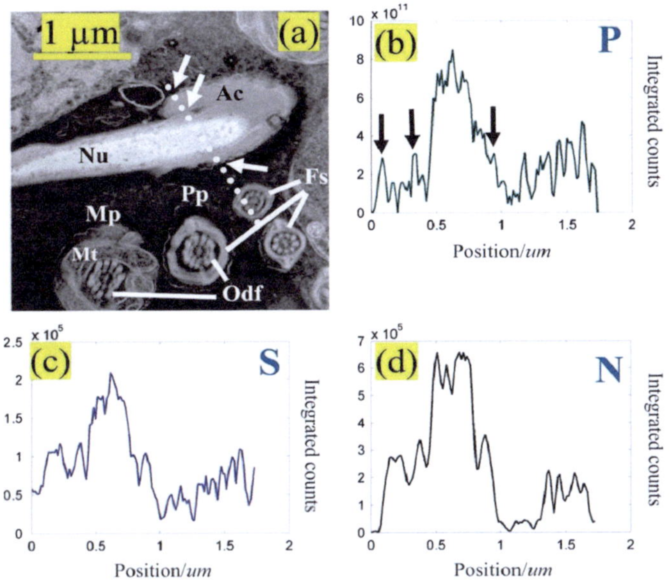

Fig. 8.14 **a** HAADF image of thin section of mouse sperm showing head and middle piece sections with white line showing region of EELS mapping, **b–d** EELS P, S, N line profile respectively (Adapted with permission from Wu et al. [19])

8.3.3.4 Challenges with EELS Analysis

In addition to versatilities capabilities of EELS analysis under TEM, still there are many challenges which need to optimize for quality analysis during specimen analysis.

Beam Damage

There is narrow difference between intensity of incident electron beam and stability of specimen surface during TEM–EELS analysis. Over exposure of electron beam will lead to damage the specimen structure brings inaccurate quantification. Knowledge of specimen nature, stability, electron beam intensity etc., factors must be known in very well way before starting EELS analysis of specimen [1, 3, 32].

Low Signal to Noise Ratio (SNR)

TEM–EELS has challenge of low SNR during precise elemental quantification for low concentration specimen or high energy loss specimen. Due to this issue, it led to misinterpretation of quantified data. Use of optimum beam intensity, beam exposure, thin specimen with contamination free sample w.r.t. optimized specimen preparation protocol and instrument alignment, facilitate precise specimen analysis [1, 3, 32].

Quantification Challenge

Even with quality signal data during TEM–EELS analysis, lack of slight misalignment w.r.t. defector positioning, detector in-efficiency, energy resolution and background subtraction factors etc., bring in- accurate quantification [1, 3, 32].

Quality Sample Preparation

Right from extraction of small amount/portion of specimen from bulk sample to specimen surface fine polishing, have probable chances of contamination from internal as well external sources of contamination. Special care must be taken to protect and preserve delicate and soft specimen during TEM–EELS analysis [1, 3, 32].

Through above stated prominent challenges w.r.t. TEM–EELS analysis, researchers/scientists will get aware about the do's and don'ts during respective sample preparation and analysis as per nature of specimen, specification and capabilities of instrument. Finally, TEM–EELS will help in analysis of any material belong to nanotechnology including semiconductor, energy materials, biological, environmental science etc., for qualitative and quantitative analysis of material. This will help in developing and upgrading the respective materials research for efficient and novel materials having efficient technologies.

NOTE: EELS empower researchers to empower to unlock the atomic secrets with identify chemical compositions and electronic structure with precision of materials.

8.3.4 STEM (BF/ADF/HAADF)

STEM will be broadly operative in bright field (BF), annular dark field (ADF) and high angle annular dark field imaging (HAADF) detectors. BF will operate in narrow electron scattering angle range (~ <0–10 mrad) through specimen whereas ADF have broad scattering angle range (~10–50 mrad). More importantly, HAADF imaging will be proceed through scattering angle ~ >50 mrad during scattering process, will provide more precise contrast-based imaging of specimen.

8.3.4.1 Principle and Working of STEM (BF/ADF/HAADF)

When high energy electron beam pass through specimen, respective beam scattered at broad and narrow angles through specimen w.r.t. samples variable atomic number-based composition. The intensity of scattered electron beam is directly depended on atomic number of respective elements in specimen.

The imaging mode of STEM includes use of ADF, HAADF, BF, annular BF (ABF) and segmented detectors for differential phase contrast (DPC) imaging. Ability of probe aberration correction in STEM technique bring converged probe size smaller than ~ 1 Å, facilitate the high-resolution atomic column imaging. Diffraction mode under STEM, utilizes pixelated probe detector to capture the diffracted probe after scattering of electron beam with specimen. Further, single probe position diffraction imaging known as convergent beam electron diffraction (CBED) or microdiffraction whereas diffraction pattering w.r.t. probe positioning classified as 4D-STEM, nanobeam electron diffraction (NBED), scanning electron nano-diffraction (SEND). STEM configuration for spectroscopic analysis, will be analyze the energy distribution of inelastically scattered electrons using EELS, XEDS, CL detectors. Under STEM-tomography configuration, imaging, diffraction and spectroscopy modes will be studied at different sample tilts. Additionally, three-dimensional reconstruction of 2D specimen projection will be converted into 3D projection through different computational algorithms. Detail of above stated modes of operation has been depicted in Fig. 8.15a–d [33]. In addition, STEM experimental setup with focused probe with and without sample has been demonstrated under Fig. 8.15e–f [34].

Under current sub-section, we have specifically discussed about high contrast imaging via inelastic scattering electron detection. The annular shape design of HAADF detector facilitate the detection of respective scattered electron at wider

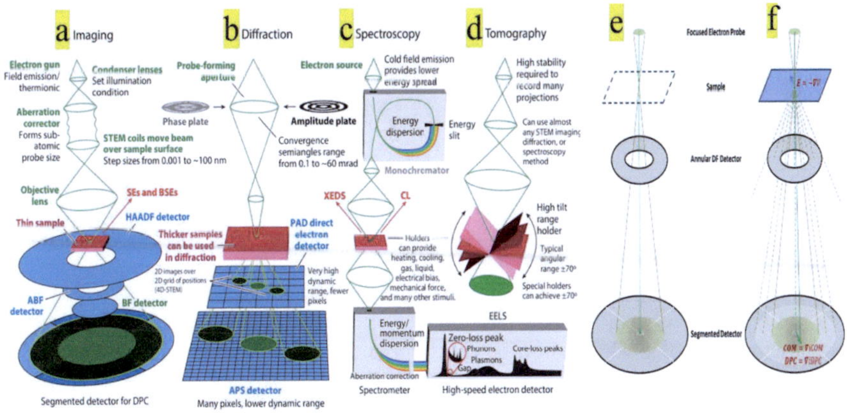

Fig. 8.15 STEM characterization mode, **a** imaging, **b** diffraction, **c** spectroscopy, **d** tomography (Adapted with permission from Ophus et al. [33] under open access), **e–f** STEM experimental setup **e** focused probe without sample, **f** focused probe with sample (Adapted with permission from Yucelen et al. [34] under open access)

angle highlighting the compositional contrast with minimizing the routine diffraction contrast.

8.3.4.2 Features of HAADF Imaging

In addition to EDS and EELS attachment in STEM for quantitative analysis of materials, HAADF mode of imaging presents as a dynamic mode of TEM operation. There are the following features of STEM-HAADF mode which are important to discuss.

Atomic Sensitivity

Due to sensitivity between atomic number of respective elements with scattering angle. This will be utilized for highlighting the presence or bondage of specific element in some other material matrix through respective contrast differentiation ability via DF and BF imaging mode w.r.t. suitability in instrument as well for specimen.

High Resolution

Due to compositional contrast feature of HAADF in STEM, atomic scale resolution of specimen will be highlighted more prominently in comparison to normal TEM or HRTEM imaging. Under similar work, Zhang et al. [24] reported the TiO_2-carbon nanotube (CNT) interface through STEM-HAADF imaging. With increase in atomic layer deposition (ALD) cycles of TiO_2 on MW-CNT from 20, 200 and 750 cycles at 220 °C shows increase in particle size whose confirmation has been presented from STEM-HAADF images at Fig. 8.16b, d, f respectively. Clear nucleation and growth mechanism of TiO_2 on the surface of MW-CNT has been elaborated with HAADF-STEM imaging [24].

High Diffraction Contrast Imaging

Due to fundamental working design of HAADF, only wider scattered electrons will be captured during respective imaging. During bright field imaging of specimen w.r.t. high angle electron scattering will be avoided due to fundamental working of respective mode. In comparison, HAADF have specialized capability in capturing or detecting respective signal for enhanced contrast imaging. This will be very useful in highlighting the compositional contrast of specimen very clearly and insightly. Satoshi Utsunomiya et al. [35] analyzed the presence of uranium inside the matrix of carbonaceous matrix through HAADF-STEM. Figure 8.17a, demonstrated the TEM configuration w.r.t. HAADF-STEM. In comparison to bright field-TEM (BF-TEM)

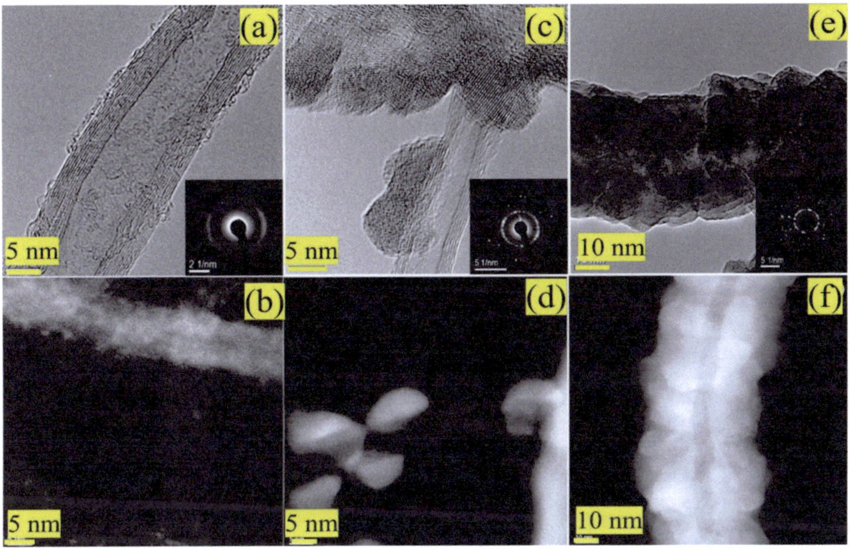

Fig. 8.16 **a**, **c**, **e** High Resolution TEM micrograph of TiO_2 deposited MWCNT using ALD 20, 200 and 750 cycles with inset shows respective selected area diffraction, **b**, **d**, **f** shows high contrast imaging of TiO_2-MWCNT via HAADF-STEM (Adapted with permission from Zhang et al. [24] under open access)

image of carbonaceous matter from Detroit (Fig. 8.17b), respective area STEM-HAADF image shows presence of bright contrast particles. The presence of uraninte phase inside the respective carbonaceous matrix has been confirmed by EDX and HRTEM images under Fig. 8.17d, e respectively [35].

From respective features of STEM-HAADF, it is widely preferred by researchers in imaging of specimen for contrast-based HR and compositional contrast imaging respectively.

8.3.4.3 Application of STEM (Imaging/Diffraction/Spectroscopy/Tomography)

STEM-HAADF will be utilized as a tool for phase identification, compositional contrast and defects analysis etc., of specimens belong to material science, nanotechnology, energy material, semiconductor industry and biological sciences etc. Under nanomaterial investigation with HAADF mode in comparison to high resolution imaging of specimen, imaging of specimen will highlight high contrast-based differentiation between different incorporated components.

Under similar explanation and analysis, Ren et al. [36] utilized STEM-HAADF for La doped Mg alloy identification and localization of respective phases at high contrast-based resolution. La 3%-Mg alloying behavior aged at 200 °C for 600 h along $[0001]_{\alpha}$, $[12\bar{1}0]_{\alpha}$, $[10\bar{1}0]_{\alpha}$ has been shows respective images at Fig. 8.18a–c whereas

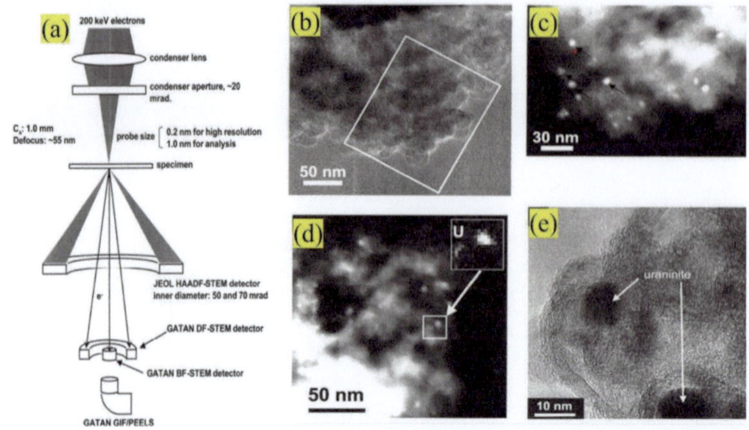

Fig. 8.17 **a** Shows TEM instrument configuration with HAADF-STEM mode, **b** BF-STEM image of carbonaceous matter, **c** STEM-HAADF image highlighting the presence of bright contrast particles, **d** STEM-HAADF with EDX analysis of uranium inside carbonaceous matrix, **e** HRTEM image of uraninite nanocrystal in carbonaceous matrix (Adapted with permission from Utsunomiya et al. [35] under open access)

red line marked area of respective specimen has been captured under Fig. 8.18d–f shows atomic contrast based differentiation between La and Mg. Further, atomic intensity profiles has been monitored for blue and purple box marked area has been demonstrated under Fig. 8.18e–f respectively [36]. Authors further analyzed and explained about tetragonal phase connected with La rich FCC structure of La 3 wt%-Mg alloy aged at 200 °C for 600 h. During respective analysis incident beam is parallel to $[0001]_{\alpha}$ orientation captured via HAADF-STEM images as shown in Fig. 8.18i, j, l whereas $[12\bar{1}0]_{\alpha}$ phase has been analyzed at Fig. 8.18k, m, n. Conclusively, La-Mg alloy analysis through HAADF-STEM, high contrast high resolution based localized positioning and structural identification and defects analysis has been reported very precisely in current study [36].

Conclusively, the fundamental of HAADF working will help in analyzing and locating the grain boundary, interface, defects, dislocation etc., dynamics of material under respective study. In addition, to ability to highlight compositional contrast of HAADF, it will be utilized for identification of active sites under catalysis science, defect analysis etc. In similar way, biological specimen will also be analyzed for study for cellular structure, proteins and viruses related various mechanisms at high resolution [37–39].

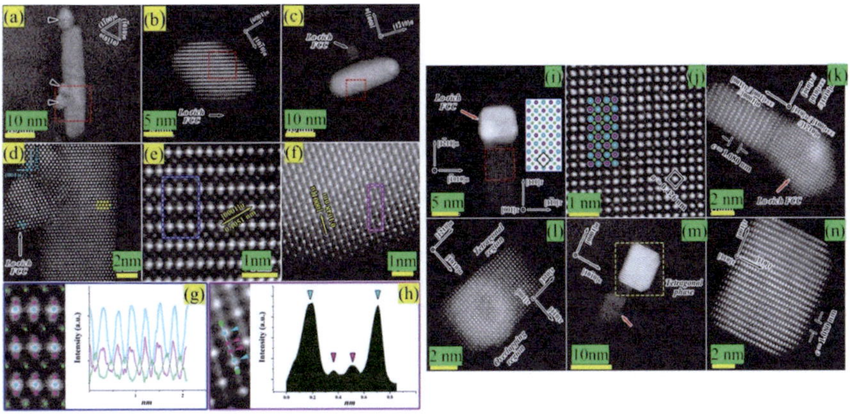

Fig. 8.18 **a** HAADF-STEM analysis of La 3 wt%-Mg alloy aged at 200 °C for 600 h for $[0001]_\alpha$, $[12\bar{1}0]_\alpha$, $[10\bar{1}0]_\alpha$, **d–f** analyzed dotted marked region for high resolution imaging of **a–c** images, **g–h** atomic column intensity profiling for **e–f** marked blue and pink area respectively; **i**, **j**, **k** HAADF-STEM images of tetragonal phase of La 3 wt%-Mg alloy for $[0001]_\alpha$ whereas **l**, **m**, **n** shows $[12\bar{1}0]_\alpha$ phase respective high contrast imaging (Adapted with permission from Ren et al. [36])

8.3.4.4 Challenges of STEM-HAADF

In addition to wide capabilities of STEM-HAADF, still there are many more operational and instrumental challenges which need to optimize during respective operation [3, 5].

Quality Sample Preparation

Quality sample preparation w.r.t. STEM-HAADF analysis, require optimum thickness, minimum impurities and defects free conditions etc. Electron transparent nature of specimen will allow maximum electron transmission generate precise representative HAADF images. The accuracy and quality of STEM-HAADF results will be severely affected by the presence of impurities and defects states of the specimen [3, 5].

Limitation of STEM-HAADF Instrumentation

The limited resolution, optimized beam alignment, beam damage effects w.r.t. STEM-HAADF operation and analysis of respective specimens, will emerge as the dominating factors. Periodically calibrated TEM instrument with well aligned electron beam having efficient electron source having minimum astigmatism and best suited detector configuration, will improve the whole specimen analysis from basic to advance level [3, 5].

Level of Interpretation

STEM-HAADF analysis will also be challenging w.r.t. precise interpretation w.r.t. natural behavior. Identifying and interpreting the specimen behavior for representative contrast mechanism, quantitative analysis and complex structure analysis, need insight understanding and expertise while explaining respective material properties. The presence of close proximity atomic number elements in specimens w.r.t. light elements etc., are the factors which need extra care and advance detection systems, to analyze and interpret respective data in more insightful manner [3, 5].

Through above discussed probable challenges w.r.t. STEM-HAADF operation, handling and analysis, researchers/scientist must have attentive during STEM instrumentation, sample preparation and precise interpretation of acquire data.

NOTE: STEM have wide capability of high contrast high resolution imaging at atomic scale.

8.4 Conclusion

The acceptability of TEM instrumentation has been widely enhanced and improved with development of different quantitative modes of operations in addition to imaging mode of TEM. Current chapter has broadly discussed about the four major quantitative techniques viz. diffraction, EDS, EELS and STEM (BF/ADF/HAADF).

Highlighting the importance of quantitative analysis of material under TEM instrumentation, has predicted about materials visualization for compositional quantity, contrast generation and crystallographic identification with chemical states confirmation. Specifically, respective analysis under diffraction mode has explained about SAED, micro-diffraction and nano-diffraction nature with its importance in research activities. In addition to structural identification (crystalline to amorphous) of material under study, factors like beam stress to specimen surface, multiphase identification, low density material analysis, instrumentation limitations etc., factors also have been explained in detail. Under EDS and EELS mode of analysis, both will work for quantitative and qualitative analysis of materials with minor detection limitations. Further improvised techniques w.r.t. EDS and EELS with new updated technologies like dual EELS, monochromated EELS, spectrum imaging and energy filtered TEM (EFTEM) have improved the respective specimen data analysis more insightly. Parallelly, STEM-BF/ADF/HAADF mode will be utilized in highlighting atomic sensitivity, high resolution and minimum diffraction contrast effects in quantitative analysis of material. During applicability of above stated quantitative modes with TEM, nanotechnology, semiconductor, energy sectors, biological and soft material, environmental science etc., have benefited with analysis of respective materials for basic to advanced technology developments.

Conclusively, from above discussion about quantitative modes of TEM analysis, researchers can use best quantitative technique for material from bulk level to nano-level investigation. This will help in minimizing the failure chances of different devices with upgrading the existing technologies through improving the holistic research.

Declaration

Author declares that there is no personal or financial conflict of interest regarding publication of this chapter.

References

1. Bozzola, J.J., Russell, L.D.: Electron Microscopy: Principles and Techniques for Biologists, 2nd edn. Jones and Bartlett Publishers, Inc. (1992)
2. Egerton, R.F.: Physical Principles of Electron Microscopy: An Introduction to TEM, SEM, and AEM, Corr. 3. print. Springer, New York (2008)
3. Ayache, J., Beaunier, L., Boumendil, J., Ehret, G., Laub, D.: Sample Preparation Handbook for Transmission Electron Microscopy. Springer, New York (2010). https://doi.org/10.1007/978-0-387-98182-6
4. Hawkes, P.W., Spence, J.C.H. (Eds.): Springer Handbook of Microscopy. Springer International Publishing, Cham (2019). https://doi.org/10.1007/978-3-030-00069-1
5. Williams, D.B., Carter, C.B.: Transmission Electron Microscopy. Springer US, Boston (1996). https://doi.org/10.1007/978-1-4757-2519-3
6. Asadabad, M.A., Eskandari, M.J.: Electron diffraction. In: Janecek, M., Kral, R. (Eds.) Modern Electron Microscopy in Physical and Life Sciences. InTech (2016). https://doi.org/10.5772/61781
7. Ganesh, K.J., Kawasaki, M., Zhou, J.P., Ferreira, P.J.: D-STEM: a parallel electron diffraction technique applied to nanomaterials. Microsc. Microanal. **16**(5), 614–621 (2010). https://doi.org/10.1017/S1431927610000334
8. Dai, Y., Zhao, S., Zhang, C.: Controlled growth of indium selenides by high-pressure and high-temperature method. Front. Mater. 8 (2022). https://doi.org/10.3389/fmats.2021.816821
9. Shen, C., Ge, M., Luo, L., Zhou, C.: In situ and ex situ TEM study of lithiation behaviours of porous silicon nanostructures. Sci. Rep. **6**, 31334. https://doi.org/10.1038/srep31334
10. Kattan, N., Hou, B., Fermín, D.J., Cherns, D.: Crystal structure and defects visualization of Cu2ZnSnS4 nanoparticles employing transmission electron microscopy and electron diffraction. Appl. Mater. Today **1**(1), 52–59 (2015). https://doi.org/10.1016/j.apmt.2015.08.004
11. Hirotsu, Y.: Application of nano-diffraction to local atomic distribution function analysis of amorphous materials. J. Electron Microsc. **50**(6), 435–442 (2001). https://doi.org/10.1093/jmicro/50.6.435
12. Gauvin, R.: What remains to be done to allow quantitative X-ray microanalysis performed with EDS to become a true characterization technique? Microsc. Microanal. **18**(5), 915–940 (2012). https://doi.org/10.1017/S1431927612001468
13. Van Borm, W.A., Adams, F.C.: A standardless ZAF correction for semi-quantitative electron probe microanalysis of microscopical particles. X-Ray Spectrom. **20**(2), 51–62 (1991). https://doi.org/10.1002/xrs.1300200204
14. Conconi, R., Ventruti, G., Nieto, F., Capitani, G.: TEM-EDS microanalysis: comparison among the Standardless, Cliff & Lorimer and absorption correction quantification methods. Ultramicroscopy **254**, 113845 (2023). https://doi.org/10.1016/j.ultramic.2023.113845

15. Longo, D.M., Howe, J.M., Johnson, W.C.: Experimental method for determining Cliff-Lorimer factors in transmission electron microscopy (TEM) utilizing stepped wedge-shaped specimens prepared by focused ion beam (FIB) thinning (1999)
16. Parisini, A., Frabboni, S., Gazzadi, G.C., Rosa, R., Armigliato, A.: Comparison of Cliff–Lorimer-based methods of scanning transmission electron microscopy (STEM) quantitative X-ray microanalysis for application to silicon oxycarbides thin films. Microsc. Microanal. **24**(3), 193–206 (2018). https://doi.org/10.1017/S1431927618000259
17. Tang, S., Tang, J., Uzuhashi, J., Ohkubo, T., Hayami, W., Yuan, J., Takeguchi, M., Mitome, M., Qin, L.-C.: A stable LaB_6 nanoneedle field-emission point electron source. Nanoscale Adv. **3**(10), 2787–2792 (2021). https://doi.org/10.1039/D1NA00167A
18. Xu, B., Ye, F., Chang, G., Li, R.: A simple and cost-effective method for producing stable surfactant-coated EGaIn liquid metal nanodroplets. Materials **13**(17), 3753 (2020). https://doi.org/10.3390/ma13173753
19. Wu, J.S., Kim, A.M., Bleher, R., Myers, B.D., Marvin, R.G., Inada, H., Nakamura, K., Zhang, X.F., Roth, E., Li, S.Y., Woodruff, T.K., O'Halloran, T.V., Dravid, V.P.: Imaging and elemental mapping of biological specimens with a dual-EDS dedicated scanning transmission electron microscope. Ultramicroscopy **128**, 24–31 (2013). https://doi.org/10.1016/j.ultramic.2013.01.004
20. Latronico, G., Singh, S., Mele, P., Darwish, A., Sarkisov, S., Pan, S.W., Kawamura, Y., Sekine, C., Baba, T., Mori, T., Takeuchi, T., Ichinose, A., Wilson, S.: Synthesis and characterization of Al- and SnO_2-doped ZnO thermoelectric thin films. Materials **14**(22), 6929 (2021). https://doi.org/10.3390/ma14226929
21. Xiong, Q., He, H., Zhang, M.: Design of flexible films based on kinked carbon nanofibers for high rate and stable potassium-ion storage. Nano-Micro Lett. **14**(1), 47 (2022). https://doi.org/10.1007/s40820-022-00791-y
22. Rai, R.S., Subramanian, S.: Role of transmission electron microscopy in the semiconductor industry for process development and failure analysis. Prog. Cryst. Growth Charact. Mater. **55**(3–4), 63–97 (2009). https://doi.org/10.1016/j.pcrysgrow.2009.09.002
23. Egerton, R.F., Malac, M.: EELS in the TEM. J. Electron Spectrosc. Relat. Phenom. **143**(2–3), 43–50 (2005). https://doi.org/10.1016/j.elspec.2003.12.009
24. Zhang, Y., Utke, I., Michler, J., Ilari, G., Rossell, M.D., Erni, R.: Growth and characterization of CNT–TiO_2 heterostructures. Beilstein J. Nanotechnol. **5**, 946–955 (2014). https://doi.org/10.3762/bjnano.5.108
25. Scott, J., Thomas, P.J., MacKenzie, M., McFadzean, S., Wilbrink, J., Craven, A.J., Nicholson, W.A.P.: Near-simultaneous dual energy range EELS spectrum imaging. Ultramicroscopy **108**(12), 1586–1594 (2008). https://doi.org/10.1016/j.ultramic.2008.05.006
26. Hachtel, J.A., Lupini, A.R., Idrobo, J.C.: Exploring the capabilities of monochromated electron energy loss spectroscopy in the infrared regime. Sci. Rep. **8**(1), 5637 (2018). https://doi.org/10.1038/s41598-018-23805-5
27. Muto, S., Yamamoto, Y., Sakakura, M., Tian, H.-K., Tateyama, Y., Iriyama, Y.: STEM-EELS spectrum imaging of an aerosol-deposited NASICON-type LATP solid electrolyte and LCO cathode interface. ACS Appl. Energy Mater. **5**(1), 98–107 (2022). https://doi.org/10.1021/acsaem.1c02512
28. Losquin, A., Zagonel, L.F., Myroshnychenko, V., Rodríguez-González, B., Tencé, M., Scarabelli, L., Förstner, J., Liz-Marzán, L.M., García De Abajo, F.J., Stéphan, O., Kociak, M.: Unveiling Nanometer Scale Extinction and Scattering Phenomena through Combined Electron Energy Loss Spectroscopy and Cathodoluminescence Measurements. Nano Lett. **15**(2), 1229–1237 (2015). https://doi.org/10.1021/nl5043775
29. Mohn, M.J., Biskupek, J., Lee, Z., Rose, H., Kaiser, U.: Lattice contrast in the core-loss EFTEM signal of graphene. Ultramicroscopy **219**, 113119 (2020). https://doi.org/10.1016/j.ultramic.2020.113119
30. Dumaresq, N., Brodusch, N., Bessette, S., Gauvin, R.: Elemental quantification using electron energy-loss spectroscopy with a low voltage scanning transmission electron microscope (STEM-EELS). Ultramicroscopy **262**, 113977 (2024). https://doi.org/10.1016/j.ultramic.2024.113977

31. Tanaka, N., Fujita, T., Takahashi, Y., Yamasaki, J., Murata, K., Arai, S.: Progress in environmental high-voltage transmission electron microscopy for nanomaterials. Phil. Trans. R. Soc. A **378**(2186), 20190602 (2020). https://doi.org/10.1098/rsta.2019.0602
32. Ribet, S.M., Murthy, A.A., Roth, E.W., Dos Reis, R., Dravid, V.P.: Making the most of your electrons: challenges and opportunities in characterizing hybrid interfaces with STEM. Mater. Today **50**, 100–115 (2021). https://doi.org/10.1016/j.mattod.2021.05.006
33. Ophus, C.: Quantitative scanning transmission electron microscopy for materials science: imaging, diffraction, spectroscopy, and tomography. Annu. Rev. Mater. Res. **53**(1), 105–141 (2023). https://doi.org/10.1146/annurev-matsci-080921-092646
34. Yücelen, E., Lazić, I., Bosch, E.G.T.: Phase contrast scanning transmission electron microscopy imaging of light and heavy atoms at the limit of contrast and resolution. Sci. Rep. **8**(1), 2676 (2018). https://doi.org/10.1038/s41598-018-20377-2
35. Utsunomiya, S., Ewing, R.C.: Application of high-angle annular dark field scanning transmission electron microscopy, scanning transmission electron microscopy-energy dispersive X-Ray spectrometry, and energy-filtered transmission electron microscopy to the characterization of nanoparticles in the environment. Environ. Sci. Technol. **37**(4), 786–791 (2003). https://doi.org/10.1021/es026053t
36. Ren, J.X., Lou, W.X., Tian, Y., Xie, G.M., Xie, H.B., Sun, B.Z., Tan, J., Xiao, N.: A novel tetragonal precipitate with multiple orientations in Mg–La alloy: an atomic scale investigation using HAADF–STEM. J. Alloy. Compd. **877**, 160238 (2021). https://doi.org/10.1016/j.jallcom.2021.160238
37. Sousa, A.A., Leapman, R.D.: Development and application of STEM for the biological sciences. Ultramicroscopy **123**, 38–49 (2012). https://doi.org/10.1016/j.ultramic.2012.04.005
38. Vanrompay, H., Skorikov, A., Bladt, E., Béché, A., Freitag, B., Verbeeck, J., Bals, S.: Fast versus conventional HAADF-STEM tomography of nanoparticles: advantages and challenges. Ultramicroscopy **221**, 113191 (2021). https://doi.org/10.1016/j.ultramic.2020.113191
39. Liu, J. (Jimmy): Advances and Applications of Atomic-Resolution Scanning Transmission Electron Microscopy. Microsc. Microanal. **27**(5), 943–995 (2021). https://doi.org/10.1017/S1431927621012125

Chapter 9
Correlative Light and Electron Microscopy (CLEM) Sample Preparation

Microscope in its highest power reveal the hidden universe, but only when our techniques match its precision
by ***Richard Feynman***

Abstract Integrated light microscope (LM) with electron microscopy (EM) hybrid version, has extended new limits of imaging and correlating of respective data at high resolution with functional insight. Chapter further proceed with basic discussion about the working, principle of correlative light and electron microscopy (CLEM) followed by importance of respective technique in current scenarios of research and development. In addition to explaining about different methods of integration between LM and EM, wide area of respective applications including biological sciences, medical and material research have been summarized. Optimized integration of CLEM with techniques like 3D tomography, super-resolution microscopy etc., have been also discussed. This chapter further, presents trending applications of CLEM dominated analysis in neuroscience, immunology and environment science etc., in addition to remediation-oriented approach of challenges faced during respective technique operation and analysis.

Keywords Light microscopy · Correlative light and electron microscopy · 3D tomography · Neuroscience · Environment science

9.1 Introduction

Correlative light and Electron Microscopy (CLEM) is the approach which bridges the gap between the microscopic and macroscopic information of materials. The complexity w.r.t. structure and functions of different materials including biological species, will be comprehensively understood and analysed via collective potentialities of light microscopy (LM) and electron microscopy (EM). The requirement of high resolution and contextual information of specimen during imaging-based study, will be satisfied via CLEM analysis more accurately.

R. Singh, *Transmission Electron Microscopy Sample Preparation*,
https://doi.org/10.1007/978-3-031-82967-3_9

In order to understand CLEM insightly, it is most appropriate to understand individually LM and EM. Light Microscopy (LM), which is known for real time analysis of living specimens' cells w.r.t. their dynamic behaviour. For example, fluorescence microscopy as a sub-unit of LM, have capabilities towards cell biology via visualization of protein and cellular components using fluorescent markers. With the rising demand and requirements of in-depth studies w.r.t. spreading of diseases, infections and respective remediation procedures, LM limited resolution found as the major limitation factor to visualize simple to complex molecular structures. On the other side, the EM atomic scale resolution ability enables the ultrastructural detailing of biological specimen including cellular system, organelles and material science specimens. Transmission Electron Microscopy (TEM) and Scanning Electron Microscopy (SEM) are dedicated EM techniques which meant for specimen internal and surface ultrastructural complementary analysis techniques to each other. Due to requirement of viewing biological specimen under EM (SEM or TEM), it need to fix, dehydrate, conductive coating, nano-slicing or staining etc., will be performed as per requirement of study. Many times, EM sample analysis default sample preparation requirement procedure will suppress the respective specimen natural conditions with dynamic features, lead to limited visualization of specimen under respective study.

CLEM, have utilizes the capabilities of both LM and EM with their integration for correlative analysis. Under hybrid approach, initially macroscopic world of living specimen will be explored for dynamic behaviour with identification of localized region of interest via fluorescent labelling. Whereas, marked region of interest located via LM study, will be examined under EM (SEM or TEM) for ultrastructural high-resolution imaging as per their capabilities. Through collaboration of both mode of operation i.e. LM and EM w.r.t. nature of sample, an inclusive visualization will be achieved for functional and structural understanding of specimen. The conventional mode of CLEM operation will be further developed via advanced imaging technologies and computational tools. For example, cryo-CLEM, will utilize the low temperature stabilization approach with fluorescence mode, allowing native state imaging of specimen at high resolution in nearly live environment. Use of CLEM technique leads to spatial organization of cellular components through protein localization will reveal complex details about different cellular processes. This approach will be directly led to development of novel therapeutic strategies, cellular investigation and complex composite structure analysis in the field of medical diagnosis.

Under current chapter, we have discussed about the basic, principle, working mechanism and application of CLEM in biological science, geological science, medical science etc. In addition, we have also explored about the historical development, current methods and future possibilities for respective advance research and technologies.

9.2 Meaning of CLEM

It is the combination of two powerful technique i.e. light microscopy (LM) and Electron microscopy (EM), which will provide complementary information through respective modes of operation. The capabilities of wide field view under live imaging of biological specimens through LM mode and high-resolution imaging analysis under EM (SEM or TEM) bring holistic imaging analysis of specimen. This will jointly try to overcome the challenges of diffraction limits w.r.t atomic or molecular resolution [1–4].

9.2.1 Principle and Working of CLEM

The principle and working of CLEM will be understood with prior knowledge of LM and EM basics, principle, strength respectively.

9.2.1.1 Fundamental of LM

Imaging process under LM proceed with the use of visible light in visualization of structure and functions of cells, tissues and material science samples. There are different simple and complex ways of contrast improvement under LM mode of operation w.r.t. nature of specimen [1–4].

Fluorescence Microscopy

The phenomenon of absorption of high intensity light via specimen molecule, follows emission of respective region of light during relaxation process, termed as fluorescence. Many time, specific fluorescent dyes will be used to locate the specific components of cellular system, live cells or proteins etc. Specifically, fluorescence microscopy will be used in cell biology, neuroscience and medical diagnostic fields for protein localization, tissue structuring and architecture with investigation of cellular communication etc. [1–4].

Confocal Microscopy

Confocal Microscopy is based on the principle of usage of spatial pinhole with pin-point illumination optics to restrict the out of focus light for improved optical resolution and contrast imaging. Collection of two-dimensional imaging of specimen at different depth transform into three-dimensional (3D) imaging known as optical sectioning. It has capabilities of high resolution, high contrast and 3D reconstruction with minimum background interference. Confocal microscopy will also be useful in thick specimen analysis. Further, the usage of current technique can be extended for development of different biological and molecular process for novel updation in respective fields [1–4].

Strength of LM Techniques with Resolution Limitation

It is a non-destructive technique w.r.t. live cell imaging process, poses as the best feature of current mode. Different dynamic processes like protein re-organization or cells dynamic behaviour etc., will be monitored in real time. In addition, LM based techniques will be compatible with different fluorescent dyes or labelling compounds during identification of specific localization study for different biological processes. Due to limited range of visible light wavelength and diffraction limit feature, respective imaging resolution is limited upto ~ 200 nm for lateral direction and ~ (500–700) nm for axial respectively. Although, with the advancement in upgraded optical instruments like stimulated emission depletion (STED), photoactivated localization microscopy (PALM), or Stochastic optical reconstruction microscopy (STORM) etc., have pushed the resolution limits down to the range of ~ (20–50) nm [1–5], in case of LM analysis also.

9.2.1.2 Fundamental of Electron Microscopy (EM)

The use of electron beam in place of light, overcome the limited resolution aspect of specimen imaging. The comparable wavelength of electron beam w.r.t. atomic arrays, allow EM in visualization of finer detail of specimen from bulk size (~micrometre etc.) to atomic scale (nanometre etc.).

Transmission Electron Microscopy (TEM)

Electron beam is transmitted through ultrathin (~ <100 nm) specimen during TEM analysis. TEM imaging proceeds with the contrast development of specimen through electron beam interaction with specimen. Atomic size equivalent wavelength facilitates high resolution internal structures of cell, organelles, protein, macromolecules or during TEM analysis. TEM applications will be extended from biological science to material science including cell biology, bacteria, viruses, protein, complex macromolecules and nanomaterial sample analysis and respective structural, functional explanations [6].

Scanning Electron Microscopy (SEM)

SEM will work on the principle of interaction of electron beam with surface of specimen in scanning mode. Different generated signal like secondary electron (SE), back scattered electron (BSE) detection produced specimen high resolution. Large size of specimen (~ like 10 mm size) can also be observed under SEM in comparison to TEM observation with large depth of field for topographical information. In similar manner to TEM, SEM analysis of specimen also belong to biological sciences, geological science or material science w.r.t. surface structure and morphological investigation [7].

Strength of EM Techniques

Through the principle of transmission of electron beam through ultrathin specimen, atomic scale resolution ~ <1 nm, will be achieved under TEM or HRTEM analysis irrespective to nature of sample and specification of instrument. Whereas in case of SEM, resolution limits w.r.t. surface information, will revolve around in the range of ~ 1–10 nm. TEM will provide ultrastructural internal detail information of samples up to atomic regime whereas SEM will elaborate about the surface structure and surface topography information [6, 7].

9.2.2 Integration of Light Microscopy (LM) with Electron Microscopy (EM)

The integration of LM and EM technique together during imaging process, benefits researchers for specimens' functional information, dynamic aspect as well resolution regime analysis. LM techniques will be helpful in locating the specimen region of interest (ROI) which can be easily transfer for high resolution imaging under EM mode [5]. Figure 9.1a–f, demonstrated the working layout of seedling plant analysis via 5-ethyl-2^1-deoxy uridine (Edu) marker for fluorescence and transmission electron microscopy (TEM) [8] study. Similarly, the atmospheric scanning electron microscope (ASEM) technique has been also used in imaging of nanogold labelled cell surface [9]. Respective process has been presented in Fig. 9.1g–i.

9.2.2.1 Importance of CLEM

There are the following gaps and limitations of w.r.t. individual LM and EM techniques, which can be overcome during collective CLEM approach.

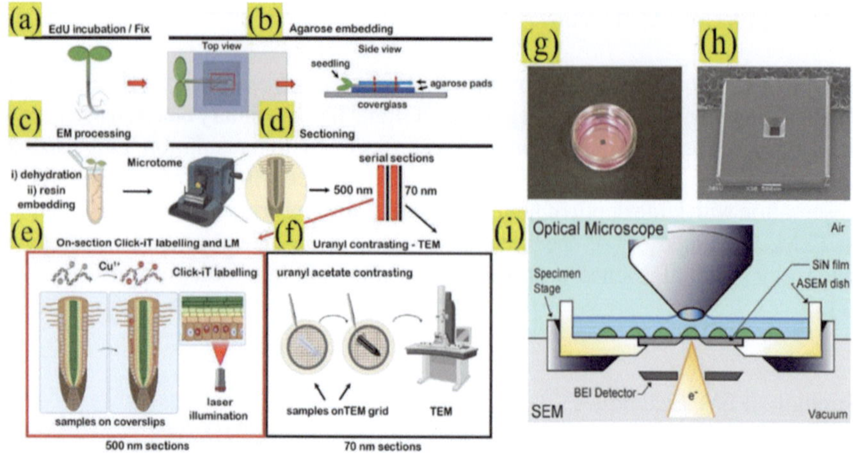

Fig. 9.1 **a–c** Labelling of Seedling plant with 5-ethyl-2^1-deoxy uridine (Edu) marker followed by fixation, dehydration, ultramicrotomy, **d** semithin section (~ 500 nm) for fluorescence microscopy with ~ 70 nm thin section for electron microscopy, **e** iT labelling of 500 nm thick section with spin disk or single molecule localization, **f** Ultrathin section were stained with 4% uranyl acetate before imaging under TEM (Adapted with permission from Franek et al. [8] under open access), **g** Atmospheric scanning electron microscope (ASEM) having removable 35 mm with 100 nm electron transparent SiN window separating vacuum and atmosphere, **h** SEM image of SiN window with scale bar ~ 500 μm, **i** ASEM schematic working diagram with fluorescence microscope arranged above the inverted SEM (Adapted with permission from Murai et al. [9] under open access)

Real Time High-Resolution Imaging

LM capabilities will image biological specimen for live functional and contextual information. In addition, with the use of fluorescent dye or protein in specific localization of cellular components, precise and localized imaging can be performed. The limited resolution due to diffraction limit in LM, will be overcome during imaging via TEM or SEM analysis. Collectively, the dynamic behaviour imaging under LM and EM mode analysis for biological specimens cellular or sub-cellular components exploration can be insightly performed [1–5].

Correlative Functional and Structural Analysis

The localized investigation of biological specimen through use of fluorescent dyes or labelling components under fluorescence or confocal microscopy, will be imaged to locate the specific sites lively. Whereas identified active sites of specific working mechanism belong to any biological or material process, will be imaged for functional and structural investigation via EM techniques. This will facilitate minimum time delay and transferring of ROI from one mode to other [1–5].

Targeted Imaging and Precision Study

Through identification of specific sites or location of life science or material species w.r.t. specific diseases, infections or defects system will be highlighted via labelling marker. Identified targeted area of interest will be analysed for high resolution mapping under TEM or SEM [1–5].

Versatile Sample Analysis

The dual nature of specimen i.e. dynamic and static, behaviour will be analysed through LM and EM mode of analysis through appropriate specimen preparation technique. Live cell imaging of specimen under LM mode will observe different dynamic processes with temporal changes. Extraction of representative specimen from parent living species for LM study will need clarity ROI, specimen size, preservation conditions and operational parameters etc. Through above study, one can understand different cellular phenomenon like cell division, migration and signalling processes etc. Moreover, the static form of specimen will be achieved via fixation, dehydration, thin slicing etc., for high resolution requirement in cellular visualization or ultrastructure investigation under TEM [1–5].

Improvised Sample Labelling

Under dual labelling mode of operation, it will use such labels or marker which are visible in both LM and EM imaging. This type of approach is very much useful in explaining the specific type of biological process. There must be need of standardized protocol of sample preparation which can preserve the integrity of specimen structure with fluorescent dyes during respective processing and imaging [1–5].

Applications in Diverse Fields

CLEM will be used in diverse field belong to biological science, medical science or material science as per objective of study. Under medical research, different disease mechanism, pathological and drug effect can be analysed at functional as well at ultrastructural level. Further, CLEM analysis will also insights into different cellular processes, protein localization and molecular interaction to understand and proposed novel remedies for existing challenges in respective field. Similarly, material science field also gets benefited to large scale with explanation of different composites and complex structure for their functional and structural analysis [1–5].

Figure 9.2, schematically presented important aspect of CLEM dominated approach.

In summary, the integration of LM and EM techniques under CLEM bring a complete and corelative understanding of biological and material science sample. It

Fig. 9.2 Schematic representation of importance of CLEM analysis

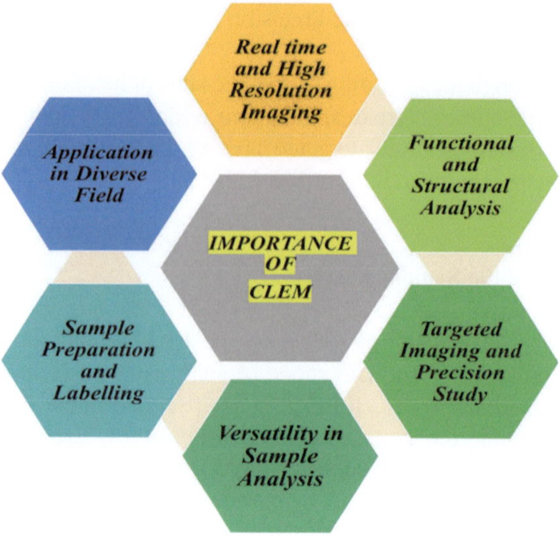

is the rarest analysis which bridge the gap between functional and structural sample analysis via imaging through two extreme ended techniques.

NOTE: CLEM technique will not only help in imaging things that how they look, but imaged for how things will work, which credits for rarest functional insights.

9.2.3 *Methods of Integration Between LM and EM*

There are following ways of integration between LM and EM technique w.r.t. CLEM instrumentation.

9.2.3.1 Sequential Imaging

Sequential imaging mode proceed sample analysis firstly under LM mode without having any deviation in natural state of specimen for live imaging. It is very much helpful in locating the region on interest (ROI) for specimen to be analysed under CLEM. Further, targeted ROI will be processed for TEM or SEM analysis. Special expertise will be desired while handling and analysing the LM and EM imaging process for same specimen in two imaging techniques [5, 10].

9.2.3.2 Simultaneous Imaging

Under this mode, researchers can use LM and EM both modes simultaneously. With switch of button, user can shift from LM mode to EM mode or can concurrently capture images for same area. Perfect alignment between LM and EM modes with operational expertise will be desired in avoiding any chance of distortion in specimen through operational conditions. Although, due to complexity in operational conditions with expensive nature of CLEM technique, it will be always challenging in performing simultaneous imaging [5, 10].

Through sequential and simultaneous imaging of specimen under respective study, it will be analysed for both dynamic and high-resolution imaging simultaneously.

9.2.4 Application of CLEM

There is the following area of research where the CLEM technique will be applied to get comprehensive insight about wide varieties of specimen with utilizing the strengths of LM and EM technique.

9.2.4.1 Biological Research

Cellular and Sub-cellular Studies

CLEM have capability of imaging individual cell for their functional and dynamic context in LM mode. Further the ultrastructural aspect of respective cellular system will be continuously analysed via required EM mode (SEM/TEM) of operation for specific highlighted/targeted area as identified by LM mode. Different mechanism like cells reorganization or modification with their transportation mechanism etc., will be imaged for dynamic function explanation. Different organelles like mitochondria, endoplasmic reticulum, Golgi apparatus etc. will also be analysed for actual functioning regime by LM with further processing for TEM analysis.

Fermie et al. [11] has demonstrated the efficient role of fluorescent bovine serum albumin (BSA)-Au(fBSA-Au) fiducial marker in endocytosed and distributed throughout the endolysosomal network of cells (HeLa Cells) via 2D and 3D cryo-CLEM analysis. HeLa cells incubation with fBSA-Au with cryo-sectioning and immunolabelling for specific site registration has been performed whose detail is comprised in Fig. 9.3a–c with fluorescence microscopy (FM) and transmission electron microscopy (TEM). Figure 9.3c highlighted the region of specific imaging cells. Figure 9.3d shows high resolution image of fBSA-Au (marked with arrow head) based organelle labelled for CD63 in all compartment from registration (1–6). Inset images under Fig. 9.3d(1–6) depicts the fluorescence visualization of CD63 and fBSA-Au. Further, Fig. 9.3d(1, 2) shows the late endosomes (LE) containing many intraluminal vesicles with higher appearance of fBSA-Au label in registration 2,

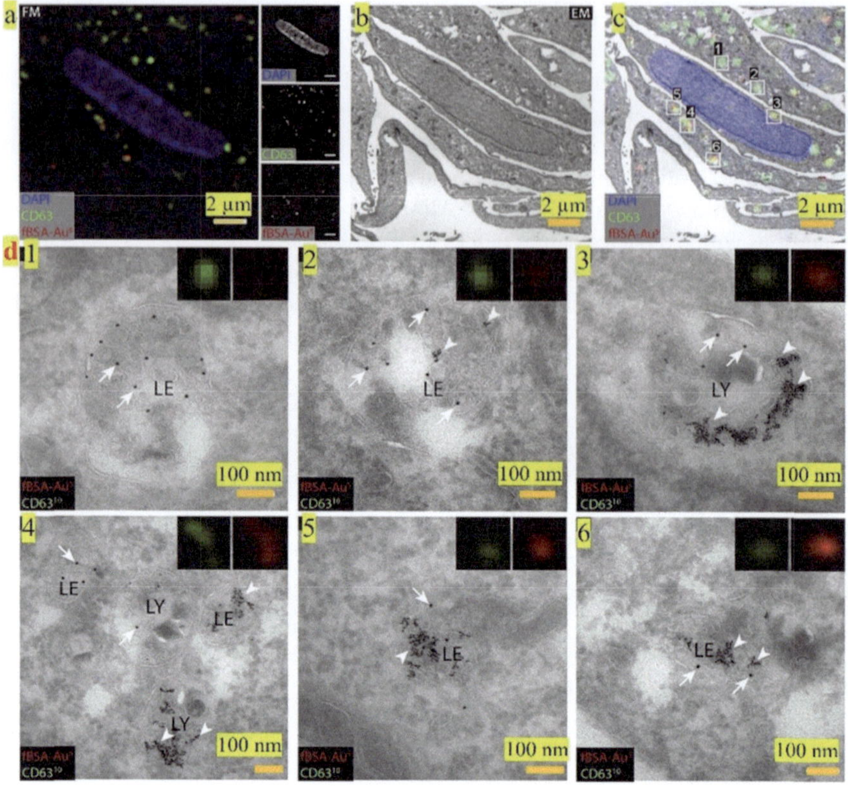

Fig. 9.3 CLEM imaging of fBSA-Au label compartments in HeLa cells, **a** Fluorescence image of ultrathin cryosections shown ROI with CD63, **b** EM image of ROI, **c** overlay image of FM and EM, **d** High resolution EM images of fBSA-Au with organelle labelled for CD63 with different site-specific region (1–6) having different late endosomes (LE) and lysosomes (LY) species presence with different gold label presence (Adapted with permission from Job Fermie et al. [11] under open access)

whereas higher concentration of gold label with lysosomes (LY) has been observed with registration 3 of respective area. Under registration 4 of same specimen, shows varying gold labels with LY and LE, whereas location 6 shows LE presence with high concentration of gold label [11].

Protein Localization Studies

The identification of specific sites in living cells w.r.t. protein interaction via fluorescent dyes will also be facilitated by fluorescent microscopy (FM). The same region of interest related to protein localization and interaction will be further visualized for ultrastructural investigation via TEM analysis. As a part of unique method development, different types of protein interaction will be studied with different species cellular system [12].

9.2.4.2 Medical Research

Pathological and Disease Mechanism Studies

Development and spreading of diseases like cancer, tuberculosis (TB), neurodegenerative disorders and infectious diseases etc., will be analysed for their insightful study via LM and EM techniques. In addition, the interaction mechanism of different viruses, bacteria or other pathogenic invaders etc., with different host cells, can also be explored more authentically. From basic to advance level tissue architecture distortion generated due to different factors, will be analysed through different pathogenic or infection factors, will also be analysed and reported through CLEM vast capabilities.

Jung et al. [13] reported mitophagy based mitochondrial quality assessment in SH-SY5Y cells with propionic acid (PPA) treatment through confocal microscopy and TEM techniques. Live cells were treated with 2 mM PPA for 24 h followed by 100 Nm Lyso Tracker staining (15 min), will be imaged under confocal microscope. In continuation, above treated specimen will be followed by fixation, dehydration, embedding, infiltration and ultramicrotomy for 60 nm thick slices were imaged under TEM. Under Fig. 9.4a, healthy mitochondria have been confirmed via green fluorescence of GFP with the presence of some red puncta. Control cells show clear contact between positive structure (blue) with red puncta as demonstrated in Fig. 9.4A3, A6. With the treatment of PPA to cellular system, damaged round mitochondria having high electron density has been observed which is shown in Fig. 9.4b. The respective co-localization through Lyso-Tracker mitophagy behaviour in mitochondrial quality [13], has been imaged from Fig. 9.4B1–B9 respectively.

Controlled Drug Delivery System

CLEM techniques will be very much useful in drug delivery assessment of drug binding, its localization individually or with some biodegradable compatible binder. In addition to efficacy of targeted drug delivery, probable side-effects on cellular functional and structural aspect, will also be analysed via dynamic and ultrastructural imaging mode of CLEM.

In similar work, Bhandari et al. [14] reported bedaquiline (BQ) based NPs drug interaction with zebrafish embryo tissue to ultrastructural level through non-invasive high resolution live and electron microscopy imaging. The reach of BQ NPs to mycobacteria infected area of zebra fish neural tube model has been demonstrated. Using fluorescence microscopy (FM), sufficient accumulation of BQ NPs has been observed in neural tube granulomas as highlighted in Fig. 9.5a, b. FM images under

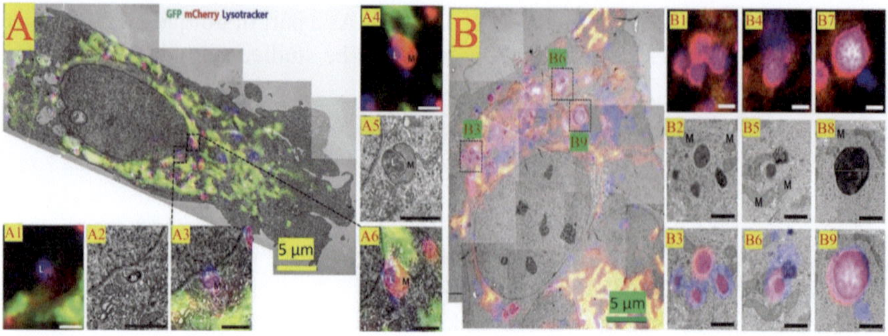

Fig. 9.4 Correlative confocal and electron microscopy images of **A** co-localized SH-SY5Y Cells with A1–A6 images (~ 1 µm) shows the mitophagy morphology, **B** Cell treated with 2 mM PPA with yellow colour indicates localization of GFP and mCherry signals. Co-localization of mCherry with Lyso Tracker has been indicated with magenta color. TEM images were captured at 1700 X for large field of view. Black dot line box indicates about the structure of magenta fluorescent puncta. Respective B1–B6 images (~ 1 µm) shows the mitophagy morphology of treated cells (Adapted with permission from Jung et al. [13] under open access)

Fig. 9.5b, shows maximum BQ NPs localization w.r.t. vascular wall of caudal vein indicating their accumulation in endothelial cells. Further, Fig. 9.5c shows all NPs (Red colour) with gold 10 nm inside the large vesicles (green colour) w.r.t. endothelial cells whereas nil interaction of respective NPs with lumen has been found. CLEM technique has mutually explained through red fluorescence behaviour of BQ NPs with respective ultrastructural imaging [14].

9.2.4.3 Material Science Research

Nanoscale Materials Characterization

The functional properties like optical, catalytic etc., behaviour of nanomaterial can be explained through fluorescence microscopy in CLEM. At same time, the ultrastructural regime of respective material also can be explored for shape, size, morphology with atomic scale exploration. The correlative explanation of targeted area of same specimen under LM and EM modes, will be very much useful in insightful understanding for novel interpretations for basic to advance applications.

Fokkema et al. [15] studied the use of fluorescent silica coated gold NPs as fiducial marker via CLEM. Fiducials marker having 81.9 nm size on the surface of 70 nm thick cryosections of HT1080 cells has been imaged through 2D CLEM widefield imaging via lamp-1 GFP. In addition to presence of fiducial marker in Fig. 9.6d, e overlay images of FM/EM show the correlation of fiducial marker with respective ultrastructural area. The high-resolution capabilities of TEM will be further utilized in identification of core–shell structure with further automatic registration of particles [15].

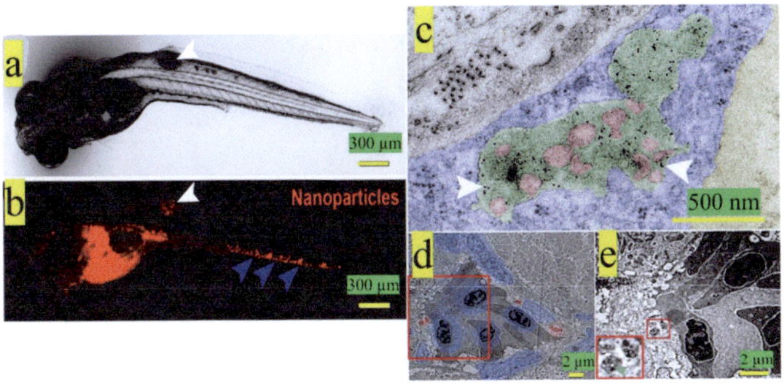

Fig. 9.5 Circulation and accumulation of NPs in zebrafish granulomas, **a** TEM image of neural tube infected embryo at 5-day post infection, **b** fluorescence imaging of same specimen after 24 h w.r.t. red fluorescent BQ NPs. White arrow head in figure (**a**, **b**) shows granuloma region with NPs accumulation region whereas blue arrow head in image (**b**) shows the NPs accumulation in caudal region endothelium, **c** 60 nm thin sections of zebra embryo fish 4 h post injected BQ NPs (Red colour) inside late endosomes (green) with 10 nm gold NPs highlighted with white arrowhead whereas blue and yellow colour highlighting the endothelial cells cytoplasm and blood lumen structure, **d** fluorescence microscopy of NPs (Red colour) inside endothelial having PCV (DAPI in blue) overlay with respective TEM image, **e** Image shows with red box highlighted region depicting presence of NPs inside late endosomes into endothelial cells near blood vessel (Adapted with permission from Bhandari et al. [14] under open access)

Analysis of Composites and Polymer Analysis

The defined composition and phase distribution of different composite and polymer materials will be explained and explored for microstructure investigation via CLEM analysis. CLEM technique will be helpful in identifying and analysing defects, interfaces, and structural inhomogeneities within composites or polymer-based bulk or nanomaterial [16].

The holistic analysis of material through CLEM technique from biological science to material specimens, will be explored and reported more deeply and authentically.

9.2.5 *Future Perspective in CLEM*

Due to wide potential capabilities in CLEM techniques during biological material to material science samples analysis and explanations, there are many key areas in development, integration related to upgradation in CLEM instrumentation [5]. In coming paragraph CLEM techniques has been explained w.r.t. advancement and integration possibilities with related techniques (SEM/TEM etc.), with probable challenges.

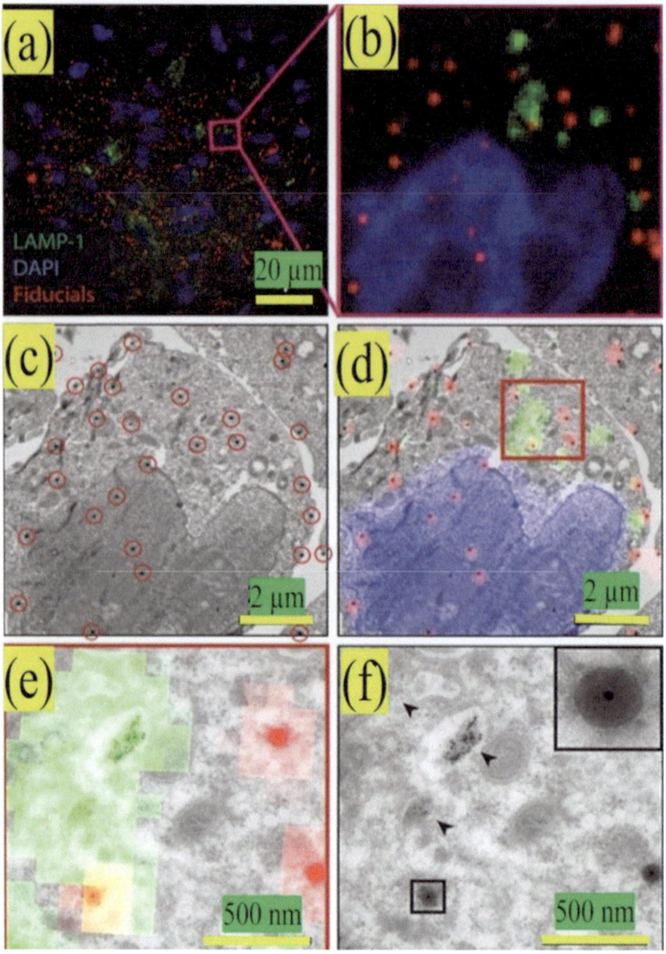

Fig. 9.6 2D CLEM of 81.9 nm fiducial on HT1080 Cell 70 nm thin cryosection, **a** widefield fluorescence microscopy, **b** Region of interest for TEM imaging, **c** TEM image of selected region with fiducial (highlighted with red colour), **d** overlay image of FM and EM, **e**, **f** high resolution images of FM and TEM with endocytosed BSA-Au NP (arrowhead mark in image **f**) presence. Inset of image **f** confirm the core shell structure of silica coated Gold NPs (Adapted with permission from Fokkema et al. [15] under open access)

9.2.5.1 Advancement in CLEM

Improved Resolution and Sensitivity

It is never easy to say that any image through any microscope (LM or EM) is perfect as there are lot of factors w.r.t. hardware, software or sample preparation, which always need further optimization. Similarly, CLEM technique also gets upgraded

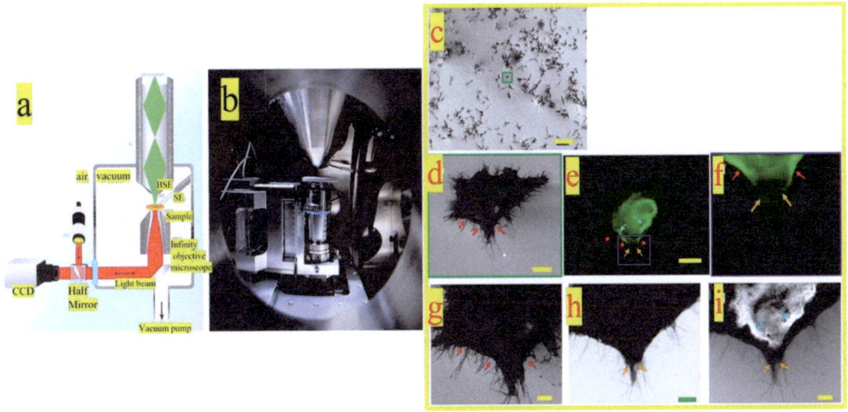

Fig. 9.7 **a** SCLEM schematic layout, **b** inside view of integrated SCLEM having objective lens underneath of sample holder and electron lens, **c** SEM image at low magnification of cortactin cancer cells, **d** respective isolated cell, **e, f** fluorescence image of marked cell from image **c** with blue, red and yellow arrow in image highlight the different type of regions having localized increase of cortactin cells density, **g** Back scattered image (BSE) at 5 keV, **h** secondary electron image at 5 keV, **i** blue marked arrow depicts cortactin cell thick region predicts enhance cell thickness (Adapted with permission from Liv et al. [20] under open access)

with advanced EM detectors and optical system for enhanced detection and sensitivity features. Integration of super resolution LM technique like STEM, PALM etc., will push existing imaging capabilities to atomic or molecular domain of specimens [17–19].

Simultaneous Imaging System

The development in the integration of LM-EM analysis will lead towards precise and correlative explanation of specimen's study in respective mode of imaging. Futuristically, CLEM can also be upgraded with spectroscopic techniques like Raman spectroscopy or X-ray spectroscopy etc., to get more information about chemical and structural analysis of material. Nalan Liv et al [20] analysed protein distribution inside cancer cell structure through simultaneous correlative light and electron microscopy (SCLEM). Figure 9.7a shows objective lens (100×1.4 NA) mounted inside SEM vacuum chamber in similar to inverted light microscope. The respective illumination and detection of optical system, can be mounted outside the vacuum chamber of EM system as shown Fig. 9.7b. Figure 9.7c–i shows the SCLEM imaging of cortactin cancer cells without transfer from FM to EM and readjustment of region on interest (ROI). Surface coverage of cancer cells on cover glass has been analysed with identification of specific area of ROI. Minimum time delay and axis alignment has been observed from SEM to FM or vice versa during current cellular fluorescence and ultrastructural analysis of specimen [20].

Automation and Data Integration

Latest software with updated data processing tools having ultrafast computational capabilities leads to quick and insight representative imaging, 3D construction etc., will be possible. Whole process will be performed within short span of time with minimum chances of errors and maximum chances of efficient data integration [17–19]. This will be helpful in saving the precious time of researchers/scientist due to manual processing/calculations during respective analysis.

9.2.5.2 CLEM Integration with Other Techniques

Cryo-electron Microscopy

The one of major challenge of losing the sample integrity during sample processing in TEM analysis during CLEM analysis, will be optimized with analysis of specimen under Cryo-TEM. It will lead to preserve the integrity of sample with minimum deviation through sample preparation/processing steps during observation of specimen dynamic behaviour [17–19].

Li et al. [10] explained very precisely about the target guided lamellae preparation through confocal microscopy and cryo-electron tomography (Cryo-ET). Custom built confocal microscope integrated with FIB-SEM has been utilized in current study. Integrated system has following instrumental component in respective layouts w.r.t. current study viz. sample loading position, LM and FIB-SEM position as shown in Fig. 9.8a–c. 3D cryogenic light, ion and electron microscopy (CLIEM) system with front view has been summarized in Fig. 9.8b, c. Respective sample holder containing three auto-grid samples and 1 mm working distance (WD) view of confocal imaging module has been depicted in Fig. 9.8d, e respectively. Further, image (h) clearly shows the contact sites of specimen with respective lamella at same position (image j). Prepared lamella image of respective cellular system (image k) has been found consistent with virtual lamella image (image h). In addition, prepared LM lamella will be used to identify on TEM grid bar (TOI) with their superposition image which is shown in Fig. 9.8l, m. Through Fig. 9.8n–p, clear identification of contact sites for LDs and mitochondria with respective tethering connection has been observed. Finally, image (q) shows consistent overlapping between LM lamella-based tomogram with respective fluorescence imaging. The current study, predicts clear correlative based study between confocal imaging with structure imaging via cryo-ET technique [10].

Super Resolution Microscopy

With the advancement in optics of LM techniques, diffraction limits get overcome for higher resolution bring exploration of unprecedented molecular structures. Real time imaging of dynamic processes in living cellular system can be studied more

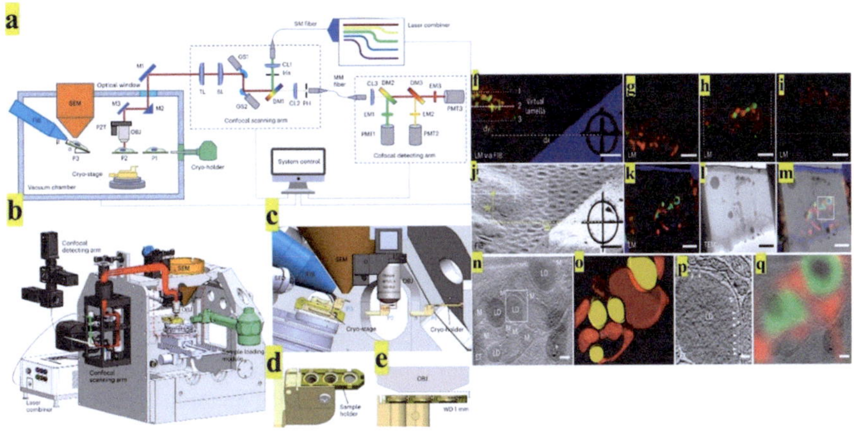

Fig. 9.8 **a** Schematic diagram of CLIEM having sample loading position (P1), LM imaging position (P2), FIB-SEM position (P3), **b** 3D rendering of CLIEM system, **c** front view of boxed area of image **b**, **d** sample holder containing three auto grid samples, **e** 1 mm working distance (WD) view of confocal imaging module, **f** LM via FIB of Hep G2 cells grown on grid having three milling positions of virtual lamella having green channel (LD-mitochondria site), red channel (mitochondria labelled with Mito Tracker Deep), blue channel (bright field), **g–i** computational generated confocal images of above three channels, **j** FIB image of same region of **f**, **k** confocal image of prepared lamella, **l** 300 kV TEM image, **m** superposition image of LM (**k**) and TEM (**l**), **n** tomographic image of HepG2 cells showing LD surrounded by mitochondria (**m**), **o** 3D rendering of LD (yellow) with mitochondria outer membrane (red), **p** tomogram of boxed region of image **n** showing contact between LD and mitochondria, **q** correlative image of LM image (image **k**) and tomographic image at **n**. Scale bar is 5 µm for **f**, **j** image and 2 µm for **b–d**, **k–m** image, 200 nm for **n**, **q** image and 50 nm scale bar for image **p** (Adapted with permission from Li et al. [10] under open access)

authentically with super resolution microscopy techniques like STEM, PALM etc. [17–19].

NOTE: Updated technologies in CLEM facilitates precise integration of LM and EM, bring improved image accuracy, automation, 3D visualization with advance data analysis of respective specimen analysis.

9.2.5.3 Potential Area of Applications and Research

There are following area of research, which can be explored with the help of CLEM technologies for precise and insightful results.

Neuroscience

Under neuroscience, synaptic functions and neural circuit etc. explanations can be studied very closely in real time with dynamic imaging feature of CLEM technique. Similarly, the neuro-degenerative disorder oriented structural alteration in cellular and sub-cellular system also can be explored very closely for functional behaviour of species study in natural state with ultrastructural aspect.

Futura et al. [21] analysed the multiscale neuronal imaging of mammalian (mouse) brain connectivity via LM/EM imaging. Figure 9.9a depicts the workflow w.r.t. LM/EM neuronal imaging of murine striatal circuitry. Mouse brain has been fixed with 4% paraformaldehyde (PFA) containing 0.2% glutaraldehyde (GA). Macroscopic and mesoscopic neural circuit mapping was conducted with controlled slow strength material (CLSM) as shown in Fig. 9.9b. Respective CLSM imaging of treated brain section shows striatofugal projection system. Specifically, dorsal CPu view in the input side of targeted neuron (Fig. 9.9C1–C4), followed by synaptic ultrastructural imaging of specific dendrite as shown in Fig. 9.9C5–C6. Further process for high resolution stacks for respective labelled neuron has been observed which is shown in Fig. 9C_1–C_3, D_1–D_3 respectively. Image re-sections were process for ABS/DAB Ni^{2+} via deposition of biotin molecule, followed by their embedding epoxy resin has been shown in Fig. 9.9C_4, D_4. Respective specimen ultrathin section has been placed at Fig. 9.9C_5, C_6, D_5, D_6 highlighted dendrite, blood vessel (BV) and axon terminal (AT) position in respective specimen.

Immunology

Challenge of sudden or slow failure of immune system of living species, will be explored very precisely through CLEM analysis. The tracking of immune cell interactions with cellular or organ system can be correlated with immune function or dysfunction behaviour. In continuation, during remediation stage of immune failure system, respective investigation and vaccine efficacy can also be visualized with immune system responses with pathogen interaction at high resolution scale.

Under similar work, Oorschot et al. [22] studied multi-resolution immuno-correlative light and electron microscopy (iCLEM) with advantages of antigenicity preservation of Tokuyasu technique. Robust and comparative protocol has been established between fluorescence microscopy (FM), scanning electron microscopy (SEM) and scanning transmission electron microscopy (STEM). iCLEM will be helpful in identification, quantification and analysis of cell population in different organism, tissue in healthy as well in their diseases state. In current study authors have investigated the neural stem and progenitor cell population of vertebrate nervous system w.r.t. adult zebrafish model.

Tokuyasu cryo-section (70–80 nm) mounted on TEM grid having immuno labelled with antibodies and fluorescent marker, brought capturing of multiple images of whole tissue hemisphere in STEM mode as shown in Fig. 9.10a–c. With reference to

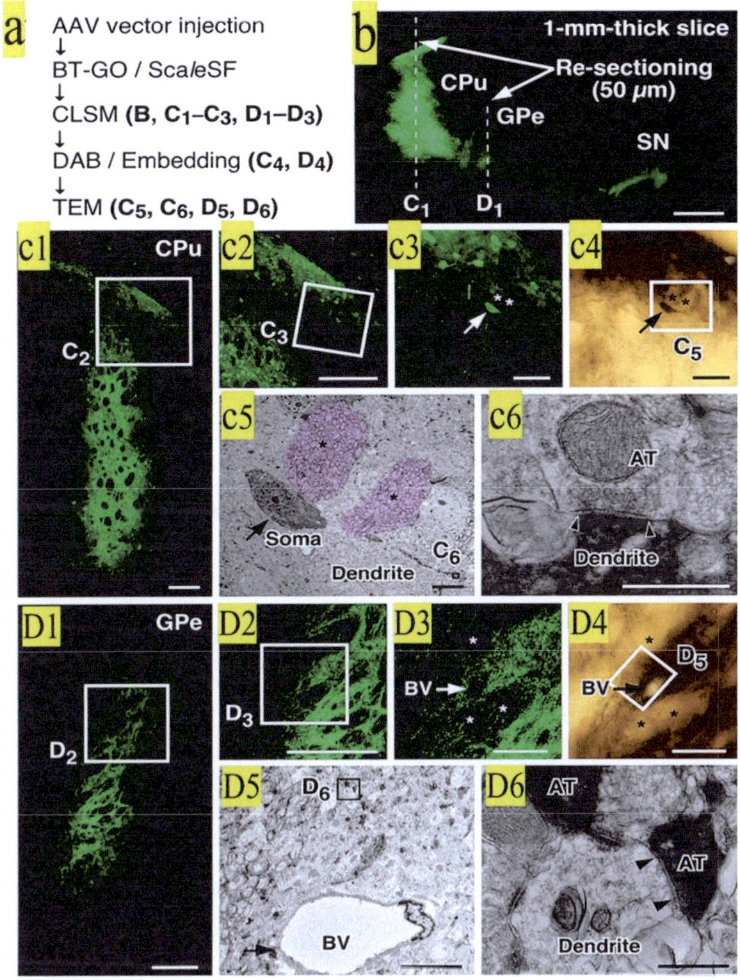

Fig. 9.9 LM/EM of neuronal imaging of mouse CPu neurons, **a** Procedure of multiscale LM/EM neuronal imaging for CPu neurons through fixation with 4% PFA and 0.2% GA, **b** 1 mm thick parasagittal brain slice cleared with scale SF. Sections cut along dotted line have thickness ~ 50 μm (**b**). Scale bar ~ 500 μm, **c**, **d** correlated fluorescence (c1–c3, D_1–D_3) with bright imaging at C4 and D4 and TEM images C_5, C_6, D_5 and D_6 at the level of CPu (C) and GPe (D), CLSM imaging-scale bar-200 μm, Images C_2, C_3, D_2, D_3 are the enlarged view of rectangles in C_1, C_2, D_1, D_2 images with scale bar 200 μm in (C_2, D_2) and 50 μm in (C_3, and D_3), (C_5 and D_5) are enlarged view of reactangle in C_4 and D_4 with scale bar 10 μm, (C_6 and D_6) images are enlarged view of (C_4 and D_4) with scale bar 10 μm. Images C_3 and C_4 have highlighted current targeted neuron whereas asterisk in (C_3–C_5), (D_3, D_4) images pointout the axonal fibers in images (C and D), images D_3–D_5 highlighted the BV position, C_6 and D_6 images indicates the postsynaptic membranes, scale bar 500 nm (Adapted with permission from Futura et al. [21] under open access)

low resolution tile set, specialized conjunction with software viz. MAPS etc., iCLEM-STEM bring zooming the specific area of interest under respective specimen region for fluorescent data as shown in Fig. 9.10d–l. Using zoom function in tile set facilitate co-labelling of radial glial cells (orange GS+/PCNA, GFP) pointed with white and black arrow) distinguished from neighbouring cycling cell (green GS/PCNA, GFP with red arrow) (Fig. 9.10g–i). With the variation in location on montage, non-cycling radial glia cells (red GS/PCNA, GFP with white, black arrow) has been observed which is shown in Fig. 9.10j–l [22].

Environment Science

In current scenario of growth and development, sustainability of ecosystem is become an utmost need in every field of research. Huge amount of organic and metallic waste generated during multiple ill and illegal practices through domestic and industrial activities, will deteriorate our ecosystem. Presence of respective harmful components have adverse impact on different biological, geological etc. processes, which can be explored and examined very precisely through CLEM technique. Further, the increasing use of microplastic and related pollutants in daily life, also need to analysed at nanoscale w.r.t. their toxicity effects [23].

9.2.5.4 Challenges and Limitation in CLEM

There are the following challenges which need to optimize during working and operation of CLEM:

Sample Preparation Complexity

Development of standardized protocols must be needed, to achieve the structural integrity with fluorescent labelling of respective specimen through LM and EM imaging. The issue of specimen compatibility with optimize concentration between labelling agent for localization and contrast enhancement etc., w.r.t. CLEM operation, need to be standardize [1–5].

Precise Correlation and Interpretation of Data

Specially in case of CLEM, the precise alignment between LM and EM mode will always be challenging to get minimum errors and deviations-based analysis. Use of updated mathematical algorithms (computational techniques) will minimize the chances of human error with saving of time. Conventional EM analysis of specimen has been compared with iCLEM on Tokuyasu prepared cryo-section in current study.

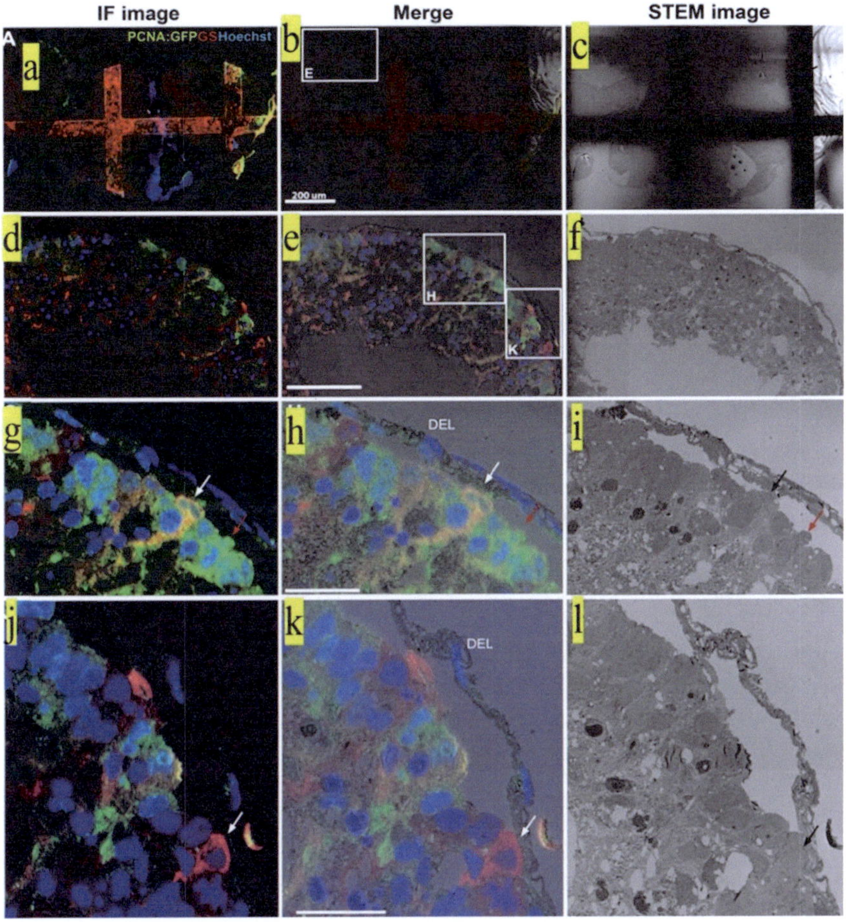

Fig. 9.10 Merged images (Middle column) of immunofluorescent (IF) (left column) and STEM images (right column) using MAPS software. **a–c** Tile set STEM images of zebrafish forebrain on TEM grid with MAPS software. Highlighted white box of image **b** has been highlighted from images **d–e** demonstrating dorsal view of zebrafish pallium having labelled cells below thin dorsal ependymal lining, highlighted box region in image **e** displayed from images **g–i** having GS+/PCNA: GFP-radial glial cell (orange white/black arrow), contrasted with GS^-/PCNA: GFP^+ cycling cell (green; red arrow), **j–l** images of GS+/PCNA: GFP-cell profile (red: white arrow). Scale bar **b** 200 μm, **e** 80 μm, **h**, **k** 20 μm (Adapted with permission from Oorschot et al. from reference [22] under open access)

It shows sharp decrease in field of view from SEM to TEM resolution whose detail has been summarized in Fig. 9.11 [22].

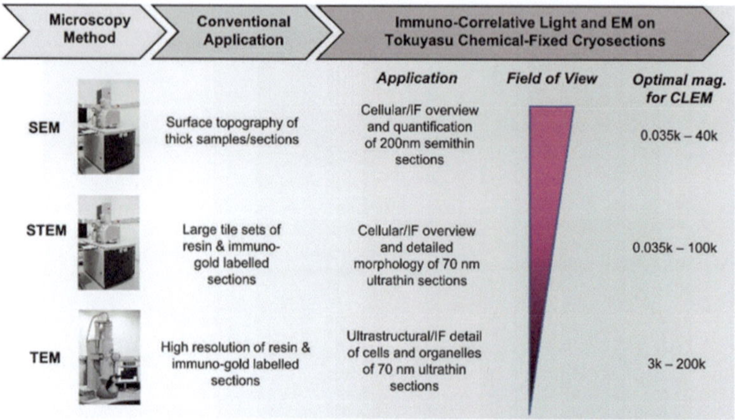

Fig. 9.11 Conventional EM application has been compared with iCLEM on Tokuyasu prepared cryo-section with decrease in field of view from SEM to TEM resolution has been demonstrated (Adapted with permission from Oorschot et al. from reference [22] under open access)

Cost and Accessibility

Due to high cost of CLEM based instrumentation with maintenance difficulty, evolves as a challenging job to maintain the respective facility for any research laboratory or institution. Obviously, purchase-installation with smooth functioning of technique like CLEM having maximum reach to researchers, is a matter of experience, finance and scientific temperament. The operational and maintenance team behind the instrument like CLEM, is always need to diversely trained qualified person. This will be really helpful in smooth operation, advance interpretation of simple to complex specimen dataset for extraordinary scientific innovations [1–5].

Conclusively, with the identification of best possible utilization of CLEM with unique integration possibilities, researchers can claim for innovative research accomplishments and findings.

9.2.6 *Sample Analysis Protocol Under CLEM*

Although, especially every biological specimen has different processing protocol for CLEM analysis, but here we have presented a novel sample preparation protocol w.r.t. Zebrafish forebrain analysis. Here, we have presented workflow for Takayasu sample preparation, iCLEM-SEM, iCLEM-STEM and iCLEM-TEM based systems as shown Fig. 9.12a–c respectively [22].

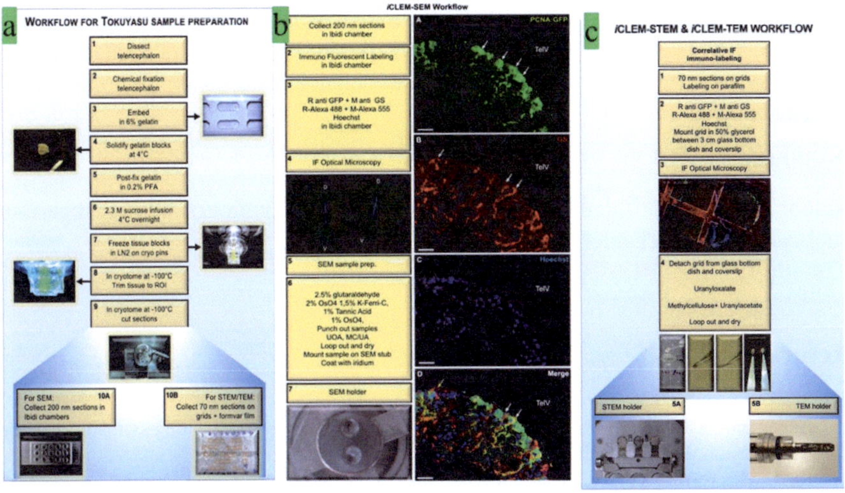

Fig. 9.12 Workflow for **a** Takayasu sample preparation, **b** iCLEM-SEM, **c** iCLEM-STEM and iCLEM-TEM based system (Adapted with permission from Oorschot et al. [22] under open access)

9.3 Conclusion

The CLEM has been emerged as the powerful technique in bridging the gaps w.r.t. imaging domain between molecular functionality and high-resolution capabilities. Through CLEM, insightful understanding has been established for simple to complex biological processes, different diseases mechanism and environmental evolutions at nanoscale.

The site-specific activity and respective visualization of molecular species through fluorescence microscopy (FM) and high-resolution ultrastructural imaging (TEM or SEM), have been revealed and interpreted in precise and accurate manner with rarest synergistic integration. The development in resolution capabilities of LM through advanced optics system, monochromatic light source etc., brings more defined and targeted imaging for contextual explanation of material. Similarly, the integrated EM (SEM or TEM) with upgraded electron source, vacuum system, lens system and detector system etc., has led to more insightful high-resolution imaging. CLEM based integrated system, leads to insightful exploration of cellular to sub-cellular species targeted behaviour in different diagnostic approaches.

CLEM emerged as the hybrid technique which has been widely utilized in different area like cell biology, neuroscience, pathology, material science etc., for routine analysis to diagnostic approach. Correlative explanation of any biological or material specimen w.r.t. molecular, structural and functional behaviour, CLEM will be very dynamic in observing and understanding the related phenomenon.

Finally, with the optimization of shortcomings under CLEM through upgraded technologies w.r.t. resolution, integration, data analysis etc., respective technique would prove to be milestone in analysis of biological as well material analysis. With the application of CLEM technique, more precise understanding and explanation for cellular system with material behaviour from diagnostic approach to device design can be achieved.

Declaration

Author declares that there is no personal or financial conflict of interest regarding publication of this chapter.

References

1. Begemann, I., Galic, M.: Correlative light electron microscopy: connecting synaptic structure and function. Front. Synaptic Neurosci. 8 (2016). https://doi.org/10.3389/fnsyn.2016.00028
2. Razi, M., Tooze, S.A.: Chapter 17 correlative light and electron microscopy. In: Methods in Enzymology, vol. 452, pp. 261–275. Elsevier (2009). https://doi.org/10.1016/S0076-6879(08)03617-3
3. Sjollema, K.A., Schnell, U., Kuipers, J., Kalicharan, R., Giepmans, B.N.G.: Correlated light microscopy and electron microscopy. In: Methods in Cell Biology, vol. 111, pp. 157–173. Elsevier (2012). https://doi.org/10.1016/B978-0-12-416026-2.00009-1
4. Guerin, C.J., Lippens, S.: Correlative light and volume electron microscopy (vCLEM): how community participation can advance developing technologies. J. Microsc. **284**(2), 97–102 (2021). https://doi.org/10.1111/jmi.13056
5. Ando, T., Bhamidimarri, S.P., Brending, N., Colin-York, H., Collinson, L., De Jonge, N., De Pablo, P.J., Debroye, E., Eggeling, C., Franck, C., Fritzsche, M., Gerritsen, H., Giepmans, B.N.G., Grunewald, K., Hofkens, J., Hoogenboom, J.P., Janssen, K.P.F., Kaufmann, R., Klumperman, J., Kurniawan, N., Kusch, J., Liv, N., Parekh, V., Peckys, D.B., Rehfeldt, F., Reutens, D.C., Roeffaers, M.B.J., Salditt, T., Schaap, I.A.T., Schwarz, U.S., Verkade, P., Vogel, M.W., Wagner, R., Winterhalter, M., Yuan, H., Zifarelli, G.: The 2018 correlative microscopy techniques roadmap. J. Phys. D Appl. Phys. **51**(44), 443001 (2018). https://doi.org/10.1088/1361-6463/aad055
6. Luo, Z.: A Practical Guide to Transmission Electron Microscopy: Fundamentals, 1st edn. Momentum Press, New York (2016)
7. Hojat, N., Gentile, P., Ferreira, A.M., Šiller, L.: Automatic pore size measurements from scanning electron microscopy images of porous scaffolds. J. Porous Mater. **30**(1), 93–101 (2023). https://doi.org/10.1007/s10934-022-01309-y
8. Franek, M., Koptasikova, L., Miksatko, J., Pospisil, J., Liebl, D., Esner, M., Macickova, E., Dvorackova, M., Fajkus, J.: In-Section Click-iT Detection and Super-Resolution CLEM: Shedding Light on Nucleolar Ultrastructure and S-Phase Progression in Plants (2023). https://doi.org/10.1101/2023.05.10.540144
9. Murai, T., Sato, M., Nishiyama, H., Suga, M., Sato, C.: Ultrastructural analysis of nanogold-labeled cell surface microvilli in liquid by atmospheric scanning electron microscopy and their relevance in cell adhesion. IJMS **14**(10), 20809–20819 (2013). https://doi.org/10.3390/ijms141020809
10. Li, W., Lu, J., Xiao, K., Zhou, M., Li, Y., Zhang, X., Li, Z., Gu, L., Xu, X., Guo, Q., Xu, T., Ji, W.: Integrated multimodality microscope for accurate and efficient target-guided cryo-lamellae preparation. Nat. Methods **20**(2), 268–275 (2023). https://doi.org/10.1038/s41592-022-01749-z
11. Fermie, J., De Jager, L., Foster, H.E., Veenendaal, T., De Heus, C., Van Dijk, S., Ten Brink, C., Oorschot, V., Yang, L., Li, W., Müller, W.H., Howes, S., Carter, A.P., Förster, F., Posthuma,

G., Gerritsen, H.C., Klumperman, J., Liv, N.: Bimodal endocytic probe for three-dimensional correlative light and electron microscopy. Cell Reports Methods **2**(5), 100220 (2022). https://doi.org/10.1016/j.crmeth.2022.100220
12. Luo, H., Jiang, C., Wen, Y., Wang, X., Wang, F., Liu, L., Yu, H.: Correlative super-resolution bright-field and fluorescence imaging by microsphere assisted microscopy. Nanoscale **16**(4), 1703–1710 (2024). https://doi.org/10.1039/D3NR04096H
13. Jung, M., Choi, H., Kim, J., Mun, J.Y.: Correlative light and transmission electron microscopy showed details of mitophagy by mitochondria quality control in propionic acid treated SH-SY5Y cell. Materials **13**(19), 4336 (2020). https://doi.org/10.3390/ma13194336
14. Bhandari, M., Soria-Carrera, H., Wohlmann, J., Dal, N.-J.K., De La Fuente, J.M., Martín-Rapún, R., Griffiths, G., Fenaroli, F.: Subcellular localization and therapeutic efficacy of polymeric micellar nanoparticles encapsulating bedaquiline for tuberculosis treatment in zebrafish. Biomater. Sci. **11**(6), 2103–2114 (2023). https://doi.org/10.1039/D2BM01835G
15. Fokkema, J., Fermie, J., Liv, N., Van Den Heuvel, D.J., Konings, T.O.M., Blab, G.A., Meijerink, A., Klumperman, J., Gerritsen, H.C.: Fluorescently labelled silica coated gold nanoparticles as fiducial markers for correlative light and electron microscopy. Sci. Rep. **8**(1), 13625 (2018). https://doi.org/10.1038/s41598-018-31836-1
16. Wang, Y., Friedrich, H., Voets, I.K., Zijlstra, P., Albertazzi, L.: Correlative imaging for polymer science. J. Polym. Sci. **59**(12), 1232–1240 (2021). https://doi.org/10.1002/pol.20210013
17. Joosten, B., Willemse, M., Fransen, J., Cambi, A., Van Den Dries, K.: Super-resolution correlative light and electron microscopy (SR-CLEM) reveals novel ultrastructural insights into dendritic cell podosomes. Front. Immunol. **2018**, 9 (1908). https://doi.org/10.3389/fimmu.2018.01908
18. Van Den Dries, K., Fransen, J., Cambi, A.: Fluorescence CLEM in biology: historic developments and current super-resolution applications. FEBS Lett. **596**(19), 2486–2496 (2022). https://doi.org/10.1002/1873-3468.14421
19. Kobayashi, S., Iwamoto, M., Haraguchi, T.: Live correlative light-electron microscopy to observe molecular dynamics in high resolution. Microscopy (Tokyo) **65**(4), 296–308 (2016). https://doi.org/10.1093/jmicro/dfw024
20. Liv, N., Zonnevylle, A.C., Narvaez, A.C., Effting, A.P.J., Voorneveld, P.W., Lucas, M.S., Hardwick, J.C., Wepf, R.A., Kruit, P., Hoogenboom, J.P.: Simultaneous correlative scanning electron and high-NA fluorescence microscopy. PLoS ONE **8**(2), e55707 (2013). https://doi.org/10.1371/journal.pone.0055707
21. Furuta, T., Yamauchi, K., Okamoto, S., Takahashi, M., Kakuta, S., Ishida, Y., Takenaka, A., Yoshida, A., Uchiyama, Y., Koike, M., Isa, K., Isa, T., Hioki, H.: Multi-scale light microscopy/electron microscopy neuronal imaging from brain to synapse with a tissue clearing method. ScaleSF. iScience **25**(1), 103601 (2022). https://doi.org/10.1016/j.isci.2021.103601
22. Oorschot, V., Lindsey, B.W., Kaslin, J., Ramm, G.: TEM, SEM, and STEM-based immuno-CLEM workflows offer complementary advantages. Sci. Rep. **11**(1), 899 (2021). https://doi.org/10.1038/s41598-020-79637-9
23. Caldwell, J., Loussert-Fonta, C., Toullec, G., Heidelberg Lyndby, N., Haenni, B., Taladriz-Blanco, P., Espiña, B., Rothen-Rutishauser, B., Petri-Fink, A.: Correlative light, electron microscopy and Raman spectroscopy workflow to detect and observe microplastic interactions with whole Jellyfish. Environ. Sci. Technol. **57**(16), 6664–6672 (2023). https://doi.org/10.1021/acs.est.2c09233

Chapter 10
Ideal TEM Imaging, Analysis and Troubleshooting Tricks

Every electron micrograph is a blend of physics, chemistry, and geometry—analysis begins by interpreting theses complex interactions
*by **Max Knoll**, co-inventor of Electron Microscope*

Abstract Current chapter comprised of basic requirements related to pre and post requisite installation of TEM including ideal imaging parameters with practical troubleshooting strategies. Chapter further, reinvestigated about the basic and advanced EM imaging operation w.r.t. quality imaging with optimization of key parameters. It includes EM standard operation, beam alignment, electromagnetic lenses astigmatism correction etc., has been summarized. Further, systematic troubleshooting for basic to advanced TEM operation has been performed w.r.t. sample artefacts, specimen-beam interaction-oriented contamination, grid handling etc. Further precise sample preparation through focus ion beam (FIB), ultramicrotomy, high pressure freezing, auto-staining, controlled grid drying procedure etc., also has been explained. Ultimately with the help of current chapter, we expect that any novice or experience electron microscopist become expert and capable in executing ideal imaging, insightful interpretation with maintaining electron-microscope for long life.

Keywords Ideal TEM imaging · Insightful interpretation · Sample artefacts · Beam alignment · Troubleshooting

10.1 Introduction

Electron microscopy (EM) technique have performed as a keystone in analysis of specimens morphological, ultrastructural and compositional exploration. EM technique will work on the principle of electron-beam interaction with specimen for ultrahigh resolution via overcoming the resolution limitation of light microscopy (LM). The capabilities of EM techniques will be only applicable at the conditions of precise sample preparation, respective instrumentation handling having profound understanding of working and principle of respective technique. Through current

R. Singh, *Transmission Electron Microscopy Sample Preparation*,
https://doi.org/10.1007/978-3-031-82967-3_10

chapter, an attempt has been made to summarize all the factors related to pre and post installation requirement w.r.t. space requirement, laboratory environment, trained manpower etc.

The journey of achieving quality imaging w.r.t. visualization and evaluation of molecular, structural or functional aspect of sample under study, will be achieved with efficient aligned instrumentation with technically and conceptually sound person behind the machine. Quality imaging of specimen belong to material science to biological science, it will be achieved through ideally aligned TEM/SEM instrumentation, standardized sample preparation with explaining each and every mechanism during static to dynamic imaging. We expect with the reading of current chapter, readers will get direct access about different minor to major technicalities related to working and operation of instruments with best practices right from installation of instrument to smooth operation, analysis and interpretation of respective results.

10.2 Pre-installation in TEM Lab Requirement

To make high-end instrumentation technique/facility working efficiently, at the initial stage it need to fulfill all the pre-installation requirement [1, 2]. Specifically, there are following pre-installation requirements w.r.t. TEM instrument.

10.2.1 Site Selection

10.2.1.1 Room Dimension and Layout

One of main criteria during the installation of TEM instrument, sufficient spacious dimension area for main instrument room, ancillary instrument room, data processing room etc., will be required. Depending upon the model of TEM instrument as per their specification, respective dimension will vary. We have tabulated generalized space requirement w.r.t. TEM instrumentation under Table 10.1. The sufficient space availability around the main room as well in ancillary instruments rooms, will make routine analysis and maintenance work smoothly w.r.t. longevity of instrument [1, 2].

Table 10.1 Detail related to space requirement for TEM installation has been summarized

Room type	Length (m)	Width (m)	Height (m)
TEM instrument main room	~ (6–8)	~ (4–6)	~ 3
Sample preparation area	~ (3–4)	~ (2–3)	~ (2.5–3)
Ancillary-equipment-room	~ (3–4)	~ (2–3)	~ (2.5–3)
Waiting area	~ (3–4)	~ (2–3)	~ (2.5–3)

10.2.1.2 Structural Integrity and Vibration Control

Floor of instrument room must have ability to support the weight of instrument, so that it will ensure minimum effect of vibration during routine working of machine. Inbuilt or externally assembled vibration damping pads must be placed at appropriate position in instrument to damp the effect of mechanical vibration from heavy machinery or foot traffic around the respective facility area etc. [1, 2].

10.2.2 Environmental Condition

10.2.2.1 Temperature and Humidity

Controlled and stable temperature range from ~ (20–24 °C) with fluctuation range from − 1 to + 1 °C, will be ideally required for smooth functioning of EM instrument operation. To avoid the development of any condensation or static electricity w.r.t. instrument room, (40–60) % humidity level must be maintained inside the laboratory [1, 2].

10.2.2.2 Electromagnetic Interference (EMI)

The TEM instrument room must be shielded from EMI due to interference from other instruments like NMR or electrical wiring etc. Minimum impact of EMI will improve the quality of normal as well high-resolution imaging [1, 2].

10.2.3 Cleanliness

Whole area around TEM instrument i.e. from laboratory inside as well from outside facility including sample preparation area must be free from dust and contaminant. Installation of efficient air filter must be installed at appropriate locations as per movement of users in and around EM facility.

10.2.4 Power Supply and Electrical Requirement

10.2.4.1 Stable Power Supply

TEM instrument will not work smoothly until we have stable, smooth and uninterrupted power supply of specification ~ (220–240) V, (50–60) Hz. Mentioned power supply requirements may vary as per geographical position of region of installation.

Sudden power surges and outages in TEM facility need be avoided with installation of suitable uninterrupted power supply (UPS) as per requirement of installed EM instrument [1, 2].

10.2.4.2 Grounding

The wiring of TEM instrument room as well main instrument wiring must be grounded appropriately. This will be very much useful in ensuring minimum electrical noise and protection of sensitive electrical component from potential damage during normal working time or sudden fluctuation [1, 2].

10.2.5 Air Supply, Vacuum and Cooling System

10.2.5.1 Compressed Air

The whole TEM operation will be based on ultrahigh vacuum, which will be maintained through pneumatic component (valve) system. Respective whole pneumatic system will be maintained through clean, dry, oil free compressed air, whose quality and conditions must be ensured from time to time.

10.2.5.2 Stablized Vacuum and Cooling System

As per specification of TEM instrument, different vacuum pump used in system like rotary pump (RP), diffusion pump (DP), turbo molecular pump (TMP) etc. Proper connections between pump to main instrument, routine exhaust facility etc., as per prevention of contamination during real time imaging inside the TEM column must be ensured time to time. High purity distilled water must be used in TEM water chiller at appropriate pressure, temperature.

10.2.6 Safety and Accessibility

The installation of fire safety alarm, fire extinguisher with display of accident handling protocol like hazardous chemical spillage or sparking inside the main machine or ancillary instrument room etc., must be displayed at appropriate place in lab. Sufficient training to concern lab staff time to time must be provided to maintain all above stated safety measure. Certain quick breakable glass windows must be installed inside the laboratory to ensure emergency exit from laboratory. The location of TEM lab must be at such place that it can be easily accessed for any equipment transportation and related maintenance work [1, 2].

10.2.7 *Operator Comfort, Convenience and Training*

10.2.7.1 Ergonomics

Workplace design w.r.t. operator of EM machine must be comfortable with adjustable seating arrangement and sufficient lightening setup. There must be availability of sufficient workstation for sample preparation, data analysis and respective documentation activities. In addition, the person going to handle and operate the machine must have sound academic background with sufficient training related to respective instrument and sample preparation. This will helpful in maintaining the EM machine lifetime for long time [1, 2].

Through fulfillment of above pre-installation conditions related to TEM/SEM instrument, installed instrument will work very smoothly for longtime with best performance.

10.3 Post-installation TEM Requirement

The optimal performance, utilization of maximum capabilities of EM instrument with satisfying all the safety guidelines, will enhance the efficient operation of instrument. There are the following factors related to post-installation of TEM facility which will improve the efficiency of EM instrument present and future performances.

10.3.1 *Regular Maintenance and Calibration*

Depending upon the load of sample analysis on TEM instrument, respective maintenance schedule must be framed. Routine cleaning of TEM sample holder, cleaning of whenhelt, greasing of mechanical parts, inspection of vacuum system etc., must be performed periodically. TEM instrument must be calibrated with appropriate standard time to time to ensure the accurate imaging and related measurements. Regular maintenance contract must be agreed between your TEM laboratory and respective instrument authorized service provider [1, 2].

10.3.2 *Regular Monitoring of Lab Environment Conditions*

Regular monitoring of humidity, temperature, EMI readings etc., in TEM lab must be documented regularly. Any sudden deviation in respective readings, will need to call respective maintenance department immediately for preventive measure.

10.3.3 User/Operator Training and Certification

Defined comprehensive training program for EM instrument operator must be scheduled regularly including all safety trainings. Training program must include training of new attachments/modes, instrument conditioning etc. Facility of re-certification course of TEM operation must also be scheduled regularly as per updation in the field credited to operators of machine to maintain high standards of TEM instrument outcomes.

10.3.4 Sample Handling and Storage

The sample preparation protocol will be varied according to nature and type of specimen. Validated sample preparation procedure through standard operating procedure (SOP) for biological to material science sample preparation must be followed. Appropriate sample preparation tools like fuming hood, cutting tool, ultrasonication etc., must be use at appropriate place in lab. Prepared specimens on TEM grid must be preserve in controlled environment w.r.t. respective viewing under TEM machine.

Figure 10.1, has elaborated about the important pre and post installation requirement of TEM instrumentation

Operation of TEM instrument prior to fulfillment of pre and post installation conditions, bring smooth operation, analysis, interpretation of EM acquired data for efficient outcomes.

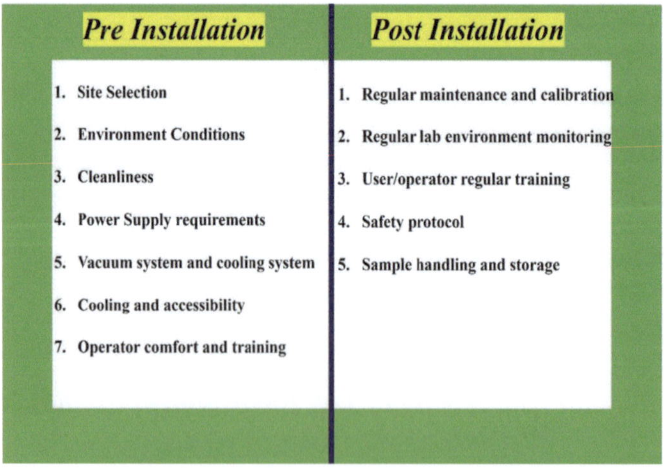

Fig. 10.1 Pre and post installation requirement of TEM instrumentation

NOTE: Pre and post TEM installation prerequisite fulfillment minimizes the different installation issues, facilitates optimal imaging with dynamic analytical capabilities bring efficient instrument performances with longevity.

10.4 Routine TEM Operation, Major Alignments and Troubleshooting

In current section, we have summarized about the standard operation of TEM with major alignments which need to performed before and during TEM operation. Although, there may be slight variation in approach or nomenclature as per nature of model to model of EM instrument or as per manufacturer guidelines (JEOL, Hitachi, Thermo Fischer, Philips, Zeiss etc.). Below written steps were prepared standard operating protocol (SOP) w.r.t. operation of JEOL 2100 Plus 200 kV TEM.

10.4.1 (Step 1): TEM Operation Window

Search and open the TEM operation window through TEM operation software from desktop which comprise detail about the accelerating voltage detail, filament current, filament biasing etc. parameters. Detail has been demonstrated in Fig. 10.2.

10.4.2 (Step 2): Use of Anti Contamination Device (ACD)

There are following steps which need to followed during ACD operation:

(i) Check the column pressure on sputter ion pump (SIP) power supply meter, which must be less than 4×10^{-5} Pascal (Pa) or better as per specification of TEM instrument available.
(ii) Before filling the ACD tank with liquid nitrogen, cover the viewing chamber, side mount camera or scanning transmission electron microscope (STEM) detector if available to avoid any contamination or damage to respective part.
(iii) Fill the ACD tank with liquid nitrogen till overflow.
(iv) Wait for 15 min, and refill ACD tank again.

Figure 10.3a, b, has demonstrated the images showing position of ACD in HRTEM.

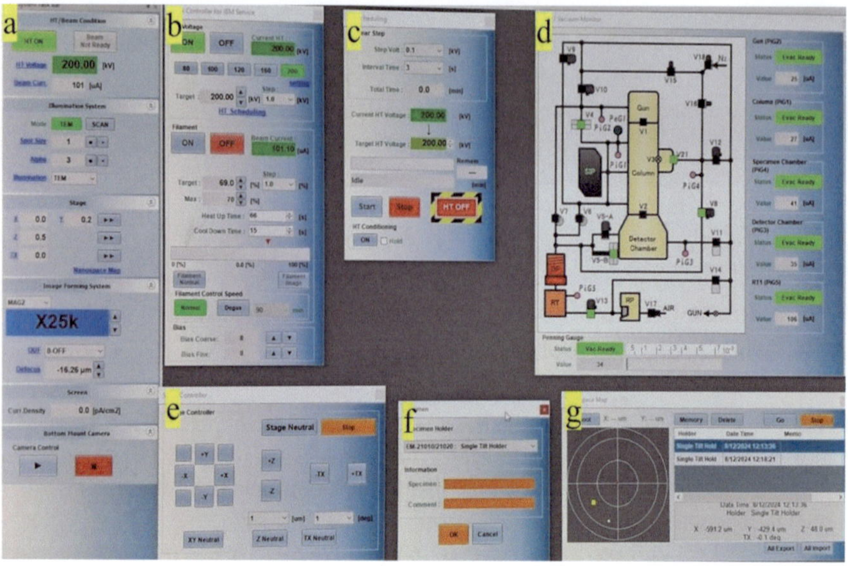

Fig. 10.2 HRTEM operation window (Image received with courtesy of Department of CIL/SAIF, Panjab University Chandigarh, India)

After filling of liquid nitrogen in ACD tank, it will take approximately 1 h to refrigerate the device.

10.4.3 (Step 3): Turn on the Accelerating (ACC) Voltage w.r.t. 200 kV

There are following steps which need to followed during **ACC** voltage **ON** operation:

(i) Open voltage control window with the help of step 1 (Sect. 10.4.1).
(ii) Click the 80 kV button and press HT button **ON**.
(iii) Repeat the step (ii) for rising HT voltage from 80 to 160 kV.
(iv) Click for HT scheduling button (label)/option. Select scheduling program w.r.t. current voltage (160 kV) to target voltage (200 kV) having step volt (like 0.1 kV) and interval time (like 0.1 kV) parameter setting.
(v) Press start button for scheduling.
(vi) At 200 kV, check the beam current value w.r.t. prescribed standard values.

Figure 10.4 has depicted detail steps about the operation and selection of desired accelerating voltage and filament current.

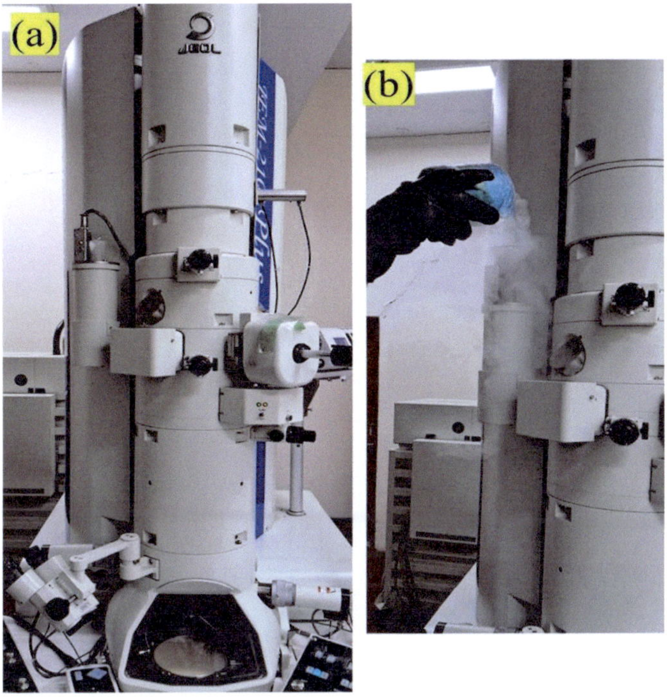

Fig. 10.3 Operation image of ACD (Image received with courtesy of Department of CIL/SAIF, Panjab University Chandigarh, India)

10.4.4 (Step 4) Loading of Specimen on Standard Holder

There are following steps which need to followed during mounting specimen grid on standard holder:

(i) Remove the cartridge from the holder.
(ii) Loosen the two screws followed with pull up and rotating the retainer.
(iii) Place the specimen grid in the hollow place at cartridge.
(iv) Return the retainer to actual position.
(v) Tighten the screws again.
(vi) Attach the cartridge to holder.

Figure 10.5a–e has demonstrated in detail about the different important component of TEM sample holder and respective sample loading procedure

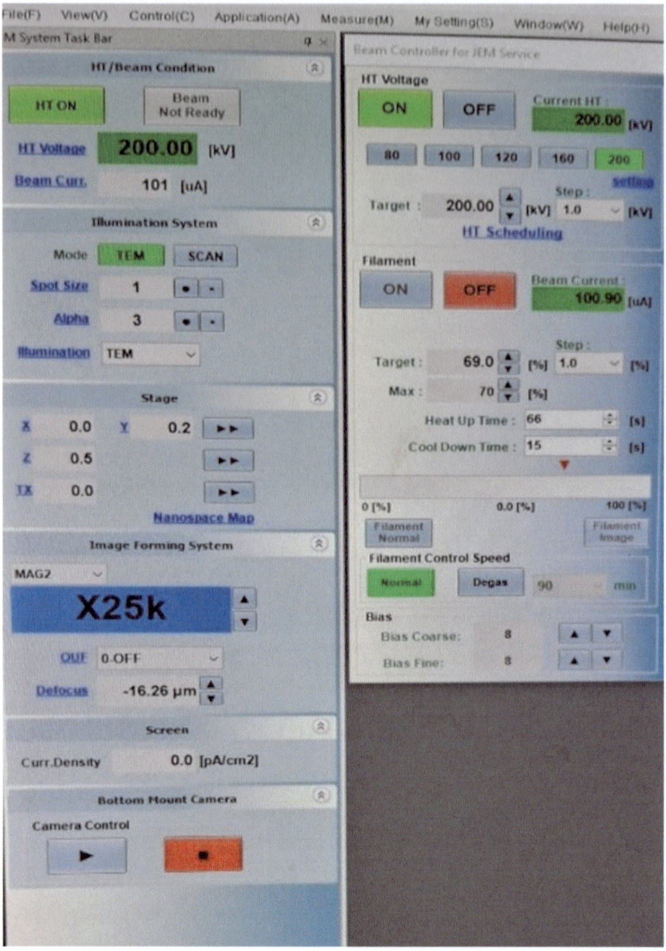

Fig. 10.4 Window image highlighting operation and selection of accelerating voltage and filament current and respective biasing etc. (Image received with courtesy of Department of CIL/SAIF, Panjab University Chandigarh, India)

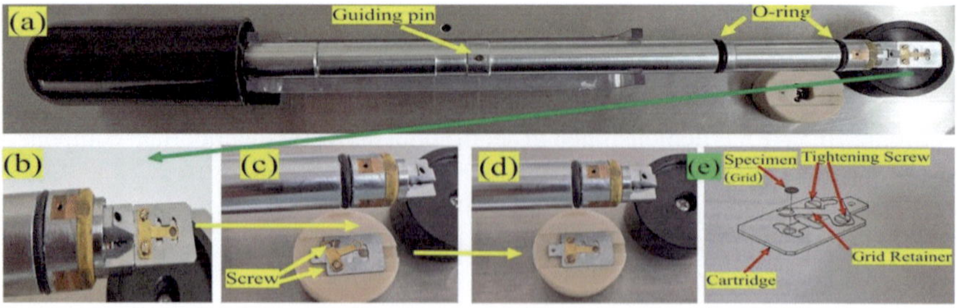

Fig. 10.5 Detail images related to TEM sample holder (Image received with courtesy of Department of CIL/SAIF, Panjab University Chandigarh, India)

10.4.5 (Step 4-Part-II) Loading of Specimen on Double Tilt Holder

There are following steps which need to followed during mounting specimen grid on double tilt holder:

(i) Loose the two screws and turn the retainer.
(ii) Remove the spacer and the plate.
(iii) Place the specimen grid in the hollow place.
(iv) Place the spacer on specimen and put the plate.
(v) Return the retainer to actual position.
(vi) Tighten the screws.

10.4.6 (Step 5) Inserting the Specimen Holder

There are following steps which need to followed during loading of specimen holder:

(i) Ensure that there must be no dust or any contaminants on O-ring of sample holder.
(ii) Align the position of guiding pin with guiding groove. Push the holder into goniometer until it stops, as shown in Fig. 10.6a.
(iii) Set the Pump/Air switch to pump.
(iv) Wait for green lamp to glow.
(v) Turn the holder little clockwise until stop, further insert it a bit.
(vi) Turn the holder fully clockwise until it stops as shown in Fig. 10.6c.
(vii) Select the type of holder which is mounted, as shown in Fig. 10.6b.

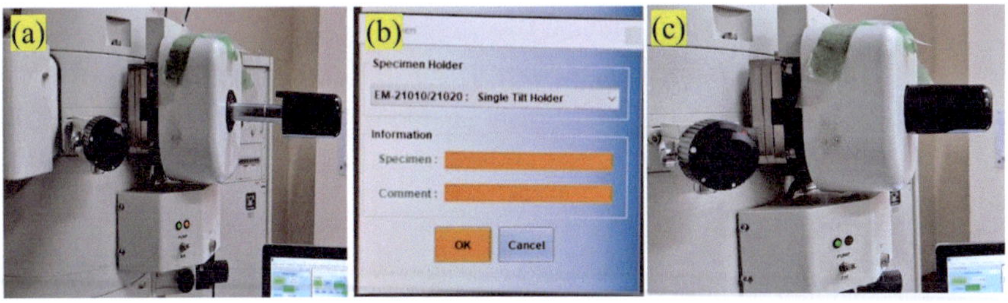

Fig. 10.6 Demonstrate the loading and unloading procedure of TEM sample holder inside TEM instrument (Image received with courtesy of Department of CIL/SAIF, Panjab University Chandigarh, India)

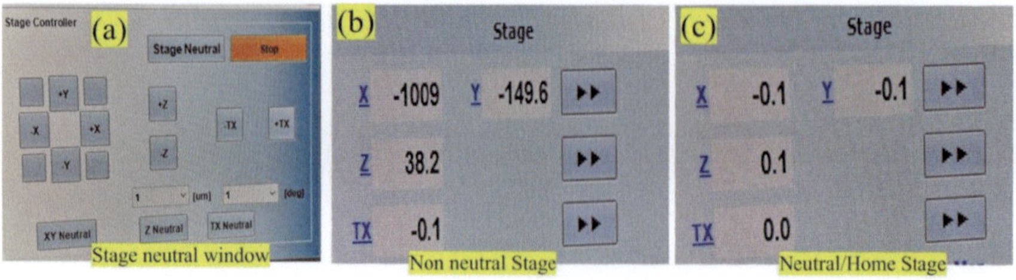

Fig. 10.7 **a–c** Pre-conditions operations needed to remove holder from TEM machine (Image received with courtesy of Department of CIL/SAIF, Panjab University Chandigarh, India)

10.4.7 (Step 6) Removing the Specimen Holder

There are following steps which need to followed during removing of specimen holder from TEM column:

(i) Turn off the electron beam. Make sure that the objective aperture and EDS detector must be retracted.
(ii) Click on X or Y button from stage window (Fig. 10.7b).
(iii) Press on the stage neutral button (Fig. 10.7a), followed by specimen movement to neutral (Fig. 10.7c).
(iv) Pull the specimen until stops.
(v) Turn the holder counterclockwise.
(vi) Pull the holder a bit and turn it fully counter clockwise.
(vii) Set Pump/Air switch to air.
(viii) Wait for the green lamp to turn off.
(ix) Pull out the holder from the goniometer.

10.4.8 (Step 7) Searching of Specimen at Low Magnification

There are following steps which need to followed during analysis of sample initially at low magnification:

(i) Check the column pressure below 4×10^{-5} pascals (Pa) or better as per mode specification.
(ii) Select the TEM **filament control** window.
(iii) Press filament **ON** button to generate the electron beam.
(iv) Objective aperture and selected area diffraction (**SAD**) aperture must be retracted.
(v) Select **LOW MAG** switch.
(vi) Adjust and illuminate specimen with **BRIGHTNESS** and **SHIFT** knob.
(vii) Set appropriate magnification with **MAG** knob and search the desired area with trackball.

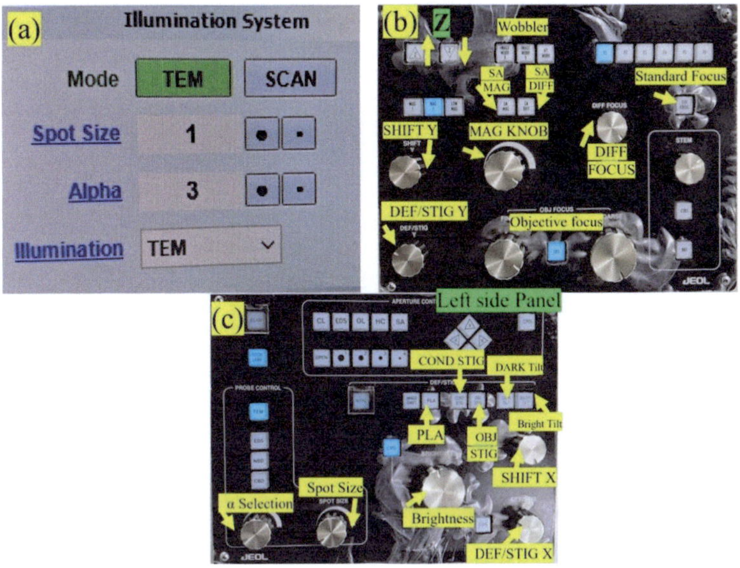

Fig. 10.8 **a** Window showing TEM illumination system, **b** TEM Right side operation panel, **c** TEM left side operation panel (Image received with courtesy of Department of CIL/SAIF, Panjab University Chandigarh, India)

(viii) Select **MAG1** for more zoom view of respective area.

The searching of specimen at low magnification will be performed with the help of operational parameters and knobs which are depicted at Fig. 10.8a–c respectively.

10.4.9 (Step 8, 9 and 10) Bright Field Imaging (< ×100 k Magnification)

10.4.9.1 Alignment of Illumination System

(i) Set spot size to 1 and alpha number to 3 (as shown in Fig. 10.9a).
(ii) Set magnification to ×50 K.
(iii) Press standard focus button and bring specimen surface in focus plane with z-switch.
(iv) Insert condenser aperture #1.
(v) Centre the aperture with condenser aperture screws.
(vi) Converge the electron beam with **BRIGHTNESS** knob followed by use of shift knob to centre the beam.
(vii) Spread the electron beam with **BRIGHTNESS** knob.

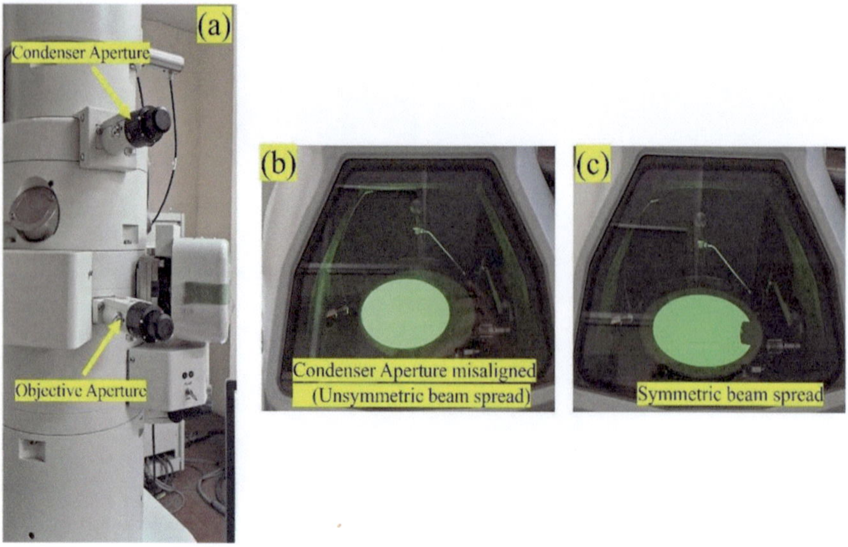

Fig. 10.9 **a** Respective position of condenser and objective aperture in HRTEM, **b, c** image of unsymmetric and symmetric beam spread during instrument alignment process (Image received with courtesy of Department of CIL/SAIF, Panjab University Chandigarh, India)

(viii) Select the **COND STIG** and remove/correct the beam distortion with DEF/STIG x and y knob.

Figure 10.9a–c demonstrated the position of condenser and objective aperture in HRTEM with unsymmetric and symmetric beam spread image during instrument alignment process.

10.4.9.2 (Step 9) Alignment of Voltage Axis

There are following steps which need to followed during aligning voltage axis:

(i) Set the magnification to ×100.
(ii) Press **STD** focus and further focus the specimen with z-switches.
(iii) Converge the beam to centre of fluorescent screen.
(iv) Spread the beam to viewing screen.
(v) Turn **HT** wobbler ON. Adjust with **DEF/STIG** x and y knob so that image will expand and contract symmetrically around the centre.
(vi) Press **HT WOBB** switch off.
(vii) Centre the beam. If not, repeat step from (iii) to (vi).

10.4.9.3 (Step 10) Alignment of Objective Aperture (OA)

There are following steps which need to followed during aligning voltage axis:

(i) Spread the beam on full fluorescent screen.
(ii) Insert third OA.
(iii) Centre the aperture with respective screws.

10.4.10 (Step 11) Recording of Image

There are following steps which need to followed during recording of quality image:

(i) Search an interesting area.
(ii) Select the desired magnification
(iii) Adjust the brightness with **BRIGHTNESS** knob.
(iv) Focus the specimen with **OBJECTIVE** focus knob with Z-switch.
(v) Finally record the image at optimum scan speed.

10.5 (Step 12) High Magnification Imaging (> ×100 k Magnification)

10.5.1 Alignment of Illumination System

(i) Set the spot and alpha < 200 k zoom(magnification): Spot-1, Alpha-2; > 200 k(magnification): Spot-2, Alpha-1
(ii) Set the magnification to ×50.
(iii) Press standard focus and adjust focus with Z switches.
(iv) Insert condenser aperture #2.
(v) Follow similar steps as mentioned in *Sect.* 10.4.8 (vi–viii).

10.5.2 (Step 13) Alignment of Voltage Axis

Follow similar steps as mentioned in *Sect.* 10.4.9.2 (Step 9).

10.5.3 (Step 14) Alignment of Objective Lens Aperture

There are following steps which need to followed during objective lens alignment:

(i) Insert selected area (SA) aperture.

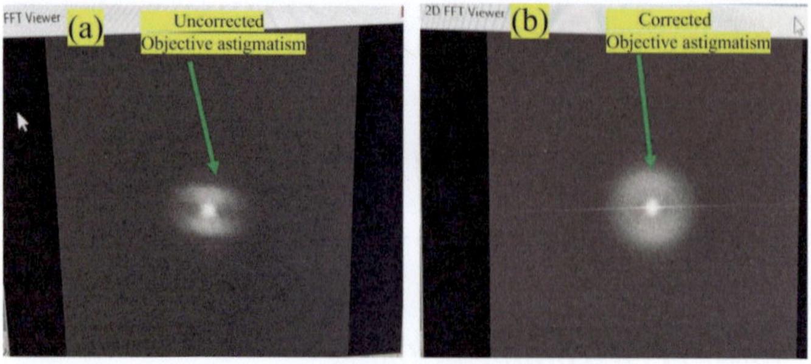

Fig. 10.10 **a** Uncorrected and **b** corrected Astigmatism image in objective lens (Image received with courtesy of Department of CIL/SAIF, Panjab University Chandigarh, India)

(ii) Press SA switch.
(iii) Insert objective aperture #1.
(iv) Sharp the beam spot with brightness knob.
(v) Focus the edge of objective aperture with **DIFF** focus.
(vi) Move the **OA** aperture so that the direct beam locates at center of aperture.
(vii) Return the **MAG1** and retract the **SA** aperture.

10.5.4 (Step 15) Correction of Objective Lens Astigmatism

There are following steps which need to followed to remove the objective lens astigmatism**:**

(i) Search the amorphous region of film.
(ii) Set the magnification to $\times$500 k.
(iii) Click the button camera control.
(iv) Click the FFT button during live camera state.
(v) Observe the 2D FFT pattern.
(vi) Focus the specimen at slight under focus state.
(vii) Correct the objective lens irregular shape to circular shape in respective FFT image.

Uncorrected and corrected astigmatism image w.r.t. objective lens has been demonstrated in Fig. 10.10a, b.

10.5.5 (Step 16) Recording of High Magnification Imaging

Follow similar steps as mentioned under Sects. 10.4.9 and 10.5 (Step 11 and 12) during recording of specimen imaging.

10.6 (Step 17) Selected Area Electron Diffraction (SAED)

There are following steps can be followed during diffraction imaging of specimen through selected area (SA) aperture:

(i) Set spot size 1 and alpha 3.
(ii) Press the **SA MAG** switch.
(iii) Select an area of interest and bring it to centre.
(iv) Focus the specimen with **STD** focus and **Z-switch**.
(v) Insert suitable **SAD** aperture followed by centre position w.r.t. beam position.
(vi) Focus the edge of **SAD** aperture with **DIFF** focus knob.
(vii) Confirm whether image is focussed or not with the help of **Wobbler**.
(viii) Press **DIFF** switch.
(ix) Set the camera length in range from (20–40) cm.
(x) Turn the **BRIGHTNESS** knob towards fully clockwise.
(xi) Focus and sharpen the diffraction spot with **DIFF** Focus.
(xii) Select the **PLA** button to make direct beam at centre.
(xiii) In case of distorted diffraction spot, respective astigmatism correction will be made through intermediate lens.
(xiv) Set the beam stopper for bottom mount camera to protect it from direct intense beam.
(xv) Record the diffraction image.

10.6.1 (Step 18) Nano Beam Diffraction (NBD)

There are following steps will be followed during Nano beam diffraction (NBD) analysis of specimen:

(i) Set spot size 1 and alpha 3.
(ii) Adjust the **DIFF FOCUS** according to **SAD** aperture as per *Sect. 10.6.1 upto (xi)*.
(iii) Switch to **MAG** mode and retract the **SAD** aperture.
(iv) Select **NBD** button.
(v) Set spot size and alpha 1.
(vi) Centre the beam with shift knob.
(vii) Switch **ON** wobbler switch. Press **BRIGHT TILT** and with the help of **DEF/ STIG** knobs make symmetric contraction and expansion of beam.
(viii) Select the **COND STIG** and correct the present beam distortion.
(ix) Bring area of interest region to centre.
(x) Insert the smallest condenser aperture.
(xi) Converge the beam on specific specimen area.
(xii) Select **SA DIFF**.
(xiii) Select the **PLA** switch and centre the beam with **DEF/STIG** knobs.
(xiv) Capture the final diffraction image.

10.7 (Step 19) Precise Gun Alignment

10.7.1 Gun Alignment

There are following steps which can be followed during TEM gun alignment [3]:

(i) Set the magnification at ×40 k.
(ii) Switch **ON** the **Bright Tilt** button (as shown in Fig. 10.11)
(iii) Set the **spot** size to 5.
(iv) Converge the beam to small spot and centre with shift knob.

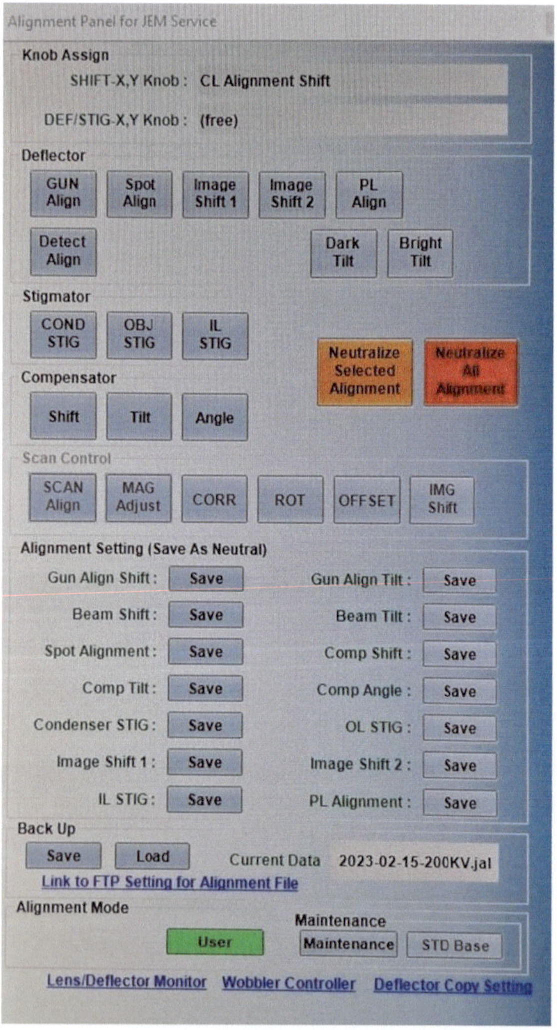

Fig. 10.11 Alignment panel of HRTEM instrument (Image received with courtesy of Department of CIL/SAIF, Panjab University Chandigarh, India)

(v) Set spot size to 1.
(vi) Press **GUN** Align on alignment window (as shown in Fig. 10.11).
(vii) Converge the beam and centre with shift knob. Repeat the step from step (ii) to step (vii) until all spots (1 to 5), will get similar position.
(viii) Click the **spot align**.
(ix) Centre the beam at spot size 2, 3, 4 with **DEF/STIG** knob.
(x) Press the filament image button on **image controller** window.
(xi) Make filament pattern clear image with **CL STIG** and **BRIGHTNESS** knob.
(xii) Press **GUN** Align button on beam alignment window (as shown in Fig. 10.11).
(xiii) Adjust the filament pattern symmetrical with **DEF/STIG** knob.
(xiv) Finally, click filament normal button and turn **GUN** Align OFF (as shown in Fig. 10.11).

Respective alignment panel window has been demonstrated at Fig. 10.11.

10.8 (Step 20) Tilt/Shift Balance

There are following steps which can be followed during Tilt/shift balance alignment [3]:

(i) Set magnification to ×40 k. Converge the beam at centre of fluorescent screen.
(ii) Use the **Wobbler** controller window.
(iii) Press **Tilt** X button.
(iv) Minimize the wobbler movement with **DEF/STIG x** knob.
(v) Centre the beam with shift X knob. Repeat step (iv) to (v) till minimum movement of beam.
(vi) Switch **OFF** the **Tilt X**.
(vii) Switch **ON** Tilt Y.
(viii) Minimize the wobbler movement with **DEF/STIG Y** knob. Repeat step (vii) to (viii) till minimum movement of wobbler.
(ix) Press the **SA DIFF** button. Select camera length to 200 cm.
(x) Turn the **BRIGHTNESS** knob clockwise till caustic spot with **DIFF** focus will be achieved.
(xi) Switch on the PLA button and centre the beam spot to centre with DEF/STIG knob.
(xii) Press Shift X.
(xiii) Minimize the wobbler movement with **DEF/STIG X** knob.
(xiv) Turn the **Bright Tilt** and centre the spot with **DEF/STIG X**. Repeat step (xii) to (ivx) till minimum movement of wobbler.
(xv) Switch **OFF** the **Shift X**.
(xvi) Switch **ON** the **Shift Y**.
(xvii) Minimize the wobbler movement with **DEF/STIG Y** knob.

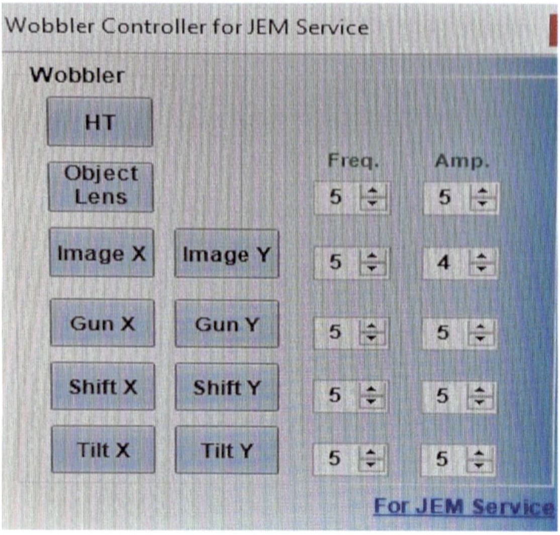

Fig. 10.12 Wobbler control window aligning shift and tilt options (Image received with courtesy of Department of CIL/SAIF, Panjab University Chandigarh, India)

(xviii) Turn the **Bright Tilt** and centre the spot with **DEF/STIG X**. Repeat step (xvi) to (xviii) till minimum movement of wobbler.

(xix) Turn **OFF** shift **Y**.

Respective wobbler control window has been depicted in Fig. 10.12.

10.9 (Step 21) Astigmatism Correction of Intermediate Lens

There are following steps which can be followed during astigmatism correction in intermediate lens:

(i) Turn on **SA DIFF** button. Set camera length to 200 cm.

(ii) Turn the **brightness** knob fully clockwise in order to obtain caustic spot with the help of **DIFF Focus**.

(iii) With help of **PLA** button, centre the beam spot through **DEF/STIG** buttons.

(iv) Select **IL STIG** from alignment panel window. Correct the respective astigmatism with **DEF/STIG** button.

(v) Turn **OFF** the **IL STIG**.

Above Sects. 10.3–10.9, an attempt has been to demonstrated about the standard operation, and alignment steps w.r.t. 200 kV LaB_6 TEM JEOL machine, which can be helpful during handling of TEM instrument with precision.

10.10 Troubleshooting w.r.t. Basic TEM Operation and Respective Sample Preparation

In coming section, we have summarized the detail about the different problems and challenges with probable solution w.r.t. sample preparation and techniques used.

10.10.1 Check Point Before Proceeding for TEM Operation

In daily routine practice, EM scientist handling TEM or HRTEM instrument before starting routine sample analysis, must have to inspect all ancillary equipment status properly. For example, the status of vacuum level of main TEM machine, working status of rotary pump and sputter ion pump (SIP) or TMP whichever present, compressor, uninterrupted power supply (UPS), water chiller, temperature and humidity etc., must be monitored and corrected as per standards. In case of operator/ scientist not able to achieved the desired reading or level of ideal working conditions w.r.t. main instrument or ancillary equipment's, contact the concern service engineer for further action or maintenance.

Fig. 10.13a–j comprised of detail of different supporting instrument used in working of HRTEM during its smooth operation.

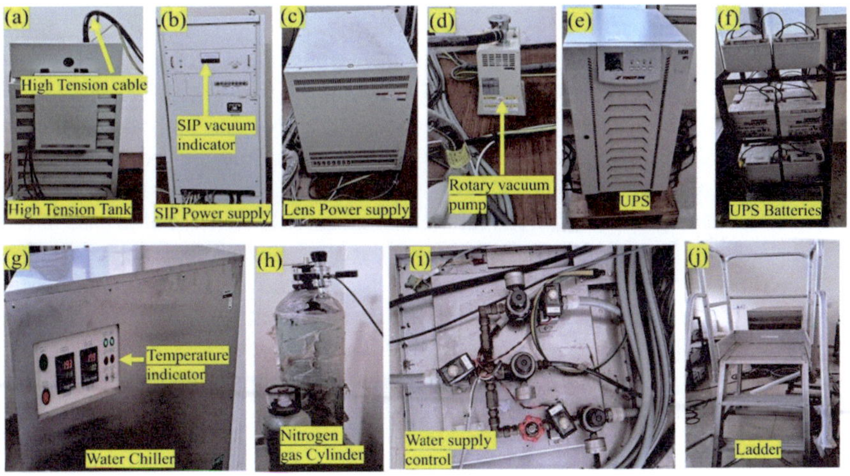

Fig. 10.13 Ancillary equipment's installed in HRTEM lab **a** HT Tank, **b** SIP power supply, **c** lenses power supply, **d** rotary vacuum pump, **e** UPS, **f** UPS batteries, **g** water chiller, **h** nitrogen gas cylinder, **i** water supply control, **j** ladder for maintenance (Image received with courtesy of Department of CIL/SAIF, Panjab University Chandigarh, India)

10.10.2 Probability of Specimen Damage

Use of improper sample preparation tool, harsh chemical like acids or organic solvents, improper fixation procedure, embedding chemicals or cutting tool etc., are the areas which has deep impact on specimen preparation, respective analysis and interpretation of data. As per nature of same sample, use of hard or soft tools, cryo-TEM/SEM, cryo-ultramicrotome, will be preferred.

10.10.3 Sample Contamination

The probability of contamination induction and respective visualization during TEM imaging will be minimized through working in neat and clean, dust free environment laboratory. The cleaning of TEM grids and related samples in plasma cleaner will be ensure minimum contaminants free imaging during final imaging process [4, 5].

10.10.4 Insufficient Contrast

Most of time researchers during and after TEM imaging, claiming and blaming for getting low or poor contrast-based images from respective TEM laboratory. Logically, if above issue will be faced in case of powder or solution-based formulation or sample having low density constituents (carbon, nitrogen, hydrogen, oxygen etc.), operator need to choose/use objective aperture, low kV accelerating voltage like 100 kV or 120 kV or staining procedure etc., as per need and availability, to improve the respective imaging contrast [6]. Non-uniformity of specimen surface due to uncontrolled synthesis conditions, will be one factor behind low contrast or poor TEM imaging. Secondly, low contrast imaging will be observed in case of thin sliced specimen (polymer or biological etc.) due to use of appropriate accelerating voltage (low voltage like 80 kV or 100 kV etc.), objective aperture, quality knife (glass knife or diamond knife) used in slicing, alignment of knife with specimen face, specimen slicing parameters, compatibility of embedding medium with specimen etc. Above stated all factors need individually monitoring and modification as per images contrast and clarity w.r.t. desired information.

10.10.5 Grid Handling and Preparation Issues

TEM grid is the one of important basic part of whole TEM operation and analysis. Right from identification of any factory manufactured defects on grid surface, handling of grid during sample preparation, use of specialized tweezer, respective grids controlled and validated drying procedure, storage conditions etc., are the factors which must be followed properly. Procedure and condition to handle and prepare the TEM grids will be varied and depend upon the nature of specimen and operation condition of TEM instrument.

10.10.6 Vacuum Issues

Ideally TEM system will operate at ultrahigh vacuum (approximately 10^{-5} to 10^{-10} Pascal or more better) due to which presence of minute contamination or volatile component during specimen-beam interaction, will deteriorate the vacuum level. Ideally, to get quality imaging, TEM column vacuum must be always stabilized. Precautionary, avoid loading of any volatile or unstable specimen inside machine for imaging. Regularly, if vacuum of TEM machine is not stable, contact the authorized service engineer for maintenance or fault finding.

10.10.7 Beam Damage During Imaging

Person going to handle TEM machine must be properly trained to handle and maintain smoothly. Selection of unsuitable accelerating voltage, over current exposure to specimen surface, over exposure time at one surface etc., factors will damage the region of interest from quality imaging. As per nature and type of specimen like metal or biological, polymer or emulsion etc., selection of TEM operational parameters (accelerating voltage beam current, exposure time etc.) will be finalized.

Through above mentioned basic information which is demonstrated in Fig. 10.13, related to TEM operation and sample preparation, scientist/operator behind the machine can perform the quality imaging. Practicing the above-mentioned points, one can enhances and improve the life of TEM machine with minimum problems and maximum productivity.

10.11 Troubleshooting Related to Advanced TEM Sample Preparation

Quality sample preparation approach will lead to improve the level of information and quality of results from respective specimen under TEM study. In coming section, we have summarized some advanced sample preparation techniques and related do's and dont's which will be performed as per need of study.

10.11.1 Focus Ion Beam (FIB) and Cryo-FIB System

Site specific and precise thinning, milling of material like semiconductor, metal etc., for TEM study will be performed by FIB technique. Formation of site-specific thin lamellae with controlled and unform thickness of specimen, will be produced with mentioned technique. In addition, thin sectioning of cryogenically stabilized water-based specimen or biological specimen can be processed by Cryo-FIB. Optimized use of operational parameters like current and voltage etc., during rough and fine thinning process of specimen must be ensured [7].

10.11.2 Cryo-ultramicrotome

In addition to ultrathin sectioning by conventional ultramicrotome, cryo-ultramicrotome will be utilized for thin slicing of cryo-stabilized or vitrified biological or unstable specimen [8].

10.11.3 High Pressure Freeze (HPF) Based Specimen Preparation

Moisture or hydrated specimen need to processed for stabilization of water content without its ice crystal formation w.r.t. EM analysis. Efficiently, it can achieve through HPF technique for vitrified specimen. There is always need of rapid and consistent freezing process so that specimen have minimum chances of ice formation [9].

10.11.4 Automatic Immunolabelling System

Conventionally, researchers using manual procedure for staining and immunolabeling which have maximum probabilities of errors, non-uniformity and lack of efficacy. Automatic staining and immunolabeling procedure will maximize the contrast and specificity of antibonding binding during respective sample preparation process. Automated stainer tool will be followed through calibrated, validated sample processing protocol through freshly prepared reagents [10], will ensure uniform and effective visualization of maximum components of biological specimen under TEM analysis.

10.11.5 Plasma Cleaning System

The refine cleaning of specimen loaded TEM grid from hydrocarbon-based contaminants will be achieved through plasma cleaning system. In addition, the presence of unstable organic constituents on specimen surface can also be cleaned through stated cleaning system. Precautionary, plasma cleaned samples and TEM grid must be stored in contamination free environment having vacuum surroundings [11].

10.11.6 Glow Discharge Unit

During operation of TEM, most of time TEM user facing issue of low distribution of sample on grid surface. This will be probably due to low sample loving nature of grid surface towards drop casted sample. Controlled treatment of TEM grid inside glow discharge unit brings maximum hydrophilic nature for solution-based specimen as well for any biological specimen. Use of fresh grids at optimized working conditions (time, pressure and type of gas etc.) w.r.t. glow discharge equipment during respective use [12, 13], will ensure maximum and uniform deposition of sample on respective support surface.

10.11.7 Use of Nano-manipulator

In case of imaging of specimen at nanoscale to get orientation specific information, handling of respective material become a difficult. With use of nanomanipulator, during sample mounting in FIB-SEM or ultra-section positioning on TEM grid, will be felicitated very smoothly with minimum contamination and damage to specimen. Although, the skill to use nanomanipulator in controlled manner, reduces the damage risk to equipment as well to sample [14].

10.11.8 Auto Grid Stainer

The automated staining sample processing will reduce the risk of contamination and mishandling during respective staining. The non-uniform contrast on specimen surface with presence of contaminants will be minimized with application of auto-stainer technique [10].

Through above utilization of advanced sample preparation equipment in TEM sample preparation has been shown in Fig. 10.14, through researchers/scientists can have maximum probability of results quality, reproducibility and precision.

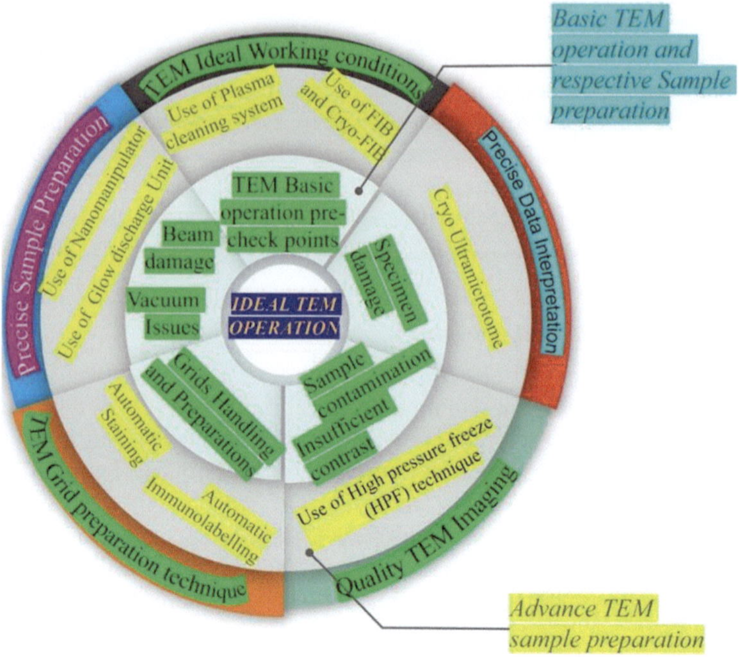

Fig. 10.14 Depicts the basic and advance TEM operation and respective sample preparation techniques

10.12 TEM Grid Preparation, Drying, Handling and Preservation

TEM grid handling and its preparation w.r.t. TEM imaging, will the one of main factor to ensure quality and precision in the TEM analysis [15]. There are following ways through which researchers can handle, prepare TEM grid skillfully.

10.12.1 How to Apply Suspension/Solution Sample on TEM Grid

Specifically, stable solution/suspension form of sample will be prepared through following steps as mention below:

Step (i): Drop cast optimum volume solution/suspension on coated side (shining side) of TEM grid using micropipette.

Step (ii): After appropriate time at step (i), remove the excess of solvent from grid surface with filter paper or blotting paper.

Step (iii): Allow air drying of TEM grid from step (ii) in air drying conditions or controlled temperature/heat conditions for 12–48 h or more as per nature and requirement of sample.

10.12.2 Mounting of Ultrathin Section on TEM Grid

This is one of crucial step during transferring of ultrathin slice from (floating surface) water surface to grid surface. There are following step which will helpful in handling and transferring sample thin slices to TEM grid surface:

Step (i): Properly fixed, dehydrate specimen must need to embedded inside stable and compatible epoxy.

Step (ii): Prior to step (i), trimmed and aligned specimen surface with suitable knife (glass or diamond) will cut for ultrathin sections under ultramicrotome or cryo-ultramicrotome as per study requirement.

Step (iii): Skilfully, ultrathin specimen slices floating on water boat or respective place as per availability of techniques (in ultramicrotome), will be mounted/transferred on actual surface of TEM grid surface suitable side.

10.12.3 TEM Grid Drying Methods

There are following ways of TEM grid drying during respective sample preparation.

10.12.3.1 Air Drying Method

This is the one of conventional method of TEM grid drying, prior to drop casting on TEM grid support surface. Current method of drying is applicable for all material including low-density specimen which are stable under air drying procedure [15].

10.12.3.2 Critical Point Drying (CPD) Method

Ideal preservation of biological and delicate specimen having water as the main components, will be dried through CPD technique. Under this technique, water of specimen will be replaced with liquid CO_2 which is further removed at its critical temperature and pressure conditions. CPD process have minimum surface side effects on specimen surface during drying [16].

10.12.3.3 Freeze Drying Method

In addition to CPD technique, freeze drying technique will be proceed on principle of direct removal of water to gaseous form via principle of sublimation under vacuum conditions. Many biological and sensitive sample will be processed under freeze drying technique [9].

Through above stated drying methods, most of samples belong from materials to biological sciences can be processed for ideal drying as per their nature and properties.

10.12.4 Handling and Preservation of TEM Grids

There are following do's and don't which need to performed during TEM grid handling and preservation process.

10.12.4.1 Handling Tool

Use of anti-static, non-magnetic and fine tip-based tweezer with neat and clean wax sheet will be preferred to pick and drop the TEM grid during their loading and unloading process. The whole process of handling of TEM grids for TEM sample preparation must be performed with hands wearing gloves in dust free environment to avoid any cross of contamination.

10.12.4.2 Storage Conditions

Use specialized contamination free grid box for storage and preservation of TEM grid box. Use of desiccator having active desiccant will be preferred for preservation of grids for short or long-time preservation. Cryo-TEM grid storage will be preserved in liquid nitrogen environment. Special care must be taken during transportation of TEM grids from one place to other.

10.12.5 What to Do and Not to Do w.r.t. TEM Operation

There are following things which must be followed during TEM operations and respective sample preparation procedure.

10.12.5.1 Rapid Heating or Cooling

Any sudden increase in temperature or cooling conditions lead to thermal stress, may harm the machine or integrity of sample. Gradual increase/decrease in processing of specimen or operation of TEM machine w.r.t. heating or cooling, will be preferred.

10.12.5.2 Rise Accelerating Voltage or Emission Current Step by Step

Avoid the use of sudden rise in accelerating voltage or emission current etc. Rise respective parameters slowly as prescribed by manufacturer recommendation. Improper handling of respective operational parameters may lead to harm the electron gun setting as well the other components of microscope.

10.12.5.3 Avoid Over Exposure of Specimen with Electron Beam

The overtime exposure of electron beam with specimen surface will may damage the surface of biological or sensitive specimen during imaging process. Normally, low dose imaging will be preferred during respective specimen analysis.

10.12.5.4 Avoid Use of Contaminated Sample

Sample must be free from any lose particles/impurities present on respective surface before mounting on appropriate sample holder. In addition, handling of specimen must be performed with gloves during loading and unloading of TEM. Presence of unwanted loose components on specimen surface may lead to contaminate TEM gun, column and may bring poor vacuum status of machine.

10.12.5.5 Do Not Ignore TEM Poor Vacuum

Condition of poor vacuum with TEM system, probably will be due to contaminated specimen, laboratory poor working environment etc. Regular check w.r.t. laboratory environment, different vacuum readings etc., must need to monitored. Working with poor vacuum conditions w.r.t. TEM operations, will deteriorate respective smooth operation and data analysis.

10.12.5.6 Avoid Rough Handling of TEM Grids

The use of specialized tweezer, wax sheet, sample preparation area etc., will be used during TEM grid handling in respective sample preparation. Routine pre-inspection of TEM grids conditions must be performed in practice before grid preparation for

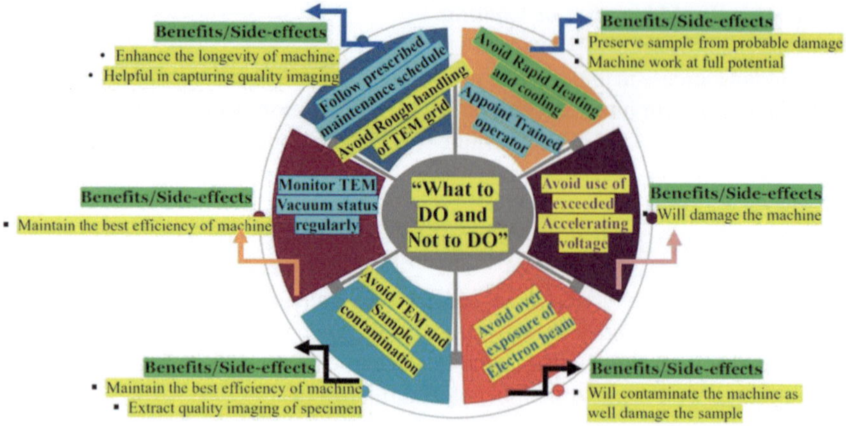

Fig. 10.15 Best practices need to follow while operation of TEM

imaging or during its loading on TEM grid holder. In similar way with minimum mishandling practices in respective samples need to followed.

10.12.5.7 Follow Prescribed Maintenance and Training Schedule

The maintenance schedule prescribe by manufacture at the time installation of machine must be followed with minimum deviation. Maintenance schedule must include routine cleaning of electron gun, column basic alignments, calibrations and servicing of other ancillary equipment's of TEM instrument with regular training to EM operation staff.

Through above stated points as shown in Fig. 10.15, any person going to handle the TEM instrument, he/she must be aware what to do and what not do w.r.t. operation of EM machine and related analysis.

10.12.6 Ways in Quality TEM Analysis and Interpretation of Results

There are following points which will ensure minimum errors during TEM operation w.r.t. TEM imaging.

10.12.6.1 Instrument Calibration

Before starting TEM analysis, instrument must be calibrate and optimized w.r.t. beam current, beam alignment and other operation related important parameters.

10.12.6.2 Image Quality Verification

Images captured during TEM imaging must be clear, sharp and have well defined features. TEM imaging must be of such area of interest which will reflect and explain the synthesis and functional mechanism of material under study. In case of poor-quality imaging, researchers need to re-evaluate the sample analysis again or prepare the whole specimen again. Contrast and brightness must be properly balanced at optimum conditions during imaging.

10.12.6.3 Probable Area of Artefacts

Specimen must be protected from artefacts generation through staining process, lens aberration or beam over-exposure etc., during sample imaging under TEM. Person operating the machine must have sound knowledge and experience to distinguish between specimen structural features with observed artefacts.

10.12.6.4 Use of Supporting Modes of TEM Operation

In addition to normal and high-resolution imaging, bright field (BF) imaging, dak field imaging (DF), selected area electron diffraction (SAED), nanoelectron diffraction, high annular angle dak field imaging (HAADF), EDS, mapping etc., modes can be utilized to support and authenticate the captured TEM imaging results.

10.12.6.5 Verification of Structural Features

Any information observed first time during TEM imaging will be claim for extraordinary theory or mechanism, need to re-confirm after proper validated or reproducible analysis. This will be applicable in case of normal imaging, HR imaging, diffraction imaging, elemental study etc., of various specimen as per their nature.

10.12.6.6 Use of Image Processing Software

In addition to quality imaging of specimen under TEM study, still there are many quantitative measurements, quality enhancements etc., processes to improve the quality assessment of specimen behaviour study. For example, measurement of particle size, respective dimension measurement, counting of particle etc., can also be evaluated through specific image processing software.

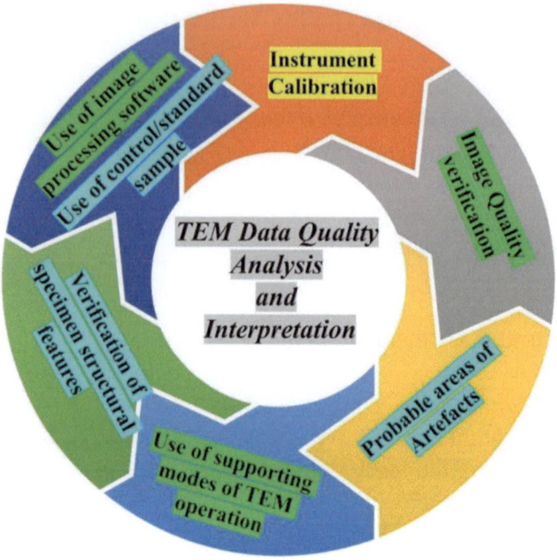

Fig. 10.16 Basics things need to perform in order to ensure TEM data quality analysis and respective interpretation

10.12.6.7 Usage of Control/Standard Samples

The quality and authenticity of TEM results will be validated through analysis of standard or control specimen initially or in between or at the end of routine analysis. Specific idea about interference of background noise during sample analysis, instrument actual capabilities w.r.t. contrast and resolution etc. can be explored, compared and improved.

Through above discussed points related to operation of TEM, sample preparation and respective data interpretation as shown in Fig. 10.16, will improve the accuracy, precision of TEM data. This will lead TEM analysis towards valid, authentic and meaningful conclusion and predictions from imaging data.

NOTE: Above troubleshooting approaches during TEM operation and analysis facilitates identification and resolving of issue related to imaging artefacts, poor resolution, sample damage, data collection and interpretation etc., via optimization of respective parameters.

10.13 Correlation of TEM Results with Other Microscopy Techniques

Ideally to understand maximum capabilities and properties of material under TEM study, respective material must also be explored under different microscopy, spectroscopy etc. techniques. Specifically, here we have quickly tried to correlate and propose best relation of TEM imaging/data with different microscopy techniques.

10.13.1 Scanning Electron Microscopy (SEM)

In contrast to TEM ultrastructural atomic resolution features of specimen, SEM will highlight about respective material surface morphology and topology features. As the both region of interest i.e. surface (SEM) and internal structure (TEM) of material will be useful during explanation of material functional behavior [17].

10.13.2 Scanning Transmission Electron Microscopy (STEM)

In addition to well-known capabilities of TEM technique, respective data further correlation can be made with STEM bright field, dark field, HAADF, EDS, EELS etc., modes of operation. This will be helpful in correlating and explaining related TEM data information to enhance and improve the quality interpretation and understanding of material [18].

10.13.3 Atomic Force Microscopy (AFM)

The correlation between TEM and AFM data, will also enhance the level of critical analysis and interpretation of material study. Ultrastructural imaging of material will be more closely authenticated and validated with AFM atomic scale high-resolution capabilities through respective modes of operations [19].

10.13.4 Confocal Microscopy

The three-dimensional imaging of living specimens through fluorescent labelling will be correlated with high resolution TEM images. The localized identification of active sites can be predicted through confined fluorescence and respective area visualization under high resolution TEM, make investigation study more convincing and dynamic [20].

10.13.5 Cryo-electron Microscopy (Cryo-TEM)

Sensitive specimen having water as the major component, require stabilized sample preparation and viewing under cryo-TEM. Depending upon the nature of sample, conventional or high-resolution TEM will also be used and respective data/images can be correlated with cryo-TEM [21].

10.13.6 X-Ray Diffraction (XRD)

This is one of basic approach through which specimen XRD data can be correlated with TEM imaging and electron diffraction data. Observed atomic plane pattern during HRTEM analysis, can be correlated with observed d-spacing of XRD spectrum w.r.t. specific peaks. Insight related to defects analysis with TEM imaging, will be correlated authenticated via respective material crystal structure or phase analysis [22].

Fig. 10.17, depicts about the correlation of TEM data with other microscopy techniques and other related instrumentation techniques.

Finally, the correlation of TEM data is not only limited with above mentioned techniques, but is depend upon the level of expertise to correlate or availability of techniques etc. Further, electron microscopy (EM) data can also be correlated with fourier transform infrared spectrometer (FTIR), ultra violet spectrophotometer

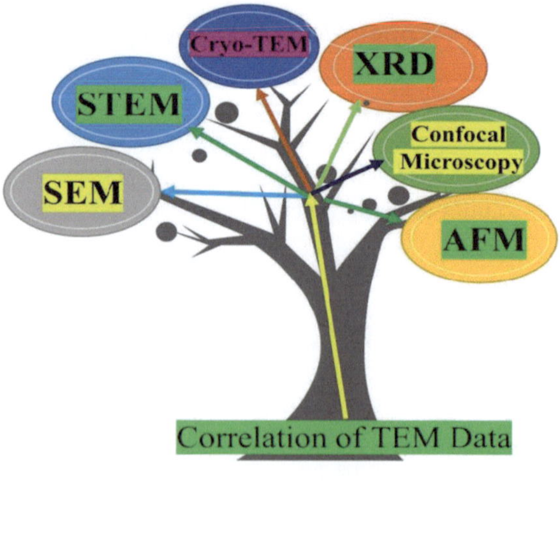

Fig. 10.17 Correlation of TEM data with other microscopy techniques

(UV–Vis.), dynamic light scattering (DLS), thermal gravimetric analysis (TGA), differential scanning calorimetry (DSC), X-ray photoelectron spectroscopy (XPS) etc. techniques.

10.14 Conclusion

TEM imaging is not confined to specific computer commands to capture respective images but functionalized through ideal operation via operational mastery, precise instrumental alignments with quality sample preparation and analysis.

The objective of ideal TEM imaging and analysis has been practiced through precise sample preparation, precise instrument working with critical data interpretation. More specifically, summary about the smooth and precise TEM operation with detailed troubleshooting and sample preparation have been also enclosed. In addition, the effect of TEM grid handling, drying, preservation and transportation conditions also has been elaborated.

The purpose of writing current chapter is to make researchers/scientist familiar and confident w.r.t. TEM instrumentation, operation, major and minor technicalities, which may be very useful during respective operation, data analysis and insight explanations. Stated approach of holistic TEM utilization, will be very much helpful in achieving the proposed scientific hypothesis for novel results and inventions.

Declaration

Author declares that there is no personal or financial conflict of interest regarding publication of this chapter.

References

1. Zechmann, B.: Facility design for, installation, and management of a 300kV cryo-transmission electron microscope. Microsc. Microanal. **30**(Supplement_1), ozae044.963 (2024). https://doi.org/10.1093/mam/ozae044.963
2. Martínez-Tejada, H.V.: General considerations for design and construction of transmission electron microscopy laboratories 23 (2014)
3. Rodenburg, J.M.: Understanding transmission electron microscope alignment: a tutorial. Microsc. Anal.
4. Höche, T., Gerlach, J.W., Petsch, T.: Static-charging mitigation and contamination avoidance by selective carbon coating of TEM samples. Ultramicroscopy **106**(11–12), 981–985 (2006). https://doi.org/10.1016/j.ultramic.2006.05.007
5. Hettler, S., Dries, M., Hermann, P., Obermair, M., Gerthsen, D., Malac, M.: Carbon contamination in scanning transmission electron microscopy and its impact on phase-plate applications. Micron **96**, 38–47 (2017). https://doi.org/10.1016/j.micron.2017.02.002
6. Minoda, H., Okabe, T., Iijima, H.: Contrast enhancement in the phase plate transmission electron microscopy using an objective lens with a long focal length. Microscopy **60**(5), 337–343 (2011). https://doi.org/10.1093/jmicro/dfr067

7. Wirth, R.: Focused ion beam (FIB) combined with SEM and TEM: advanced analytical tools for studies of chemical composition, microstructure and crystal structure in geomaterials on a nanometre scale. Chem. Geol. **261**(3–4), 217–229 (2009). https://doi.org/10.1016/j.chemgeo.2008.05.019
8. Thompson, R.F., Walker, M., Siebert, C.A., Muench, S.P., Ranson, N.A.: An introduction to sample preparation and imaging by cryo-electron microscopy for structural biology. Methods **100**, 3–15 (2016). https://doi.org/10.1016/j.ymeth.2016.02.017
9. Butler, M.K., Prow, T.W., Guo, Y.-N., Lin, L.L., Webb, R.I., Martin, D.J.: High-pressure freezing/freeze substitution and transmission electron microscopy for characterization of metal oxide nanoparticles within sunscreens. Nanomedicine **7**(4), 541–551 (2012). https://doi.org/10.2217/nnm.11.149
10. Yang, R., Wang, S., Wang, J., Luo, X., Zhao, W., Zhang, Q., Nan, Z., Yang, L., Wang, S.: Comparison of manual and automatic processing of biological samples for electron microscopy. Microsc. Res. Techniq. **80**(6), 570–577 (2017). https://doi.org/10.1002/jemt.22832
11. Thanu, D.P.R., Srinadhu, E.S., Zhao, M., Dole, N.V., Keswani, M.: Fundamentals and applications of plasma cleaning. In: Developments in Surface Contamination and Cleaning: Applications of Cleaning Techniques, pp. 289–353. Elsevier (2019). https://doi.org/10.1016/B978-0-12-815577-6.00008-6.
12. Brackmann, V., Hoffmann, V., Kauffmann, A., Helth, A., Thomas, J., Wendrock, H., Freudenberger, J., Gemming, T., Eckert, J.: Glow discharge plasma as a surface preparation tool for microstructure investigations. Mater Charact **91**, 76–88 (2014). https://doi.org/10.1016/j.matchar.2014.02.002
13. Kazan, R., Bourgeois, G., Carisetti, D., Florea, I., Larquet, E., Maurice, J.-L., Mechulam, Y., Ozanam, F., Schmitt, E., Coureux, P.-D.: Grid batch-dependent tuning of glow discharge parameters. Front. Mol. Biosci. **9**, 910218 (2022). https://doi.org/10.3389/fmolb.2022.910218
14. Fahlbusch, St., Mazerolle, S., Breguet, J.-M., Steinecker, A., Agnus, J., Pérez, R., Michler, J.: Nanomanipulation in a scanning electron microscope. J. Mater. Proces. Technol. **167**(2–3), 371–382 (2005). https://doi.org/10.1016/j.jmatprotec.2005.06.022
15. Michen, B., Geers, C., Vanhecke, D., Endes, C., Rothen-Rutishauser, B., Balog, S., Petri-Fink, A.: Avoiding drying-artifacts in transmission electron microscopy: characterizing the size and colloidal state of nanoparticles. Sci. Rep. **5**(1), 9793 (2015). https://doi.org/10.1038/srep09793
16. Hawkins, D.M., Ellis, E.A., Stevenson, D., Holzenburg, A., Reddy, S.M.: Novel critical point drying (CPD) based preparation and transmission electron microscopy (TEM) imaging of protein specific molecularly imprinted polymers (HydroMIPs). J. Mater. Sci. **42**(22), 9465–9468 (2007). https://doi.org/10.1007/s10853-007-1806-4
17. Inkson, B.J.: Scanning electron microscopy (SEM) and transmission electron microscopy (TEM) for materials characterization. In: Materials Characterization Using Nondestructive Evaluation (NDE) Methods, pp. 17–43. Elsevier (2016). https://doi.org/10.1016/B978-0-08-100040-3.00002-X
18. Kübel, C., Voigt, A., Schoenmakers, R., Otten, M., Su, D., Lee, T.-C., Carlsson, A., Bradley, J.: Recent advances in electron tomography: TEM and HAADF-STEM tomography for materials science and semiconductor applications. Microsc. Microanal. **11**(5), 378–400 (2005). https://doi.org/10.1017/S1431927605050361
19. Gujrati, A., Khanal, S.R., Pastewka, L., Jacobs, T.D.B.: Combining TEM, AFM, and profilometry for quantitative topography characterization across all scales. ACS Appl. Mater. Interfaces **10**(34), 29169–29178 (2018). https://doi.org/10.1021/acsami.8b09899
20. Keene, D.R., Tufa, S.F., Lunstrum, G.P., Holden, P., Horton, W.A.: Confocal/TEM overlay microscopy: a simple method for correlating confocal and electron microscopy of cells expressing GFP/YFP fusion proteins. Microsc. Microanal. **14**(4), 342–348 (2008). https://doi.org/10.1017/S1431927608080306

21. Hurbain, I., Sachse, M.: The future is cold: cryo-preparation methods for transmission electron microscopy of cells. Biol. Cell **103**(9), 405–420 (2011). https://doi.org/10.1042/BC20110015
22. Schwenzer, B., Hu, J., Wu, Y., Mishra, U.K.: Elucidation of the correlation between atomic-level defects in GaN nanoparticles and photoluminescence properties by NMR, XRD and TEM. Solid State Sci. **8**(10), 1193–1201 (2006). https://doi.org/10.1016/j.solidstatesciences.2006.06.002

Chapter 11
Unique Case Studies in TEM Instrumentation, Analysis and Interpretation

The task is not so much to see what no one has yet seen, but to think what nobody has yet thought about that which everybody sees
by ***Erwin Schrodinger***

Abstract This chapter present a series of unique case studies highlighting critical aspect of transmission electron microscopy (TEM) instrumentation requirements, ideal imaging and related interpretation aspect. Mentioned case studies has dedicatedly explained about minutiae details w.r.t. TEM smooth operation including major and minor installation requirements, low temperature stabilized specimen analysis, EM ancillary instrumentation requirement, resolving technical challenges etc. It has presented an optimized sample analysis and interpretation approach towards reproducible and insightful data. Finally, this chapter will serve as a practical manual for EM users during establishment of sophisticated EM laboratory, user friendly troubleshooting guide with enhancing the understanding of TEM capabilities in refining EM instrumentation and analytical data outcomes.

Keywords Unique case study · Installation requirement · Ancillary instruments · Troubleshooting guide · Technical skill

11.1 Introduction

The objective to write current text book on transmission electron microscopy (TEM), is to practicing systematic sample analysis on electron microscopy (EM) and related techniques. This will train and equip EM users/researchers, from colleges, universities and industries, with instrumental skills related to respective instrument operation and data analysis. The explanation about the use of TEM technique in samples morphological visualization (shape and size) at high resolution, quantification analysis etc., has been briefly described. Specifically, in current chapter, case studies related to insight capabilities of TEM technique, presented the use of basic to advance EM instrumentation, cutting edge sample preparation with novel interpretation and

R. Singh, *Transmission Electron Microscopy Sample Preparation*,
https://doi.org/10.1007/978-3-031-82967-3_11

explanations, has been presented. Systematic analysis and understanding of any research and development hypothesis can be approached towards optimization of different material's novel fabrication and design, remediation of diseases mechanism and upgradation in instrumentation technologies.

The ultimate objective of this chapter is to make users of TEM capable in understanding the basic to advance requirements related to TEM with exploring and explaining respective material under study, beyond their limits. This approach will train person behind the machine in extracting and learning in-depth intricacies related to material analysis, developing microscopic vision in exploring material behavior w.r.t. material failure or efficient performances.

11.2 Why to Study Case Studies w.r.t. TEM

There are following general reasons which will promote the study of specific case study w.r.t. TEM instrumentation, operation, sample analysis and respective interpretation of data.

11.2.1 To Understand the Insight Instrumentation

Study of work related to TEM operation and working during routine sample analysis, will be helpful for researchers in exploring different EM instrument parameters in precise operation. This may include optimum electron beam characteristics, electron beam alignment, vacuum status, water supply etc. [1, 2].

11.2.2 Specialized Investigation

Research investigation from generalized analysis to targeted area, would lead to develop insights in respective topic/study. Special expertise in respective field will be developed through analyzing specific fields material/specimens like biological, material science or nanotechnology etc. This approach will be useful in finding remedies of existing device failure or environmental remediation via development of novel technologies.

11.2.3 Error Identification with Problem Solving Skill

During analysis of any material belongs to biological to non-living category, TEM study will be helpful in identifying the probable failure/errors/defects during synthesis of respective samples. Study of specific case studies w.r.t. material growth, device failure etc., through identification of inbuilt or process-oriented defects, will be helpful in rectifying the respective limitations in subsequent formulations or devices [3]. All stated factors guide researchers/scientist, to use TEM effectively and efficiently in different research commitment.

11.2.4 Critical Analysis Approach

With the precise analysis of previous publish literature w.r.t. TEM technique, one can find strengths, challenges and scopes in respective area of research. TEM analysis will guide researchers for novel sample preparation techniques, modification in existing material for efficient performances etc. This will save energy, time and enhance the efficiency of whole approach towards sustainable efficiency.

Through above stated points as demonstrated in Fig. 11.1, one can easily understand and correlate, the usage and importance of studying specific case studies w.r.t. TEM operation, working, maintenance and usage of updated techniques with insightful interpretation of respective data.

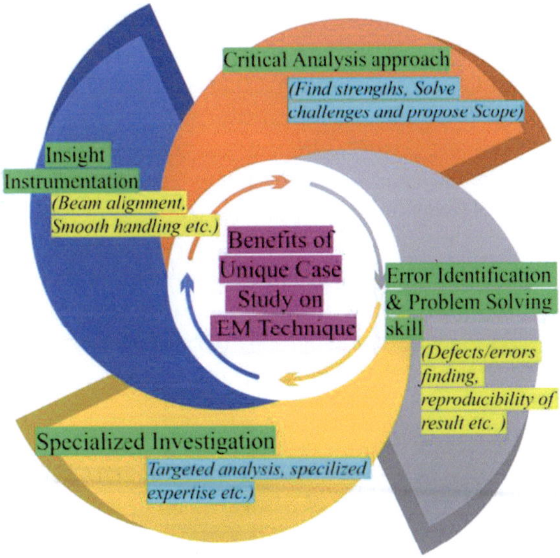

Fig. 11.1 Pictorial representation of importance of studying specific case study

11.3 Case Studies

In coming section, we have described and explained materials analysis w.r.t. TEM centric application and explanations.

11.3.1 Case Study: Setup and Operation of Cryo-EM Laboratory

The objective of current study deals with setup of cryo-electron microscopy (cryo-EM) laboratory for visualization of subcellular structure to sub-nanometer resolution of structural biology of different macromolecules assemblies. As per author of current publication, different EM techniques (electron microscopy and cryo-electron microscopy) related instrumentation, installation, sample preparation, operation and maintenance requirements etc., has been evolving as per *revolution in resolution* [4].

The information and data provided in current article is totally based on personal experience of author *Deryck J Mills,* who had dedicated experience of four decades in electron microscopy field. With the increasing demands in the field of material analysis at atomic or molecular scale, author found need to procure, and maintain the sophisticated cryo-EM laboratory at his workplace. Interestingly, journey of author *Deryck J Mills* in field of EM started with installation of first EM facility at University of Brimingham, UK in department of biological sciences and Paediatrics in 1980. Author performed duties all over the globe initially as an application engineer in Siemens and Oxford Company's instrument. Author worked with reputed laboratory named European Molecular biology laboratory (EMBL) with the Max Haider's electron optics development group for many years. Most importantly, author also worked with Max Planck institute of Biophysics in Frankfurt am main, Germany. From year 2003, author moved to Riedberg university campus which evolved over the years to till date into state of art facility globally. Currently, the EM laboratory has single particle EM, cryo-electron tomography (Cryo-ET) with focus ion beam (FIB)-SEM, correlative light and electron microscopy (CLEM) with total eight electron-microscopes [4].

11.3.1.1 Highlights of Study

Instrumental, Operational and Working Conditions in Cryo-EM Laboratory

As per author, conventional transmission electron microscope (TEM) will be dedicated for multiple samples analysis and respective data collection in air drying condition, whereas low temperature stabilized biological or hydrated sample will be processed at 300 kV cryo-TEM. As per author, mainly two companies all over the globe manufacture high resolution cryo-EM namely Thermo Fischer Scientific (who take up FEI) (300 kV Titan Krios, 200 kV Talos Arctica) and JEOL (Cryo-ARM series). Efficient data collection of specimens during EM imaging will be facilitated by use of direct electron detector namely Falcon 3 or 4, Gatan K2 or K3, Direct Electron (DE16 or DE64). Dedicated TEM instrument for screening of samples will be utilized which must be equipped with CMOS detectors (like Gatan one view, TFS Ceta, TVIPS F416 etc.). In addition, the presence of energy filters will also be required for thick specimen analysis in contrast enhancement purpose [4].

Specifically, through single particle analysis or Cryo-ET techniques, resolution upto 1 Å can be achieved. Condition of low temperature (80 K or less) stabilized specimen having minimum specimen drift rate (1 nm min^{-1}), camera's low electron flux (0.5 electron/pixel/second) etc., need to maintained during respective EM working and analysis. The performance of specimen analysis in cryo-ET is equally good with cryo-stage specimen having tilt upto $\pm 60°$ in term of resolution, specimen drifting etc., conditions.

Procedure During Screening of Specimen

Every biological sample require standardized vitrification and processing protocol to acquire precise sample analysis under appropriate EM. Figure 11.2, shows pictures of JEOL 3200 FSC microscope with author of current publication. Ideally, biological specimen must be screened under less expensive low accelerating instrument viz. Talos Arctica or Glacios and Titan krios from TFS TEM instrument, which has been demonstrated in Fig. 11.2c, d. Above mentioned instrument, can be utilized before proceeding for high resolution Cryo-EM 300 kV or Cryo-ARM instrument (Fig. 11.2b). The cost of screening samples through EM instrument is two third and floor area requirement is half in comparison to Cryo-TEM 300 kV requirements. Satisfactorily cryo-processed TEM grid with specimen, will be transferred to high end EM instrument for detailed data collection study (hours to several days).

The probable chances of disintegration, aggregation or heterogeneity aspect w.r.t. biological specimen [5], also can be analyzed under staining procedure having side entry 120 kV TEM with LaB_6 filament. Such instruments can be easily handled with low maintenance cost. Specifically, TFS Talos L120C or JEM 1400 Flash JEOL fitted with 4 k × 4 k CMOS detector are the good example for above mentioned category [4].

Requirements of Camera and Detectors, Energy Filters w.r.t. Cryo-TEM

Data recording or imaging in modern cryo-EM, will be proceed with direct electron detectors having, high readability and sensitivity to low dose electron images via low electron flux features. The feature of high detection quantum efficiency (DQE) will be facilitated via direct counting cameras like Gatan K2 and K3 or TFS Flacon 3 and 4. The problems of mechanical drift and beam induced specimen damage, will be overwhelmed through above specified instruments [6].

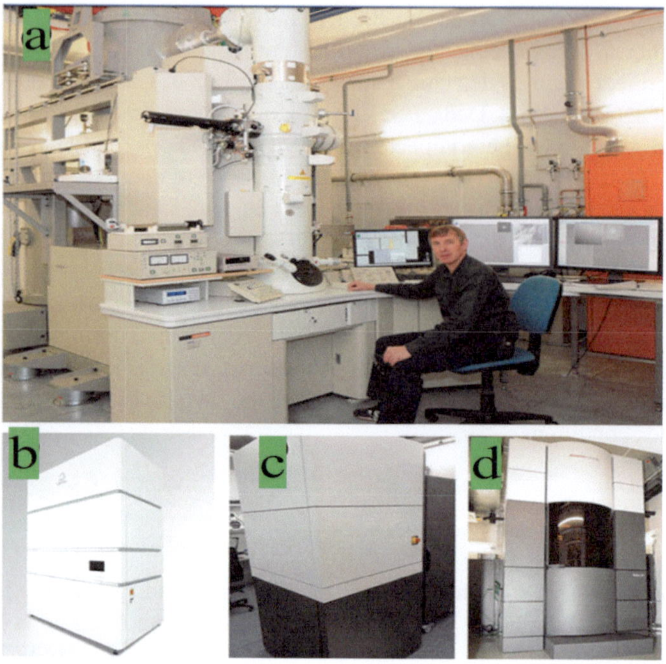

Fig. 11.2 **a** JEOL 3200 FSC microscope (3.75 m high with ceiling height must be 4.1 m) with the Author, **b** Cryo-ARM300 (JEOL), **c** Glacios from TFS (respective box have 2.52 m high and ceiling height must be 2.8 m), **d** Titan krios from TFS (Adapted with permission from Mills [4] under open access)

Thick specimen will face high inelastic scattering having noisy signal bring interference during high resolution imaging. Issue of noise generation will also be encountered during Cryo-ET imaging due to tilting of specimen. Presence of energy filter will confiscate the electron which have lost their energy and may diminish the respective noise. As per manufacturer design and specification, JEOL have in-column energy filter (Omega filter) whereas TFS microscope have post column filters built by Gatan [7].

Cyro FIB-SEM and CLEM (Correlative Light and Electron Microscopy)

Thin specimen preparation with optimized conditioning of biological specimen through FIB-SEM and cryo-FIB SEM will be prepared for cryo-TEM (300 kV) tomography study. Thin slices lamellae of biological specimen under cryo-FIB SEM [8], will be smoothly achieved without damaging individual organelles. The sight specific processing of biological specimen can be performed with incorporation of fluorescent probes through CLEM [9].

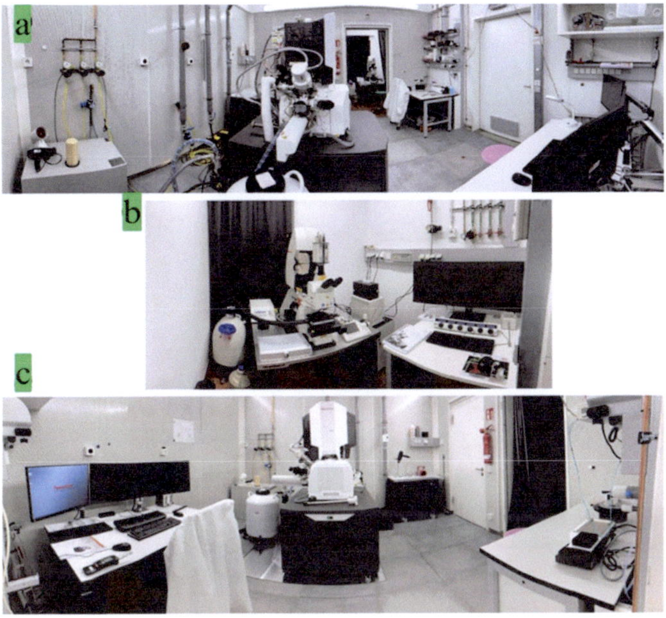

Fig. 11.3 CLEM room **a** Cryo-FIB SEM with Leica SP8 confocal cryo-CLEM, **b** cryo-CLEM, **c** Front image of Aquilos FIB-SEM (Adapted with permission from Mills [4] under open access)

Requirement in Cryo-EM Lab w.r.t. Quality Specimen Preparation

There is always a challenge in analyzing quality specimen from raw form to precise phase through high specification electron microscope. There are following requirements related to basic to advance equipment's, which must be procure/present in any cryo-EM laboratory (for example CLEM lab contains (a) Cryo-FIB SEM with Leica SP8 confocal cryo-CLEM, (b) cryo-CLEM and (c) Aquilos FIB-SEM as shown in Fig. 11.3a–c).

(a) **Carbon evaporator**: It will be utilized to produce high quality carbon thin film support for routine imaging and in negative staining [4].
(b) **Glow discharge unit**: It is used to transform different carbon support viz. lacy carbon, holey film back coated, amorphous carbon or graphene etc., into hydrophilic nature. This will transform grid support surface into supportive and loving nature w.r.t. specimen, which is to be placed (slices) or drop casted etc. [4].
(c) **Light microscopy (LM)**: LM technique will be engaged during investigation of integrity aspect of carbon coated or holey carbon supported grids [4]. In addition, LM will also be exploited in different pre-identification or screening of specimen before precise preparation procedure.

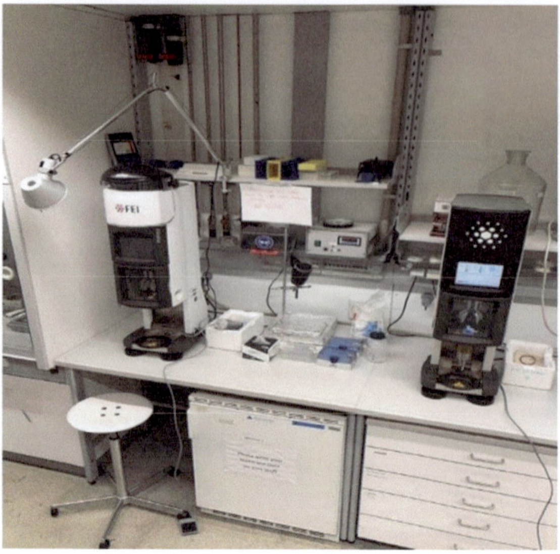

Fig. 11.4 Image of vitrification processing instrument from TFS (Adapted with permission from Mills [4] under open access)

(d) **Robotic plunge freezer**: Robotic plunge freezer technique will be used in vitrification of biological samples. Fundamentally, vitrification process of specimen proceeds in liquid ethane, subsequently followed by warming and removal through proper safety guideline (in presence of fume hood). Image of commonly used plunge freezer is Vitrobot from TFS [4] which is shown in Fig. 11.4.

(e) **Area for loading/mounting TEM grids**: Dedicated spacious area during grid loading on high end TEM instrumentation like Krios, Glacios or cryo-ARM, must be allocated nearby to main instrument room [4].

(f) **Cryo-specimen holder**: TEM instrument without inbuilt cryo-stage must have cryo-specimen holder with specialized sample loading station. Respective facility also must have liquid nitrogen dewars facility to store the frozen grids. This will avoid the specimen from ice contamination during preservation span.

(g) **Water distillation plant**: Triple water distillation assembly must be present/installed in electron microscopy laboratory for use in different synthesis and cleaning work.

(h) **Liquid Nitrogen supply**: Facility of adequate supply of liquid nitrogen must be present in premises of EM laboratory, to ensure uninterrupted working of EM instrument.

Further, Fig. 11.5a–d demonstrated the cyro-grid preservation, storage dewar, four slot box for cryo-grid storage, eight slot designed aluminum box for cryo-grid and two slot designed aluminum box for Polara cartridge respectively.

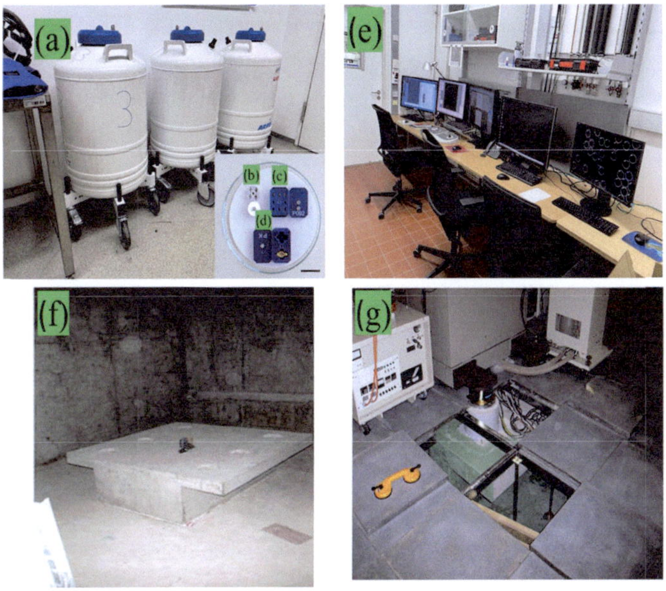

Fig. 11.5 Cyro-grid preservation **a** Storage dewar, **b** four slot box for cryo-grid storage, **c** eight slot designed aluminum box for cryo-grid, **d** two slot designed aluminum box for Polara cartridge (Adapted with permission from Mills [4] under open access)

Cryo-EM Room Requirements

There are following requirements w.r.t. cryo-TEM instrument facility for smooth functioning, as explained by Mills [4], whose detail have been summarized in Table 11.1.

Table 11.1, has summarized in detail about the physical criteria/requirements for main EM instrument and ancillary rooms, flooring, wiring, safety guidelines, staff requirements with maintenance schedule for cryo-TEM laboratory.

11.3.1.2 Outcomes

Above discussed articles explained and guided about the importance of current and futuristic upgradations w.r.t. Cryo-EM instrumentation, operations, analysis etc., through '***Resolution Revolution***'. Upgradation in existing electron microscopes lead to coherent electron source, stable electron optics, cryo-stage with eucentric tilting for tomogram data collection, direct electron counting cameras etc. As per author vast experience in EM operation, maintenance and analysis, there is immense need of specialized optimization in cryo-TEM grid freezing techniques analysis for insightful studies as per nature and properties of sample under study. Major frontier targets from

Table 11.1 Summary w.r.t. requirements, specifications related to Cryo-TEM lab [4]

Name of room/condition	Specifications/requirement
300 kV Cryo-EM (room dimension)	(i) Floor area: ~ 6×6 m^2, Height: ~ 4 m (ii) Powerful air conditioning
Microscope for screening of samples (room dimension)	(i) 120 kV TEM: ~ 4×4 m^2, Water cooler room: ~ 1.5×2 m^2 (ii) 200 kV TEM: ~ 4×5 m^2 and ~ 3 m high
Ancillary Room (water coolers, vacuum pumps, data acquisition and data storage etc.) (as shown in Fig. 11.5)	~ (2×3) m^2
FIB-SEM room	(i) ~ 4×4 m^2 and ~ 2.5-m height (ii) Cryo-light microscope = ~ (2×2)m (iii) Relative humidity: < 20%
Remote control room	~ 2×4 m^2 (Adjacent to main room or at a 15 m distance from main room)
EM storage room (two dedicated room)	(i) **Room 1** (Storage of measuring equipment like lead detector, vacuum gauges or electronics meters, service tools, spare parts etc.) = ~3 m × 4 m × 3 m (ii) **Room 2** (packing and unpacking of old or new instrument): ~ 6 m × 6 m × 4 m (if possible)
Temperature and humidity	(i)Temp. = 22 °C ± 0.5 °C, Humidity < 20%
Liquid nitrogen supply requirement	(i) ~ 3000-L water free liquid nitrogen tank (ii) Storage tank should be connected main instrument room
Flooring and noise level w.r.t. 300 kV cryo-EM room	(i) Low noise level and vibration free floor (ii) Concrete plinth = (4×4) m^2 and 1 m height
Distance between EM power supply and high voltage tank	~ 1.5 m from EM column
Air delivery system in EM room	Installation of wind socks (Fig. 11.6a)
Alaram in the lab	Installation of oxygen sensor and fire alarm
Shielding of ancillary equipment and main EM instrument	(i) Acoustic paneling over the ancillary equipment (Fig. 11.6b) (ii) To avoid any mechanical vibration, microscope enclosure must be fitted (Fig. 11.6c)
Data collection server	Respective system must be placed inside the sound proof cabinet
Electrical wiring and large power cables	Fixing of large cables and wiring need to fix through ground level to avoid electromagnetic interference (EMI)
EM column maintenance or filament exchange	Availability of overhead gantry crane

(continued)

Table 11.1 (continued)

Name of room/condition	Specifications/requirement
EMI generation	In case of electromagnetic field > 80 nT (peak to peak in TEM lab) generated from outside facility room **Remedies**: Installation of active field compensator
Safety guidelines	(i) Use of safety googles or visor (ii) **Liquid nitrogen use**: Good ventilation, activation of oxygen alarm if oxygen level is < 19.5%, in case of nitrogen spillage (iii) **Ethane Handling**: Procced liquification process as well any discarding, inside the fume hood (iv) **Handling of SF_6**: (i)Used for electrical insulation in high tension tank as well in field emission gun (ii) SF_6 is harmful greenhouse gas, respective sensor must be installed in lab with extra ventilation
Discarding of toxic chemical	(i) Chemicals like uranyl acetate, uranyl formate, lead citrate or phospho-tungstate (PTA) must be handled with care (ii) Any chemical waste must be disposed in dedicated container under proper discard policy
Staff requirements	(i) Qualified lab manager will ensure minimum downtime, precise operation and work at highest standard during imaging and data analysis (ii) Smooth working of main EM with ancillary instrument must be ensured by lab manager with coordination of all supporting staff
Maintenance	(i) **Routine maintenance** of main EM as well ancillary instrument must be performed by qualified service engineer (ii) **Performance Check**: High Resolution check of EM instrument must be proceeded through standard holey carbon film having gold island and graphitized carbon. Single data collection will be proceeded through standard cryo-sample named apoferritin (iii) **Smooth cooling supply to EM**: Improper supply have adverse effect on data quality

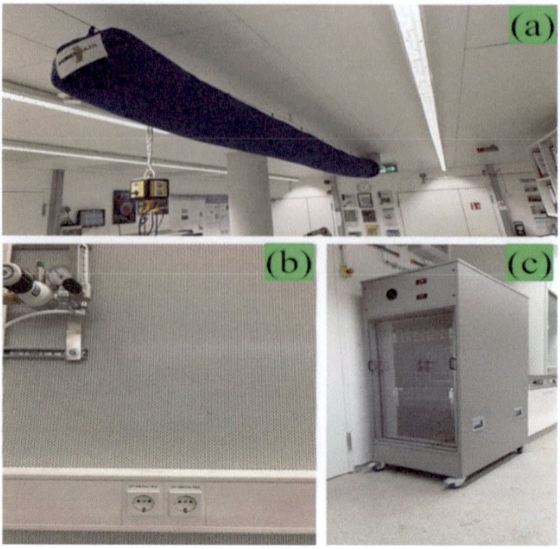

Fig. 11.6 Reduced vibration in EM laboratory, **a** Wind sock, **b** acoustic paneling, **c** soundproof cabinet for data servers (Adapted with permission from Mills [4] under open access)

Cryo-TEM, is to achieve resolution beyond 1 Å with biological specimen is expected from future.

11.3.2 Case Study: Quality Assessment of EM LaB_6 Field Emission Electron Source

Requirement for improved spatial resolution and analytical capabilities-based electron microscopy, will be mainly dominated through quality electron source. Under current study, LaB_6 nanotip electron source has been analyzed and observed as a stable, efficient and effective field emission option in TEM imaging [10].

11.3.2.1 Highlights of Study

There are the following major highlights of study.

Why to Develop LaB_6 Nanoneedle as Field Emission Source

The quality and performance of any electron source will be decided through (a) energy spread through temporal coherence and chromatic aberration, (b) stable electron beam, (c) high brightness of electron beam. High work function energy and high energy spread (eV) of tungsten (W) filament, bring clear path of research and

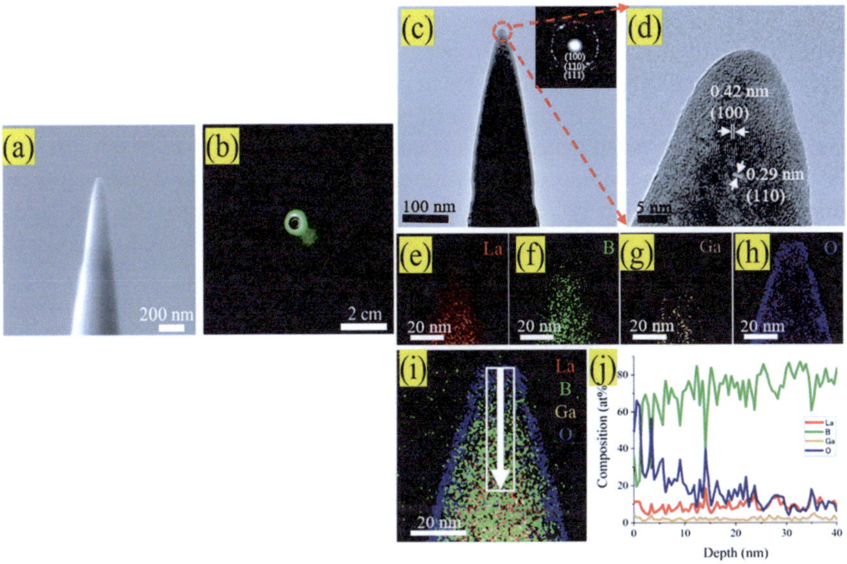

Fig. 11.7 **a** SEM image of LaB6 nanoneedle tip having 11 nm of radius of curvature, **b** respective source image single spot emission in axial direction, **c** Nanoneedle TEM tip image, **d** Tip with hemispherical apex having 7.5 nm radius, **e–i** elemental distribution of **e** Lanthanum, **f** Boron, **g** gallium, **h** oxygen, **i** La + B + Ga + O, **j** depth profiling of nanoneedle area along arrow direction (Adapted with permission from Tang et al. [10] under open access)

development work for LaB_6 as an efficient electron emission option. In current work, authors has uniquely reported LaB_6 nanoneedle as a mechanically and structurally robust, stable field emitter having low work function (~ 2.1 eV) and high melting point [11, 12] etc., features confirmed through SEM and TEM.

Ultrastructural Analysis of LaB_6 Nanoneedle

The conditioning of LaB_6 nanoneedle will be designed through low voltage FIB milling refinement. LaB_6 electron source (Fig. 11.7a), shows single spot emission in comparison to tungsten (W) multiple spot emission [13] features, whose confirmation has been demonstrated in Fig. 11.7b. In addition, respective filament shows confined electron emission having respective area of 4.4 nm^2 with current density $1.4 \times 10^{10} Am^{-2}$ at 57 nA emission current in field emission microscope [10].

Further Tang et al. (2012) has reported ultrastructural high-resolution imaging of LaB_6 nanoneedle image with elemental mapping, which has been depicted in Fig. 11.7c–j. Crystalline nature (as shown in-set of Figs. 11.7c) of respective filament tip area highlighted in Fig. 11.7c with high resolution lattice fringes having lattice spacing values 0.42 and 0.29 nm without presence of any mechanical vibration [14], has been observed. Further, detailed chemical distribution for filament material has been presented from Fig. 11.7e–i. In addition to presence of Lanthanum (La), Boron (B), Gallium (Ga), oxygen (O) elements w.r.t. nanoneedle structure, respective composition depth profiling also has been performed. Figure 11.7j, shows increase in concentration of boron from outer surface to inner side and saturated at ~ 10 nm distance whereas oxygen concentration decreases and saturated at 30 nm distance. Due to different facet composition at different location have bring variation in work function values [15]. Specifically, La/B value at the surface of tip is much higher than 1/6 ratio, predicts surface is rich in La content bring preferential for emission regardless to its orientation.

In addition, a comparative study between LaB_6 and W (310), also has been presented w.r.t. current decay and emission noise parameters. It shows current diminishes to 80% value after 10 h., for W filament whereas LaB_6 shows stable current emission [16]. Similarly, W (310) cold field emission source shows 18.5% noise level whereas LaB_6 have respective (1–2) % noise level [17].

11.3.2.2 Outcomes

Current study guided development of field emission source having minimum energy spread, noise stability features. This study will also play a torch-bearer role during development of new generation electron sources for smart electron microscope like atomic resolution microscopes (ARM) or aberration (C_s) corrected TEM.

11.3.3 Case Study: Comparative Analysis Between Standard TEM and Cryo-TEM for Liposomes Formulation

The nature of nanoparticle or material under electron microscopy (EM) study, will affect the insights of explanations. In current work, authors have uniquely studied and reported comparative analysis of entrapped drug nanocrystal with liposomes through TEM and cryo-TEM technique [18].

11.3.3.1 Highlights of Study

Importance of Normal TEM Versus Cryo-TEM w.r.t. Liposomes Formulations

Both electron microscopes i.e. normal TEM and cryo-TEM, have depth of information during their respective analysis. Due to high demand and applicability of liposomes-based drug delivery formulations, directed focus on exploration of respective material analysis. Many times, due to low stability of lipid nanoparticles under EM imaging process, will disintegrate the specimen's actual structure and behavior.

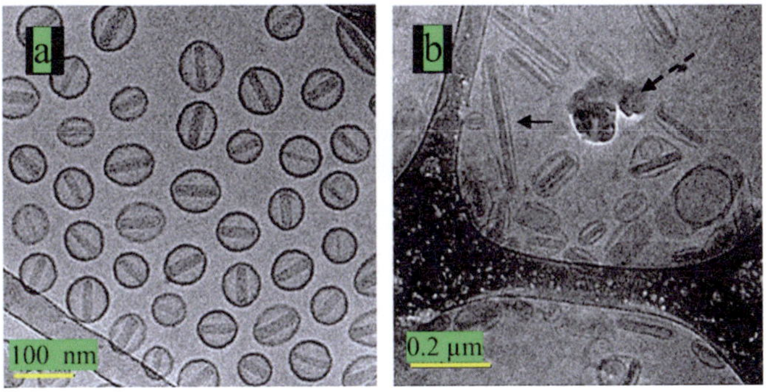

Fig. 11.8 **a** Commercial Doxcil liposomes cryo-TEM image (Adapted with permission from Barenholz [20]), **b** Liposomal ciprofloxacin formulation through freeze thaw having presence of ice artefacts during freeze drying (Adapted with permission from Li et al. [18] under open access)

It will direct for vitrified specimen preparation via low temperature stabilization (plunge freezing etc.). TEM grid preparation techniques having minimum artefacts generation possibilities [19], must be preferred during respective analysis.

Cryo-TEM Imaging of Standard Doxil Liposome and Ciprofloxacin Entrapped Liposomes

First FDA approved liposomes formulation containing doxorubicin sulphate nanocrystal has been analyzed through cryo-TEM analysis as shown Fig. 11.8a. Respective nanocrystal has been clearly entrapped inside intact bilayer of lipid as shown in Fig. 11.8b. Normally, current observed liposomes structure will be collapsed during normal TEM imaging and specimen air drying procedure [18].

TEM Grid Preparation Protocol for Standard TEM and Cryo-TEM

(a) **Grid Preparation Procedure for Standard TEM**

Continuous carbon coated TEM 200, 300 or 400 mesh, were plasma cleaned for 2 min in presence of oxygen/argon gas. Drop of 2 μl sample solution will be casted on TEM grid with 1 min adsorption time. It will be followed by blotting of extra solvent removal with Whatman 541 filter paper and air-drying procedure for 10 min. Properly dried grid will be examined under FET Tecnai G^2 T20 microscope (200 kV) at best suitable parameters.

(b) **Grid Preparation Procedure for Cryo-TEM**

Lacey carbon film 200 mesh TEM grid will be treated under glow discharge instrument in presence of nitrogen gas. It will ensure specimen have maximum deposition on grid surface. Sample solution of 4 μl pipetted on TEM grid for 30 s, followed by blotting time through Whatman 541 filter paper for 2 s. Further, low temperature freezing of TEM grid, will be proceed with plunging into liquid ethane in presence of liquid nitrogen. Imaging of processed grids will be proceed with loading of respective grid into Gatan 626 cryo-holder followed by viewing of specimen under Tecnai 12 120 kV under electron low dose imaging mode [18].

Comparative Analysis of TEM and Cryo-TEM Imaging

The negatively stained liposomal nanocrystal was adversely affected the visualization between liposomes and ciprofloxacin nanocrystal. During standard TEM imaging without staining of specimen, imaging was performed at 13,000× with the use of objective aperture at sufficient defocus (Fig. 11.9a–f). Approximately, 500 nanocrystals were imaged for 20–30 images during normal TEM imaging. Due to basic density difference between nanocrystal and liposomes, face difficulty in visualization of liposomes during imaging. In addition, respective nanocrystal aggregation through coffee ring effect also has been observed. Respective phenomenon brings accumulation of nanocrystal towards the perimeter of solution droplet on grid support surface [21].

Cryo-TEM imaging of respective specimen has enable the observation of both components i.e. liposomes as well ciprofloxacin nanocrystal as shown in Fig. 11.9g–i. Due to lack of optimized sample preparation w.r.t. thawed temperature procedure, restricted its use in quantitative data analysis due to observation of limited number of nanocrystals. Clear confirmation and correlation of nanorod morphology of nanocrystal encapsulation inside liposomes through cryo-TEM has been validated and confirmed. Similar images via standard TEM imaging also has been observed [18].

In addition, with increase in thawing temperature (4, 20, 50 °C), crystal growth has been decreased to smaller size. The size of respective nanocrystal formulation at 50 °C have smaller dimension as compared to large dimension at 4 °C. Observed variable aspect ratio behavior of material under current study, is solely not due to thawing temperature factor, but will also be affected through lipid composition and bilayer rigidity factors [18]. Different dimension of respective liposomes nanocrystal and aspect ratio data are presented in Fig. 11.10a–c.

11.3.3.2 Outcomes

Current study has uniquely highlighted the importance of both standard TEM as well cryo-TEM data analysis w.r.t. drug nanocrystal loaded liposomal formulation. The quantitative particle size distribution will be efficiently analyzed by standard TEM analysis whereas cryo-TEM has highlighted individual components at high contrast and resolution conditions. Through integrated analysis with standard TEM and cryo-TEM techniques, can contribute efficiently for current and futuristic liposomal nanocrystal drug delivery system developments.

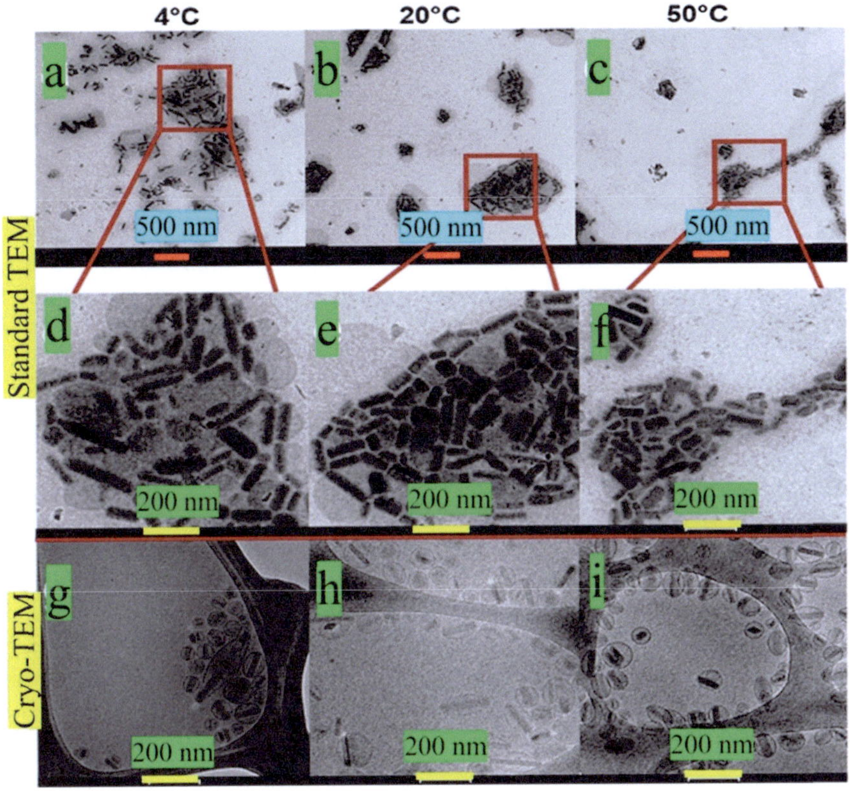

Fig. 11.9 Comparison of imaging of liposomal ciprofloxacin nanocrystal with lipid bilayer at different thaw temperature through standard TEM (figure **a**–**f**) and cryo-TEM (figure **g**–**i**). Respective liposomes specimen thawed at 4, 20, 50 °C respectively (Adapted with permission from Li et al. [18] under open access)

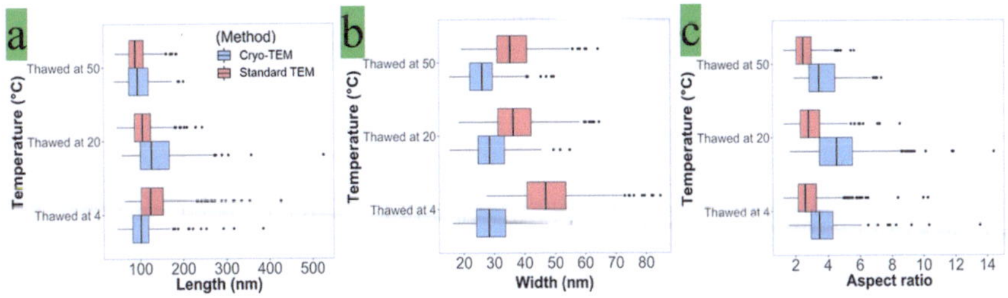

Fig. 11.10 Size arrangement of liposomal ciprofloxacin nanocrystal through standard TEM and cryo-TEM **a** length, **b** width, **c** aspect ratio between length to width. Respective liposomes specimen thawed at 4, 20, 50 °C respectively (Adapted with permission from Li et al. [18] under open access)

11.3.4 Case Study: Mo-W-S-Se Sliding Contact Induced by FIB and In-Situ Micro-tribometer: Analysis by TEM

Current work specifically analyses the behavior of solid lubrication, wear scar surface and contact interface of Mo-W-S-Se thin film. Novel micro-tribometer was operated for respective study in FIB microscope. In current study, cross-section TEM specimen has been prepared w.r.t. contact point without tip/film separation technique. In-situ FIB micro-tribometer technique, is efficiently used in investigation of intact structure of lubricant film used in stated process [22].

11.3.4.1 Highlights of Study

Synthesis of Mo-W-S-Se Thin Film

Mo-W-S-Se thin film were synthesized by pulse laser deposition (PLD) method on silicon (100) wafer. Specifically, laser will operate at pulsed beam of 248 nm wavelength, 20 ns duration at 400 mJ energy conditions. The laser target was made-up of MoS_2 and WSe2 mixing in 75:25 ratio, shaped into compact disk of 25.6 mm disk. Respective material plasma plumes, will be produced by laser ablation having vacuum inside deposition chamber of order of ~ 10^{-9} torr [22].

Results

The tribological properties of Mo-W-S-Se composite thin film were analyzed in dry nitrogen and humid environment. With switching from dry to humid environment, in addition to increase in friction coefficient, respective endurance of specimen surface also has been observed.

(a) **SEM and Raman Spectroscopy Observation**

SEM images of wear track were observed at the load of 100 g in air with 50% relative humidity (at 10,000 cycle test), having dark contrast than surrounding coatings as shown in Fig. 11.11a. In addition, Raman spectroscopy analysis shows the fingerprint of MoS_2 for wear scar surface having peak position at 269, 374, and 404 cm^{-1} as shown in Fig. 11.11b [22].

(b) **TEM Analysis**

FIB microscope will be used in preparation of thin foil having width ~ 30 μm with depth of 7 μm (as shown in Fig. 11.12a), through etching from inside of wear track with Ga^+ ion bombardment. Figure 11.12b demonstrated the precise TEM grid preparation procedure through welding of foil on grid finger by Pt deposition.

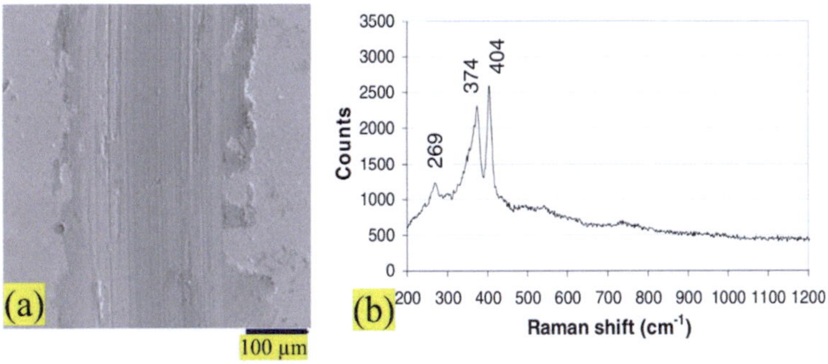

Fig. 11.11 **a** SEM image of wear track after 10,000 cycle tests with load of 100 g in air at 50% relative humidity, **b** respective area observation through micro-Raman spectrum. (Adapted with permission from Hu et al. [22])

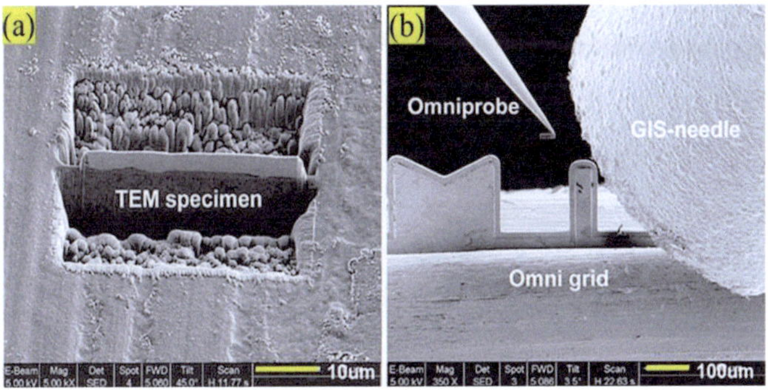

Fig. 11.12 **a** SEM image of specimen wear track area prepared for TEM analysis through FIB technique, **b** respective TEM specimen lift out process using Omniprobe manipulation system (Adapted with permission from Hu et al. [22])

Respective specimen surface will be finished to electron transparent nature through ion beam technique [22].

Further, Fig. 11.13 shows respective Mo-W-S-Se thin film specimen cross section TEM image as well as the corresponding elemental mapping. Presence of expected elements Mo, W, S, Se has been observed between Pt protection cap and steel substrate. In addition, confirmed micro-cracks has been observed parallel to wear scar surface as highlighted by white arrow in Fig. 11.13. Through high resolution image, (002) basal planes were arranged parallel to surface as shown in Fig. 11.14. The basal plane re-orientation has been further confirmed through observation of two diffraction spot w.r.t. (002) plane via selected area electron diffraction (SAED) imaging, as shown in Fig. 11.14 [22].

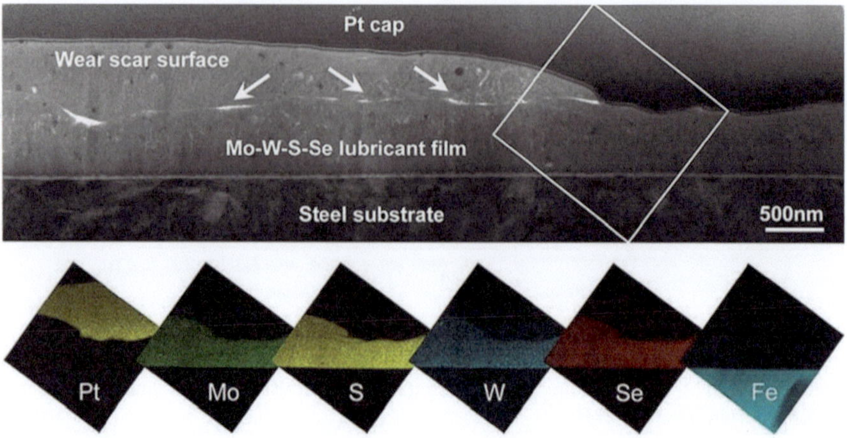

Fig. 11.13 Specimen cross-section TEM image and respective elemental mapping. White box highlighted was analyzed for EDS mapping (Adapted with permission from Hu et al. [22])

Fig. 11.14 Cross-section TEM image with selected area electron diffraction image for wear scar surface (Adapted with permission from Hu et al. [22])

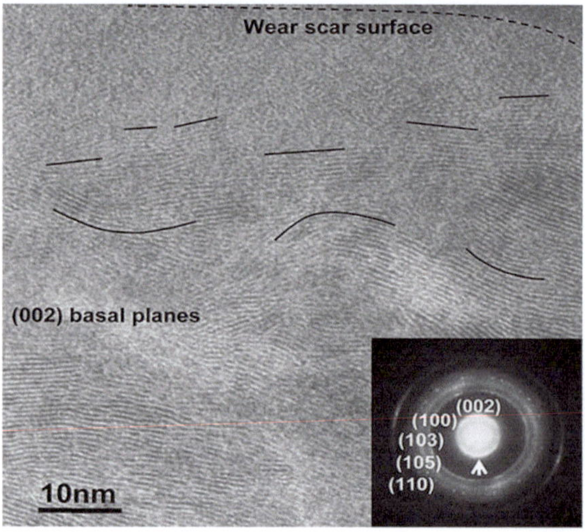

11.3.4.2 Outcomes

Current study has presented a cross-sectional microstructure analysis of Mo-W-S-Se thin film through FIB and TEM techniques. Uniquely installed micro-tribometer with FIB, work very efficiently during monitoring of insitu-tribological processes. The interfacial microstructure of lubricant film has been found intact as confirmed by microscopic techniques. Respective lubricating film has been observed and imaged between sliding tip and sample surface. Further, current study also confirms about the recrystallization and reorientation of (002) basal plane of respective material with low shear stress motion [22].

11.3.5 *Case Study: Sample Preparation and Imaging for Structural Biology by Cryo-electron Microscopy*

Current study has highlighted the analysis approach of different specimens belong to eukaryotic cells to individual protein > 150 kDa. Era of resolution revolution, in present study highlighted about the different sample preparation strategies, EM analysis modes and respective imaging processing software. Whole approach will work around to solve and simplify the unique challenges related to structural biology [23].

11.3.5.1 Highlights of Study

Importance of Quality Sample Synthesis

Ideally quality imaging of specimen, will be ensured through homogenous nature of specimen. Practically, compositional and conformational inhomogeneity probably due to binding of compound or sub-units respectively. Compositional homogeneity will be ensured through purified form of used protein, chemicals etc., whereas conformation purity will be ensured through ligand-ligand stabilization, ultimately leads to stable complex formation. Commonly, problem is to transfer the sufficient number of proteins molecules or specimen particles/nanoparticles onto 3.05 mm TEM grid surface through limited sample volume of (2–5) μl, with optimum solution concentration. Controlled sample deposition on grid support surface will always need to optimized during respective preparation [23].

Preparation of Quality TEM Grid

There are following points/ways which need to fulfill/followed while performing quality TEM grid preparation:

(a) **Stabilization of specimen**: The biological specimen must be stabilized in his native state with optimized protocol. Specimen must be sufficient thin through suitable technique. This will be helpful in describing the actual description of specimen during respective analysis [23].
(b) **Description of Grid**: Normally, TEM grid is of 3.05 mm diameter having mesh body made up of Copper (Cu), gold (Au), Nickel (Ni), Molybdenum (Mo), or Rhodium (Rh) etc. Mesh size of grid will be depend upon the number of meshes present. For example, 200 mesh grid have 20 square or 400 mesh grids have

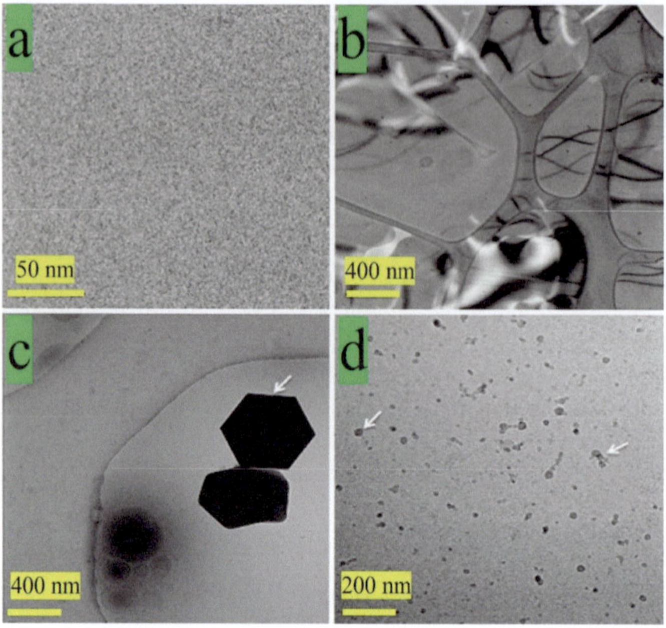

Fig. 11.15 **a** Empty vitreous ice, **b** hexagonal ice, **c** large ice crystal, **d** probable ethane contamination (Adapted with permission Thompson et al. [23] under open access)

40 squares in one direction respectively. Higher number mesh grid has benefits of good support and strength, but may interfere during tilt series analysis mode [23].

(c) **Grid staining**: In order to improve the contrast of specimen, negative or positive staining will be preferred to investigate factors like non-homogenous, impurity or conformational flexibility etc., aspect of specimen. Typically, specimen is adsorbed on carbon support thin film (~ 10 nm), followed by specified exposure time of heavy metal i.e. 1–2 (w/v) uranyl acetate or uranyl formate etc. Analysed specimen and respective concentration, stain concentration, washing of grid etc. factors, need to validate at optimum level, to achieve highest contrast with high signal to noise (SNR) ratio [24].

(d) **Vitrification**: Normally, embedding and staining process will be utilized during biological specimen preparation under EM imaging, have probabilities to modify/alter specimen nature from its native environment state. Vitrification process will freezes the water content of specimen at 10^6 °C/s rate, into vitreous state as shown in Fig. 11.15a, b. Any deviation during freezing like ethane contamination (Fig. 11.15d) w.r.t. processing temperature ~ −137 °C, lead to ice crystal formation (crystallization) as shown in Fig. 11.15c. Precisely, plunge freezing, high pressure freezing etc. techniques, will be exploited in respective cryo-sample preparation [23].

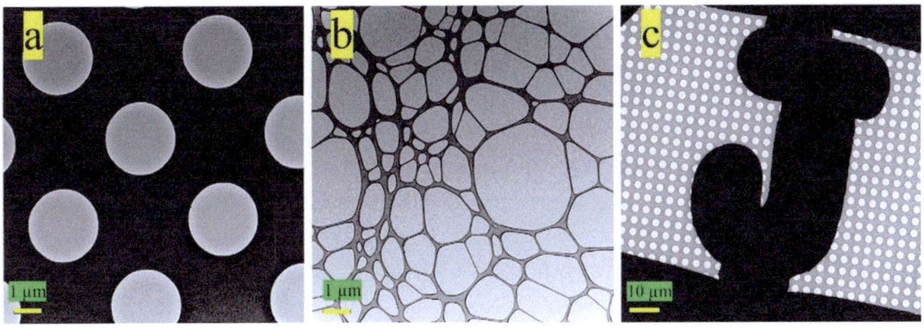

Fig. 11.16 EM support film **a** Holey carbon (Quantifoil R2/2-2 µm hole separated by 2 µm), **b** lacy carbon film (irregular carbon film), **c** Finder grid (Quantifoil R2/2-2 µm hole separated by 2 µm) (Adapted with permission Thompson et al. [23] under open access)

(e) **Type of TEM grid support film**: Current study has highlighted the importance of nature of grid support film, during specimen imaging. Perforated carbon film or continuous carbon thin film will be employed in negative staining application. In addition, perforated amorphous carbon thin film have regular array of holes with Quantifoil and C-Flat grids whereas lacy carbon has irregular pattern [23] as shown in Fig. 11.16.

The challenges of low affinity support thin film towards specimen, will be improved through exposure to UV radiation, glow discharge or detergent treatment etc. The amorphous carbon film will also be used with challenges like instability w.r.t. beam induced effects, blurring of specimen imaging etc. Continuous research work is on the track with full pace in overcoming in above stated challenges w.r.t. support thin film of gold, graphene or silicone carbide material. This will also be very much useful in non-tilt and tilted cryo-TEM data collection.

Factors Related to Quality EM Imaging

There are following factors in term of electron source, electron detector etc., which are very much helpful in quality imaging:

(a) **Electron source**: The quality electron source will be very much helpful in insightful explanation of experiment under performance. Normally, the thermionic and field emission gun (FEG) loaded tungsten (W) and LaB_6 filament source will be used [25], in respective TEM analysis. Thermionic emission of electrons will be proceeded through W and LaB_6, operated between 80 to 200 kV. In case of FEG emission, fine tip ZrO_2 coated W filament will be operated via field emission between 200 and 300 kV at 1800 K temperature [25]. Respective high coherency and brightness specification of FEG gun, will be preferred in high-resolution investigations whereas basic imaging and negative staining analysis process, will be executed through thermionic source under suitable EM.

(b) **Electron Detectors**: Detector quantum efficiency (DQE) has key role, which ensure the efficient capturing of emitted signal from specimen [26]. Normally, photographic films, charged couple devices (CCD) or direct electron detector (DED) etc., will be used in recording of respective data. For example, low density specimen like emulsion, have maximum contamination during beam exposure, will be minimized through use of pre-desiccation and anti-contamination device (ACD). Large field view of film-based specimen imaging has expensive and time-consuming factors promotes CCD fast data collection feature. In addition, the challenge of lowered sensitivity, point spread function w.r.t. CCD, has extended resolution to sub nanometer range in comparison to film-based imaging [27]. DED technologies are one more step ahead in comparison to CCD and film detection setups through principle of direct detection of electrons with minimum back scattering of electrons. Prominently, FEI, Gatan and Direct Electron are the leading manufacture of DED based EM technologies [26]. Overall, DED have high frame rate, correction in specimen movement during imaging in comparison to existing EM detection technologies.

(c) **Energy filters and phase plate**: Beam sensitive and low-density specimen need to analyzed under low-dose imaging mode, which subsequently face challenge of poor signal to noise ratio (SNR) or low contrast etc. Optimization of improved SNR signal via maximum elastic scattered electrons will be achieved via use of phase plate and energy filters. Low SNR during EM imaging, will be interfered through inelastic scattered electrons, which will be deflected via two energy filters named Omega filter (Ω) and post-column Gatan energy filters (GIF) [25]. Phase plate is also one more technological upgradation which is also useful in improving the contrast of specimen. It will work on the principle of introducing additional phase shift w.r.t. strongly scattered electron beam. Specifically, zernike phase plate (ZHP) [28] and volta potential phase plate (VPPP) [29] are the carbon-based specialized design, which can be used in enhancement of respective image contrast.

(d) **Data collection**: The challenge of low SNR signal during imaging, representation of multiple number of images of specimen for respective structure via single particle study [30], will also improve the data insights. Due to variation in different captured images in term of orientation, symmetry etc., automated data collection as well processing will be performed for more better representative 3D images. For example, FEI has developed related automated data collection system named E Pluribus Unum (EPU), with one source data programs like Leginon [31], Serial EM [32]. Further, the automated tilt series data collection system viz. Serial EM, Xplore 3D etc., also has been developed.

Other Supporting Methods w.r.t. EM Analysis

In addition to routine data analysis under EM, other correlative data analysis techniques are immensely desired to make critical observation of material under study. In current study, new emerging methods has been developed and discussed in order to provide extra dimension for existing EM structural data viz. correlative light electron microscopy (CLEM) and time resolved EM:

(a) **CLEM**: Specially any biological specimen exact behavior cannot be predicted through simple morphological study alone. Fluorescence microscopy uses different fluorescent markers for exact positioning and tracking of proteins or other cellular components during respective material analysis [33]. Under CLEM technologies, identified area of interest through fluorescent markers under LM will be transferred to EM mode [34]. Method of correlation in CLEM will be analyzed efficiently through integrated microscopes where minimum shifting of specimen with no cross-contamination has been ensured. Commercially FEI manufactured FEI iCorr system, having fluorescence microscope (FM) integrated with Tecnai [2]. Design-wise FM mounted perpendicular to electron beam in vacuum system of EM. Whereas in second design, separate imaging will be performed for FM and EM mode. Practically, fiducial marker will be used to locate the area of interest in second mode of imaging.
(b) **Time Resolved EM**: Ultrafast conformational changes occurs within different macromolecules over varying time scale (< 10 ms) under external stimuli [35]. Different precise sample preparation techniques like plunge freezing etc. during cryo-TEM analysis, will freezes all the conformational changes during mixing/reaction under time resolved mode of analysis. Respective time resolution insight will be achieved with spraying technique w.r.t nature of specimen. Under one way, first reactant is sprayed on grid followed by second reactant before freezing [36], whereas in second method both mixed reactants will be spray on grid just before vitrification process.

Computational Aspect in EM Analysis

In case of in-depth biological or material science specimen atomic or molecular structure analysis, single particle analysis or tilt series-oriented tomography study through direct electron detection (DED) with high frame rate, has revolutionized the cryo-EM generated data, data storage as well respective interpretation aspect. For example, in comparison to conventional CCD camera images, a high-end CCD camera (32-bit 4 k × 4 k MRC format) image have ~ 64 Mb in size. Further, to capture 10,000 particles dataset, per image 100 particle micrograph, represent 6.4 Gb raw image dataset. In continuation, DED 4 k × 4 k camera (Falcon 2 FEI) operated at 17 Hz, will capture in 2 s exposure 35 frame movies having 2.2 Gb size. Although, 8 k × 8 k Gatan K2 summit camera, will capture images at frame rate in the range of 40 Hz.

EM facility running 24 h. unattended, will collect captures ~ 1800 exposure movies having ~ 4 (terabyte) Tb data space. With continuous 300 working days in laboratory, 1.2 petabyte raw data will be generated. During designing of data storage facilities in respective laboratory, 10 Gbit ethernet connection and 40 Gbit is desirable. With respect to computational facilities for image processing packages, RELION package in Ranson laboratory using single or multiple core servers can be used. For example,

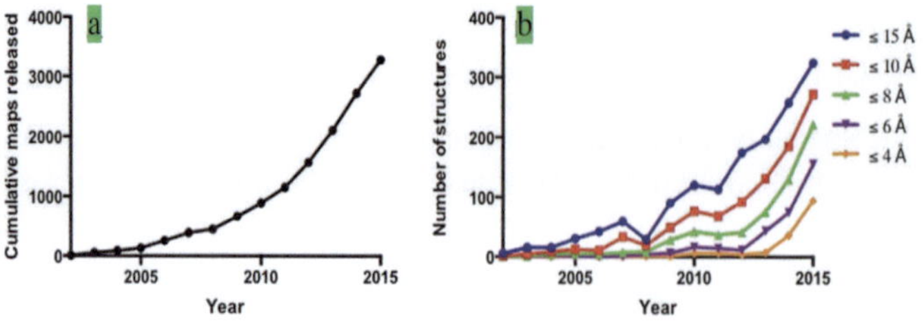

Fig. 11.17 Studied and reported in EMDB **a** cumulative map releases from 2002 to 2015, **b** map released between 2002 and 2015 w.r.t. given resolution (Adapted with permission Thompson et al. [23] under open access)

64 core, 256 Gb server was used to determine the 480 × 480 × 480 volume to 3 Å resolution with respective movies detail [37]. As per author advise, laboratory which do not have sufficient storage for cryo-EM processing data, cloud computing will be flexible and cost-effective option [38], keeping in mind the safety policies for respective data protection.

11.3.5.2 Outcomes

The EM data analysis demand w.r.t. biological specimen from basic imaging to single particle analysis through conventional EM to cryo-EM is increasing very rapidly whose detail is depicted in Fig. 11.17a, b. Specifically, under electron microscopy data bank (EMDB) more than 2500 density map through single particle analysis, reconstruction and electron diffraction study has been published with many latest high-resolution studies being going to release.

With the latest developments in cryo-EM, single particle processing and cryo-electron tomography with unique methodologies, brings understanding of different macromolecule complexes insightly in the range of < 10 Å. Through insightful determination of different structural estimation of biological processes with latest complimentary techniques, resolve the solution for unsolved and unclear questions in the sphere of EM observations.

"Science cannot solve the ultimate mystery of nature, and that is because, in the last analysis, we ourselves are part of mystery that we are trying to solve"
Max Planck

11.4 Conclusion

The objective of present chapter is to upgrading the expertise of EM users in respective instrumentation, sample preparation and respective data interpretation. This will be helpful for researchers in getting skill-based knowledge to use basic to advance instrumentation techniques, quality specimen preparation methods with insightful explanation in respective material field via updated EM technologies.

More importantly, current studies highlighted the basic to advanced requirements and practices of EM instrumentation including installation, smooth operation, analysis and interpretation. Ultimately, with this chapter, students/researchers/scientists get more interest and sensitivity towards EM technique insightful analysis. This approach will be very much helpful in improving the existing devices/systems/ formulations performances towards novel material with efficient device development.

Declaration

Author declares that there is no personal or financial conflict of interest regarding publication of this chapter.

References

1. Schröder, R.R.: Advances in electron microscopy: a qualitative view of instrumentation development for macromolecular imaging and tomography. Arch. Biochem. Biophys. **581**, 25–38 (2015). https://doi.org/10.1016/j.abb.2015.05.010
2. LaGrange, T., Reed, B.W., Santala, M.K., McKeown, J.T., Kulovits, A., Wiezorek, J.M.K., Nikolova, L., Rosei, F., Siwick, B.J., Campbell, G.H.: Approaches for ultrafast imaging of transient materials processes in the transmission electron microscope. Micron **43**(11), 1108–1120 (2012). https://doi.org/10.1016/j.micron.2012.04.010
3. Rai, R.S., Subramanian, S.: Role of transmission electron microscopy in the semiconductor industry for process development and failure analysis. Prog. Cryst. Growth Charact. Mater. **55**(3–4), 63–97 (2009). https://doi.org/10.1016/j.pcrysgrow.2009.09.002
4. Mills, D.J.: Setting up and operating a cryo-EM laboratory. Quart. Rev. Biophys. **54**, e2 (2021). https://doi.org/10.1017/S003358352000013X
5. D'Imprima, E., Floris, D., Joppe, M., Sánchez, R., Grininger, M., Kühlbrandt, W.: Protein denaturation at the air-water interface and how to prevent it. eLife **8**, e42747 (2019). https://doi.org/10.7554/eLife.42747
6. Campbell, M.G., Cheng, A., Brilot, A.F., Moeller, A., Lyumkis, D., Veesler, D., Pan, J., Harrison, S.C., Potter, C.S., Carragher, B., Grigorieff, N.: Movies of ice-embedded particles enhance resolution in electron cryo-microscopy. Structure **20**(11), 1823–1828 (2012). https://doi.org/10.1016/j.str.2012.08.026
7. Nakane, T., Kotecha, A., Sente, A., McMullan, G., Masiulis, S., Brown, P.M.G.E., Grigoras, I.T., Malinauskaite, L., Malinauskas, T., Miehling, J., Uchański, T., Yu, L., Karia, D., Pechnikova, E.V., De Jong, E., Keizer, J., Bischoff, M., McCormack, J., Tiemeijer, P., Hardwick, S.W., Chirgadze, D.Y., Murshudov, G., Aricescu, A.R., Scheres, S.H.W.: Single-particle cryo-EM at atomic resolution. Nature **587**(7832), 152–156 (2020). https://doi.org/10.1038/s41586-020-2829-0

8. Zachs, T., Schertel, A., Medeiros, J., Weiss, G.L., Hugener, J., Matos, J., Pilhofer, M.: Fully automated, sequential focused ion beam milling for cryo-electron tomography. eLife **9**, e52286 (2020). https://doi.org/10.7554/eLife.52286
9. Sartori, A., Gatz, R., Beck, F., Rigort, A., Baumeister, W., Plitzko, J.M.: Correlative microscopy: bridging the gap between fluorescence light microscopy and cryo-electron tomography. J. Struct. Biol. **160**(2), 135–145 (2007). https://doi.org/10.1016/j.jsb.2007.07.011
10. Tang, S., Tang, J., Uzuhashi, J., Ohkubo, T., Hayami, W., Yuan, J., Takeguchi, M., Mitome, M., Qin, L.-C.: A stable LaB_6 nanoneedle field-emission point electron source. Nanoscale Adv. **3**(10), 2787–2792 (2021). https://doi.org/10.1039/D1NA00167A
11. Singh, G., Bücker, R., Kassier, G., Barthelmess, M., Zheng, F., Migunov, V., Kruth, M., Dunin-Borkowski, R.E., Purcell, S.T., Miller, R.J.D.: Fabrication and characterization of a focused ion beam milled lanthanum hexaboride based cold field electron emitter source. Appl. Phys. Lett. **113**(9), 093101 (2018). https://doi.org/10.1063/1.5039441
12. Zhang, H., Tang, J., Zhang, Q., Zhao, G., Yang, G., Zhang, J., Zhou, O., Qin, L.-C.: Field emission of electrons from single LaB_6 nanowires. Adv. Mater. **18**(1), 87–91 (2006). https://doi.org/10.1002/adma.200500508
13. Tang, S., Tang, J., Wu, Y., Chen, Y.-H., Uzuhashi, J., Ohkubo, T., Qin, L.-C.: Stable field-emission from a CeB_6 nanoneedle point electron source. Nanoscale **13**(40), 17156–17161 (2021). https://doi.org/10.1039/D1NR04907K
14. Zhang, H., Tang, J., Yuan, J., Yamauchi, Y., Suzuki, T.T., Shinya, N., Nakajima, K., Qin, L.-C.: An ultrabright and monochromatic electron point source made of a LaB6 nanowire. Nat. Nanotech. **11**(3), 273–279 (2016). https://doi.org/10.1038/nnano.2015.276
15. Bellucci, A., Mastellone, M., Girolami, M., Serpente, V., Generosi, A., Paci, B., Mezzi, A., Kaciulis, S., Carducci, R., Polini, R., Orlando, S., Santagata, A., De Bonis, A., Meucci, M., Mercatelli, L., Sani, E., Trucchi, D.M.: Nanocrystalline lanthanum boride thin films by femtosecond pulsed laser deposition as efficient emitters in hybrid thermionic-photovoltaic energy converters. Appl. Surf. Sci. **513**, 145829 (2020). https://doi.org/10.1016/j.apsusc.2020.145829
16. Sawada, H., et al.: Super high resolution imaging with atomic resolution electron microscope of JEM-ARM300F. JEOL New **49**(No. 1), 51–58 (2014)
17. Kasuya, K., Katagiri, S., Ohshima, T., Kokubo, S.: Stabilization of a tungsten ⟨310⟩ cold field emitter. J. Vac. Sci. Technol., B: Nanotechnol. Microelectron.: Mater., Process., Meas., Phenom. **28**(5), L55–L60 (2010). https://doi.org/10.1116/1.3488988
18. Li, T., Nowell, C.J., Cipolla, D., Rades, T., Boyd, B.J.: Direct comparison of standard transmission electron microscopy and cryogenic-TEM in imaging nanocrystals inside liposomes. Mol. Pharmaceut. **16**(4), 1775–1781 (2019). https://doi.org/10.1021/acs.molpharmaceut.8b01308
19. Milne, J.L.S., Borgnia, M.J., Bartesaghi, A., Tran, E.E.H., Earl, L.A., Schauder, D.M., Lengyel, J., Pierson, J., Patwardhan, A., Subramaniam, S.: Cryo-electron microscopy—a primer for the non-microscopist. FEBS J. **280**(1), 28–45 (2013). https://doi.org/10.1111/febs.12078
20. Barenholz, Y. (Chezy).: Doxil®—the first FDA-approved nano-drug: lessons learned. J. Control. Release 160(2), 117–134 (2012). https://doi.org/10.1016/j.jconrel.2012.03.020
21. Deegan, R.D., Bakajin, O., Dupont, T.F., Huber, G., Nagel, S.R., Witten, T.A.: Capillary flow as the cause of ring stains from dried liquid drops. Nature **389**(6653), 827–829 (1997). https://doi.org/10.1038/39827
22. Hu, J.J., Wheeler, R., Zabinski, J.S., Shade, P.A., Shiveley, A., Voevodin, A.A.: Transmission electron microscopy analysis of Mo–W–S–Se film sliding contact obtained by using focused ion beam microscope and in situ microtribometer. Tribol. Lett. **32**(1), 49–57 (2008). https://doi.org/10.1007/s11249-008-9360-z
23. Thompson, R.F., Walker, M., Siebert, C.A., Muench, S.P., Ranson, N.A.: An introduction to sample preparation and imaging by cryo-electron microscopy for structural biology. Methods **100**, 3–15 (2016). https://doi.org/10.1016/j.ymeth.2016.02.017
24. Berner, S., Horne, R.: A negative staining method for high resolution electron microscopy of viruses. **34**, 103–110 (1959)

25. Williams, D.B., Williams, C.B., Cater, C.B.: The Transmission Electron Microscope, pp. 3–17. Springer (1996)
26. McMullan, G., Faruqi, A.R., Clare, D., Henderson, R.: Comparison of optimal performance at 300 keV of three direct electron detectors for use in low dose electron microscopy. Ultramicroscopy **147**, 156–163 (2014). https://doi.org/10.1016/j.ultramic.2014.08.002
27. Cheng, L., Zhu, J., Hui, W.H., Zhang, X., Honig, B., Fang, Q., Zhou, Z.H.: Backbone model of an aquareovirus virion by cryo-electron microscopy and bioinformatics. J. Mol. Biol. **397**(3), 852–863 (2010). https://doi.org/10.1016/j.jmb.2009.12.027
28. Danev, R., Nagayama, K.: Transmission electron microscopy with zernike phase plate. Ultramicroscopy **88**(4), 243–252 (2001). https://doi.org/10.1016/S0304-3991(01)00088-2
29. Danev, R., Buijsse, B., Khoshouei, M., Plitzko, J.M., Baumeister, W.: Volta potential phase plate for in-focus phase contrast transmission electron microscopy. Proc. Natl. Acad. Sci. U.S.A. **111**(44), 15635–15640 (2014). https://doi.org/10.1073/pnas.1418377111
30. Cheng, Y., Grigorieff, N., Penczek, P.A., Walz, T.: A primer to single-particle cryo-electron microscopy. Cell **161**(3), 438–449 (2015). https://doi.org/10.1016/j.cell.2015.03.050
31. Carragher, B., Kisseberth, N., Kriegman, D., Milligan, R.A., Potter, C.S., Pulokas, J., Reilein, A.: Leginon: an automated system for acquisition of images from vitreous ice specimens. J. Struct. Biol. **132**(1), 33–45 (2000). https://doi.org/10.1006/jsbi.2000.4314
32. Mastronarde, D.N.: Automated electron microscope tomography using robust prediction of specimen movements. J. Struct. Biol. **152**(1), 36–51 (2005). https://doi.org/10.1016/j.jsb.2005.07.007
33. Chang, Y.-W., Chen, S., Tocheva, E.I., Treuner-Lange, A., Löbach, S., Søgaard-Andersen, L., Jensen, G.J.: Correlated cryogenic photoactivated localization microscopy and cryo-electron tomography. Nat. Methods **11**(7), 737–739 (2014). https://doi.org/10.1038/nmeth.2961
34. Paez-Segala, M.G., Sun, M.G., Shtengel, G., Viswanathan, S., Baird, M.A., Macklin, J.J., Patel, R., Allen, J.R., Howe, E.S., Piszczek, G., Hess, H.F., Davidson, M.W., Wang, Y., Looger, L.L.: Fixation-resistant photoactivatable fluorescent proteins for CLEM. Nat. Methods **12**(3), 215–218 (2015). https://doi.org/10.1038/nmeth.3225
35. Shaikh, T.R., Yassin, A.S., Lu, Z., Barnard, D., Meng, X., Lu, T.-M., Wagenknecht, T., Agrawal, R.K.: Initial bridges between two ribosomal subunits are formed within 9.4 milliseconds, as studied by time-resolved cryo-EM. Proc. Natl. Acad. Sci. U.S.A. **111**(27), 9822–9827 (2014). https://doi.org/10.1073/pnas.1406744111
36. Berriman, J., Unwin, N.: Analysis of transient structures by cryo-microscopy combined with rapid mixing of spray droplets. Ultramicroscopy **56**(4), 241–252 (1994). https://doi.org/10.1016/0304-3991(94)90012-4
37. Hesketh, E.L., Meshcheriakova, Y., Dent, K.C., Saxena, P., Thompson, R.F., Cockburn, J.J., Lomonossoff, G.P., Ranson, N.A.: Mechanisms of assembly and genome packaging in an RNA virus revealed by high-resolution cryo-EM. Nat. Commun. **6**(1), 10113 (2015). https://doi.org/10.1038/ncomms10113
38. Cianfrocco, M.A., Leschziner, A.E.: Low cost, high performance processing of single particle cryo-electron microscopy data in the cloud. Biophys. Struct. Biol. **4**, e06664 (2015)

MIX
Papier aus verantwortungsvollen Quellen
Paper from responsible sources
FSC® C105338

If you have any concerns about our products,
you can contact us on
ProductSafety@springernature.com

In case Publisher is established outside the EU,
the EU authorized representative is:
Springer Nature Customer Service Center GmbH
Europaplatz 3, 69115 Heidelberg, Germany

Printed by Libri Plureos GmbH
in Hamburg, Germany